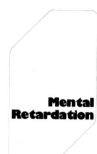

**Mental
Retardation**

Karger Continuing Education Series

Editor: Irene Jakab,
Pittsburgh, Pa.

Mental Retardation

77 figures and 43 tables, 1982

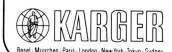KARGER

Basel · München · Paris · London · New York · Tokyo · Sydney

Karger Continuing Education Series, Vol. 2

Topics covered in the Karger Continuing Education Series are selected to help improve clinical skills and introduce the reader to health-related areas undergoing exceptional growth. Produced as compact instructive texts, volumes set forth information which serves to heighten the general awareness and command of current medical procedures and practice. The concise textbook format enhances the value of these books as convenient teaching and training tools for medical scientists, medical clinicians, and health professionals.

National Library of Medicine, Cataloging in Publication
    Mental retardation
    Editor, Irene Jakab. – Basel; New York: Karger, 1982
    (Karger continuing education Series; v. 2)
    1. Mental Retardation   I. Jakab, Irene
    WM 300 M584 (P)
    ISBN 3–8055–3433–7

Drug Dosage
    The authors and the publisher have exerted every effort to ensure that drug selection and dosage set forth in this text are in accord with current recommendations and practice at the time of publication. However, in view of ongoing research, changes in government regulations, and the constant flow of information relating to drug therapy and drug reactions, the reader is urged to check the package insert for each drug for any change in indications and dosage and for added warnings and precautions. This is particularly important when the recommended agent is a new and/or infrequently employed drug.

Contents

**Basic Science Research and
Its Application in Prevention and Treatment**

Contents

Diagnostic and Treatment Procedures

I. Jakab

Psychology

C. Latham and R. Yando

R. Yando

V.T. Harway and E. Shapiro

Neurology

R.S. Kandt and B.J. D'Souza

E. Niedermeyer

Psychiatry

P.B. Henderson

Social Services to Retardates and Their Families

B. Hanley

M. Gerber

Disorders Frequently Associated with Mental Retardation

L.A. Bloom

D. Linn

Contents   X

List of Contributors

Allard, Mary Ann, MPA, Research Associate, Human Services Research Institute, Boston, Mass. (USA)

Andrulonis, Paul A., MD, Associate Director, Department of Child Psychiatry, The Institute of Living; Assistant Professor, Child Psychiatry, University of Connecticut, School of Medicine, Hartford, Conn. (USA)

Bentz, George H., DDS, MS, Assistant Professor of Pedodontics, Dental School, University of Pittsburgh, Pittsburgh, Pa. (USA)

Bloom, Lawrence A., PhD, Director, Department of Communication Disorders, Children's Hospital, University of Pittsburgh, Pittsburgh, Pa. (USA)

Bradley, Valerie J., MA, President Human Services Research Institute, Boston, Mass. (USA)

D'Souza, Bernard J., MD, Assistant Professor, Departments of Pediatrics and Neurology, Johns Hopkins University School of Medicine, Baltimore, Md. (USA)

Gerber, Magda, Director RIE, Pacific Oaks College, Pasadena, Calif. (USA)

Glor-Scheib, Susan, M.Ed., Research Assistant, Learning Research and Development Center, University of Pittsburgh, Pittsburgh, Pa. (USA)

Hanley, Barbara, ACSW, Senior Social Worker, John Merck Program, Western Psychiatric Institute and Clinic, Department of Psychiatry, University of Pittsburgh, Pittsburgh, Pa. (USA)

Harway, Vivian T., PhD, Associate Professor of Child Psychiatry, University of Pittsburgh, Pittsburgh, Pa. (USA)

Henderson, Peter B., MD, Associate Professor of Child Psychiatry, University of Pittsburgh, Pittsburgh, Pa. (USA)

Jakab, Irene, MD, PhD, Professor of Psychiatry, Department of Psychiatry, University of Pittsburgh; Director, Graduate Course in Mental Retardation, University of Pittsburgh School of Medicine, Pittsburgh, Pa., and Lecturer, Harvard Medical School, Boston, Mass. (USA)

Kandt, Raymond S., MD, Instructor, Department of Pediatrics and Infectious Disease and the Department of Neurology, University of Michigan Medical Center, Ann Arbor, Mich. (USA)

Katz-Garris, Lynda, PhD, Assistant Professor of Psychiatry and Education, Department of Psychiatry, University of Pittsburgh, Pittsburgh, Pa. (USA)

Kepes, John J., MD, Professor of Pathology, College of Health Sciences and Hospital, University of Kansas School of Medicine, Kansas City, Kans. (USA)

Latham, Craig, PhD, Instructor in Psychology, Department of Psychiatry, Harvard Medical School, Staff Psychologist, Judge Baker Guidance Center, Boston, Mass. (USA)

Linn, Dorothy, LPT, Physical Therapist, John Merck Program,
    Western Psychiatric Institute and Clinic; Department of Psychiatry,
    University of Pittsburgh, Pittsburgh, Pa. (USA)
Moser, Hugo, W., MD, Director, John F. Kennedy Institute for Handicapped Children,
    and Professor of Neurology and Pediatrics, Johns Hopkins University, Baltimore,
    Md. (USA)
Niedermeyer, Ernst, MD, Associate Professor of Neurology, Electroencephalographer-
    in-Charge, The Johns Hopkins University, Baltimore, Md. (USA)
Shapiro, Edward S., PhD, Assistant Professor of Psychology, Department of Psychology
    and Human Development, Lehigh University, Bethlehem, Pa. (USA)
Steele, Mark W., MD, Associate Professor of Pediatrics, University of Pittsburgh
    School of Medicine, Pittsburgh, Pa. (USA)
Yando, Regina, PhD, Associate Professor of Psychology, Department of Psychiatry,
    Children's Hospital Medical Center, Harvard Medical School,
    and Chief Psychologist, Judge Baker Guidance Center, Boston, Mass. (USA)

Foreword

It is rare indeed for the first edition of a scholarly textbook to hit the press with its utility already established. Yet, such is precisely the case for *Irene Jakab's* 'Mental Retardation'. The separate chapters have been developed on the basis of direct experience in teaching a postgraduate training course, which Dr. *Jakab* has led each year for almost a decade and in which she has taught for even longer. Classroom interactions with students and their evaluations of the modules have resulted in progressive shaping of topic and focus in order to increase the relevance of the material to the needs of clinical practice. The authors who have contributed to this book have been chosen not only because of their expertise and leadership in the field but also because of their teaching skills. Thus, in writing the foreword of this book, I can confidently state: 'Practitioners who deal with the problems of the retarded can turn to this book with assurance that they will find useful and practical information.' The statement rests on more than opinion; it reports what has been demonstrated in action.

This book is much needed. Most health workers, including physicians, receive only the most rudimentary education about the syndromes of mental retardation. It is unconscionable that this should be so, given the prevalence of these disorders, their chronicity and the morbidity associated with them. Certain of the forms of mental retardation can be entirely prevented by vigorous public health campaigns employing the best of contemporary scientific knowledge; others can be minimized by appropriate social and educational measures [1]. Yet, there is a considerable lag between what we know and what we do. In part, this results from insufficient education for professionals about what can be done; in part, from priorities for public funding which undervalue preventive measures.

For those youngsters with afflictions we do not yet know how to prevent – or failed to prevent in time – there is still much which can be done in order to enhance the development of the patient's residual abilities and to support families which must carry the burdens of a chronically handicapped member. Success in general medicine has increased the longevity of the severely retarded; thus, understanding the psychosocial and educational needs of the adult retardate takes on added importance. Perhaps most neglected of all have been the doubly handicapped: those who suffer simultaneously from mental retardation and emotional disorder [2]. Traditional agencies have defined their aims as being directed at one or the other problem; they have been uninterested in, and incompetent at, managing the doubly handicapped. Dr. *Jakab* has been a pioneer in addressing the needs of this important group of patients, and several chapters in this volume deal with how they can be helped.

If this book is widely read – and if its lessons are taken to heart – it can help change professional attitudes. There is a long and sad history of neglect of retarded patients and their families by physicians. When I entered the field in the 1950s, child psychiatry clinics, with few exceptions, dismissed the problems of the mentally retarded as falling outside the boundaries of the field. Similar attitudes characterized pediatrics and child neurology. Despite the efforts of a *Howard Potter* [3], a *Grover Powers* [4] and a *George Jervis* [5], most of their confreres remained indifferent, if not disdainful. The catalyst for change was provided by the parents of the retarded through the National Association for Retarded Children (now, the National Association for Retarded Citizens). Their grass roots work in the community and their lobbying with legislators made it possible to capitalize on the accident that an elected President (John F. Kennedy) had a severely retarded sister and was prepared to exert leadership for that class of citizens.

For the first time, considerable sums of public money for care and for research became available. This led to a period of unseemly professional claims for hegemony as pediatrics, neurology and psychiatry, so indifferent just a few years earlier, each insisted on leadership. As funding receded, the claims were less vociferous. It became evident that no single specialty is adequate to the task and that each is needed for comprehensive care.

The advances in the past decade have been considerable, even if far short of the challenge. This volume epitomizes the main developments as well as the remaining areas of ignorance. The practitioner familiar with its contents will be well equipped for patient care. What a book alone cannot supply is the need for a moral commitment to serve as advocate for the retarded.

No parable better conveys what a committed professional can do on behalf of the retarded than what *Leo Kanner* accomplished by careful outcome research to investigate suspected exploitation of handicapped citizens. In the mid-1930s, *Kanner* undertook a follow-up study of 166 patients who had been released from Maryland State Training Schools for the Retarded over a 20-year period by habeas corpus writs [6]. Three-quarters of these releases had been obtained by enterprising attorneys who, for a substantial fee, secured unpaid domestic servants for affluent Baltimore households. Of the 166, *Kanner* was able to locate 102, of whom only 13 were making even a modestly satisfactory adjustment at the time of the study; 11 had died before the age of 30 from illness or neglect; 17 had tuberculosis, syphilis, or gonorrhea; 20 were prostitutes; 8 had been committed to mental hospitals; and 6 were in prison. These released patients had produced 165 children, of whom 18 had died from neglect, 30 had been committed to orphanages, and 108 tested at a feeble-minded level when examined. The most common sequence had been a period of domestic servitude, followed by peremptory release when they proved to be inadequate as house servants, and then a sad peregrination through the whorehouses and flophouses of the slums.

Presentation of the paper resulted in a double row of inch-high headlines across the front page of the *Baltimore Sun* on April 8, 1938 and led to prompt community action to end the despicable collusion of attorneys and judges. Clinical skill joined to social conscience had resulted in immediate benefit for a neglected minority. Professor *Kanner* went on to do many distinguished things in his career, but none which spoke with greater eloquence of his humanity.

That bit of history goes back more than 40 years. Does it have any relevance today? The habeas corpus writ may no longer be in use to produce domestic slaves but facilities for the retarded are still deplorable in most states; 'the least restrictive alternative' in the community all too often means exploitation in welfare hotels and flophouses. There is much to be done. It will require heart as well as mind.

Leon Eisenberg
MD, Maude and Lillian Presley Professor and Chairman,
Department of Social Medicine and Health Policy,
Harvard Medical School, Boston, Mass.

References

1   Eisenberg, L.: A research framework for evaluating the promotion of mental health and prevention of mental illness. Publ. Hlth Rep., Wash. *96:* 3–19 (1981).
2   Reiss, S.; Levitan, G.W.; McNally, R.J.: Emotionally disturbed mentally retarded people: an underserved population. Am. Psychol. *37:* 361–367 (1982).

3   Potter, H.W.: Mental retardation: the Cinderella of psychiatry. Psychiat. Q. *39:* 537–
     549 (1965).
4   Powers, G.F.: John Howland Award Address. Pediatrics, Springfield *1953:* 217–
     226.
5   Jervis, G.A.: Phenylpyruvic oligophrenia. Proc. Ass. Res. nerv. ment. Dis. *33:* 259–
     282 (1954).
6   Kanner, L.: Habeas corpus releases of feebleminded persons and their consequences.
     Am. J. Psychiat. *94:* 1013–1033 (1938).

Preface

This textbook is the product of an NIMH Grant supported postgraduate training course for physicians called the Graduate Course in Mental Retardation (GCMR) (Grand No. 5 TO1 MH13794–08).

The need for a Graduate Course in Mental Retardation was already evident two decades ago, especially in view of the lack of formal training in mental retardation in medical schools, as well as in psychiatric, pediatric and neurology residency training programs throughout the United States. This well-documented need has led to the organization of and NIMH grant support for, the Letchworth Village Graduate Course in Mental Retardation, established in 1959 and directed for 12 years by Dr. *Howard Potter.* The course has responded to the need of physicians for a comprehensive learning experience based on sound theoretical foundation, while at the same time providing up-to-date practical guidelines for the diagnosis, treatment and rehabilitation of mentally retarded persons and of the many conditions associated with retardation.

This writer has been a lecturer at the Letchworth Village Graduate Course since 1964. Dr. *Potter,* who had been contemplating his retirement for a while, asked me to take over the direction of the course for the last academic year of its grant period at Letchworth Village (1970–1971). During that year, the interest and feasibility of setting up such a program in the Boston area, involving the Harvard Medical School (where I was on the faculty), the McLean Hospital, and the Walter E. Fernald School, became evident. Indeed, the course in Boston opened in 1971 in time to provide continuity of education, based on the same philosophy as the Letchworth Village Course. The funding was provided by NIMH through a Grant to the McLean Hospital.

The long waiting list of the Letchworth Village Course has been taken over by the Boston Course, which also remained continuously oversubscribed.

The enthusiastic response from the highly qualified academic staff of the Harvard Medical School, and the genuinely felt need and support for such a program by local professional organizations for the treatment and rehabilitation of retardates, made this traditional and unique course in Mental Retardation well known throughout the country.

In 1974, the decision to move the course to Pittsburgh, Pa., was based on the fact that this writer (the program director of the Graduate Course in Mental Retardation in Boston) moved from the Harvard Medical School to the University of Pittsburgh Medical School.

The merits of this course are most evident in the increased involvement of our alumni in programs for retardates. A survey made by Dr. *Potter* following the first 10 years of experience with the course at Letchworth Village, revealed that as many as 70% of those who have taken the course became involved in the actual management and treatment of retardates, or became consultants to such programs.

A survey made by this author, after the second 10 years of experience with the Graduate Course in Mental Retardation, was extended to include the trainees who have completed the course at Letchworth Village and those who attended it in Boston and in Pittsburgh. The statistical data have revealed that about 60% of the trainees have actually started activities related to the services for retarded persons, or have expanded their former field of involvement.

The course, regardless of its geographical site, responds to the need for an updated professional education in the field of retardation. The curriculum includes lectures delivered by the best possible specialists in the field of retardation. The course is, indeed, well known throughout the country, and as one of the site visitors remarked, at the last grant renewal, 'this course has become somewhat of a national institution'.

As Director of the GCMR for the last 10 years, I became aware of the need for a comprehensive textbook in the field of mental retardation for physicians and other professionals involved in the diagnostic assessment and the day-to-day treatment, rehabilitation and counselling of retardates.

This publication was made possible through the support of our NIMH Grant and the collaboration of the co-authors, who are on the faculty of the Graduate Course in Mental Retardation. We all hope that the readers will gain up-to-date theoretical and practical information, and experience an upsurge of motivation to be involved in the treatment, the counselling and the program management of retardates.

Irene Jakab, Editor
MD, PhD, Professor of Psychiatry, University of Pittsburgh,
Director, Graduate Course in Mental Retardation

This book is dedicated
To all retarded persons and their families
With our desire to better their lives.

To Be Retarded Is a Handicap, Not a Disgrace.
Irene Jakab

Basic Science Research and Its Application in Prevention and Treatment

1 Mental Retardation due to Genetically Determined Metabolic and Endocrine Disorders

Hugo W. Moser

Surveys of large and representative groups of mentally retarded people indicate that genetically determined metabolic or endocrine disorders are the cause of 3–7% of severe mental retardation [25, 33, 51]. Identification of these disorders is of importance because it provides a precise etiological definition of a serious disability, the opportunity for genetic counseling and, occasionally, specific therapy.

Diagnosis is complicated by the fact that there may be more than a thousand separate disorders which can cause mental retardation [52], their phenotype may not be distinctive, and some diagnostic tests are highly specialized, expensive and/or not generally available. At present there are two major pathways to the diagnosis of genetic or endocrine disorders associated with mental retardation: (a) Diagnosis by mass screening. These are important public health measures. The practicing physician deals with the consequences of these surveys, but is not directly involved otherwise. (b) Diagnostic studies undertaken on the basis of clinical indications. It is here that the practicing physician has the central role. The main purpose of this chapter is to help the physician responsible for mentally retarded people, to identify and to treat persons who have genetically determined metabolic or endocrine disorders, and also to be aware of opportunities for genetic counseling.

Diagnosis by Mass Screening of the General Population

Diagnosis by mass screening involves new public health techniques which have already made significant contributions toward the prevention of mental retardation or neurological deficits. The most widely used screening techniques involve mass screening of newborn infants for treatable metabolic diseases, such as phenylketonuria or hypothyroidism. On a more restricted basis, screening techniques are being used to identify carriers of recessively inherited disorders [20], and to detect women at risk of bearing children with neural tube defects [46].

The first newborn screening test was introduced by *Centerwall* [14] in 1957, and consisted of a modified ferric chloride test applied to the infants' diaper. *Guthrie's* [26] bacterial inhibition assay was first introduced in 1963. This revolutionary technology utilizes a 'dried blood spot', that is a special filter paper impregnated with a blood sample obtained from a capillary heel puncture. The amount of blood per unit area of filter paper is remarkably constant, and the sample is stable so that it can be transported by regular mail without refrigeration. The phenylalanine level in the 'blood spot' is quantitated by a bacterial inhibition assay and the initial screening results can be interpreted by personnel with only limited training. Finally, the same blood spot can be used to test for other disorders including congenital hypothyroidism [31, 49, 68], galactosemia [8], maple syrup urine disease and homocystinuria [26]. Table I lists the estimated frequency of various metabolic disorders detected by the Massachusetts mass screening program [42]. These results are comparable to those in other parts of the world. Screening for hypothyroidism is currently attracting world-wide interest. This is of importance since its incidence is higher than any other of the genetic metabolic disorders associated with mental retardation: in England the incidence was 1:3,363 [31] and 1:3,800 in New England [49]. Methods have been developed recently which have overcome an earlier problem with a high 'noise' level, that is, a large number of false-positive tests on the initial screen. Presently, the 'blood spot' assay includes measurement of the T_4 level, followed by measurement of thyroid-stimulating hormone (TSH) levels for those samples with reduced T_4 level [49]. With this approach, over 75% of children identified as hypothyroid suspect by the screening test, were indeed found to have the disorder. The ethical aspects of newborn screening are an issue of concern [38, 48]. It is recommended that a clear demonstration of the therapeutic benefits of testing should precede state-supported mass testing of infants [38]. Such evidence is available for hypothyroidism, phenylketonuria, galactosemia, maple syrup urine disease and several other disorders.

Diagnosis in Follow-Up to Specific Clinical Indications

The physician who is responsible for developmentally disabled children has to face many pressures and take many decisions, be it in his office, clinic, school or institution. Detailed knowledge about the thousand or so

Table I. Metabolic disorders and their estimated frequency among newborns in Massachusetts

Disorder	Estimated frequency
Hypothyroidism[1]	1:3500
Phenylketonuria (classical)[1]	1:14,000
Phenylketonuria (atypical)[2]	1:16,000
Phenylketonuria and PMH (maternal)[2]	1:30,000
Iminoglycinuria[2]	?1:11,000[3]
Cystinuria[2]	1:13,000
Hartnup disorder[2]	1:18,000
Histidinemia	1:20,000
Histidinemia (atypical)	1:290,000
Histidinemia (maternal)[2]	1:100,000
Galactosemia[1]	1:75,000
Maply syrup urine disease[1]	1:290,000
MSUD (intermeidate variant)[1]	1:600,000
Argininosuccinicacidemia[1]	1:70,000
Argininosuccinicacidemia (atypical)	<1:500,000
Cystathioninemia	1:65,000
Homocystinuria[1]	1:290,000
Hyperglycinemia (non-ketotic)	1:190,000
Hyperprolinemia[2]	1:290,000
Methylmalonicacidemia[1]	1:75,000
Propionicacidemia[1]	<1:500,000
Hyperlysinemia[2]	1:290,000
Sarcosinemia[2]	1:275,000
Hyperornithinemia[2]	<1:500,000
Carnosinemia	<1:500,000
Urocanicaciduria	<1:500,000
Hyperglutamicaciduria	<1:500,000
Fanconi syndrome	<1:500,000
Rickets (Vitamin D dependent)[1]	<1:500,000

This table summarizes the experience of the Massachusetts screening program up to 1977 [42].
[1] Disorders with definite clinical complications.
[2] Disorders that may or may not be associated with clinial disease.
[3] The number of cases and incidence for iminoglycinuria may be falsely high since carriers for this disorder who only have hyperglycinuria later in life may have iminoglycinuria as young infants.

Table II. Symptoms associated with inborn errors of metabolism in high-risk infants and children [from Berry, 7]

Newborn period	Older children
Cataracts at birth	Mental retardation
Seizures	Seizures
Vomiting, diarrhea	Delayed development, mental, motor,
Jittery	physical
Floppy	Hematologic abnormalities, anemias
Acidosis	Behavior problems
Persistent jaundice	Central nervous system disorders
Unusual odor	Hepatomegaly, splenomegaly, or both
Failure to thrive	Renal defects, renal calculi
	Blindness, cataracts, dislocated lens,
	optic atrophy,
	Other eye defects
	Recurrent infections
	Speech defects
	Failure to grow
	Fever of unknown origin
	Skeletal disorders, dwarfism,
	osteomalacia, osteoporosis
	Rickets
	Skin lesions
	Unusual facies

genetic disorders that may be associated with mental retardation cannot be a top priority: the disorders in the aggregate account for only a relatively small proportion of the children served by the clinic, and in many instances, no specific therapy is available. Yet, when these disorders do exist, correct diagnosis has profound implications both for the child and the family. It is our plan here to offer a set of guidelines which may help the busy physician to deal with this part of his or her practice.

Clinical Settings Which May Be Associated with Inborn Errors of Metabolism in High-Risk Infants and Children

Table II lists signs or symptoms that may be associated with inborn errors of metabolism, and the presence of these features should alert the physician to this possibility.

Since the disorders under discussion are genetically determined, suspicion would be heightened if more than one member of the family is affected.

Most of the disorders follow an autosomal recessive mode of inheritance, so that it is most common for sibs to be affected. Even though table II emphasizes unusual facies as one of the signs, most persons with inborn errors of metabolism do not have an unusual general appearance. This sets them apart from persons with Down's syndrome or other disorders in which abnormalities in number and appearance of chromosomes can be demonstrated with the light microscope. In these 'chromosomal' disorders, abnormalities may exist in nearly every organ. The inborn errors of metabolism are due to a single mutation, and all other processes function normally, and this may account for the children often having a normal appearance. While in 'chromosomal' disorders, the abnormalities of appearance are present at birth, in the inborn errors of metabolism, if present at all, they usually develop postnatally. Thus, in the mucopolysaccharidoses, there is gradual postnatal accumulation of polysaccharides in the skin, visceral organs and bones, due to the genetically determined deficiency of one specific enzyme. The abnormal facies is a progressive postnatal phenomenon, related to the extent of polysaccharide accumulation.

Acidosis, which may be intermittent, or intermittent coma, are clear indications for a search for metabolic disorders. Intermittent acidosis is a frequent feature in disorders of fatty acid metabolism, such as maple syrup urine disease, methylmalonic aciduria, isovaleric acidemia and propionic acidemia. Intermittent coma occurs frequently in disorders of the urea cycle, and is usually due to elevated blood levels of ammonia.

Many of the inborn errors of metabolism present with progressive loss of mental or neurological function. This loss may become evident within the first few months after birth, such as in Tay-Sachs disease, or the 1st to 3rd year, as in metachromatic leukodystrophy, or in the early school years, adolescence or even later, such as in Wilson's disease, Batten's disease, adrenoleukodystrophy or Huntington's disease. It may be difficult to distinguish between a progressive disorder and those deficits associated with static lesions, such as those due to anoxia at times of birth: the manifestations of the static lesion may be progressive during the first few years of life; precise serial observations of psychomotor performance may be lacking; symptoms of a dementing illness in a child may be attributed to stress at home or in school. These and other features make the detection of inborn errors of metabolism in developmentally disabled children a challenging task. *Rapin* [60] has written a very helpful article about the clinical manifestations of the progressive genetic-metabolic disorders of the nervous system.

Table III. Qualitative urine metabolic screening tests [from *Schmidt* [71]; see also ref. 12, 66 and 72 for detailed descriptions of these tests]

Test	Quality of substance detected	Condition suspected
Odor	mousey	phenylketonuria
	maple syrup	maple syrup urine disease
	sweaty feet	isovaleric acidemia
Color	black-brown on standing or with addition of alkali	alkaptonuria
Density	1,006 or less	diabetes insipidus
Labstix	glucose	diabetes mellitus
		renal glycosuria
		Fanconi symdrome
	protein	
	ketones	α-keto acids
	occult blood	
Phenistix of ferric choloride	phenylpyruvic acid	phenylketonuria
	imidazole pyruvic acid	histidinemia
	p-hydroxyphenylpyruvic acid	transient tyrosinosis
Clinitest	reducing substances	diabetes mellitus
		galactosemia
		fructose intolerance
		essential fructosuria
		congenital lactosuria
		essential pentosuria
	ending in brown or black color (homogentistic acid)	alkaptonuria
Brand test	cystine, homocystine	cystinuria
		homocystinuria
Millon test	tyrosine, *p*-hydroxy-phenylpyruvic acid	tyrosinemia
		Wilson's disease
		Hartnup disease
		galactosemia
2,4-Dinitrophenylhydrazine	α-keto acids and ketones	phenylketonuria
		maple syrup urine disease
		histidinemia
Azure A	mucopolysaccharides	mucopolysaccharidosis

A 'Safety Net' Provided by Simple Metabolic Screening Tests

There is no economically feasible method to screen for all metabolic disorders in all developmentally disabled children, hence the continued need for clinical judgment. However, there are two 'safety nets' – the first is the mass screening program of newborn children, described in the second section. The newborn screening programs can detect most children with congenital hypothyroidism, or with phenylketonuria, the two most common and important treatable causes of genetically determined mental retardation.

However, it is unwise to place complete reliance on these programs. In respect to phenylketonuria, the Guthrie test would miss 16% of infants with this disorder if the test was performed before the infant was 24 h old, and 4% if it was performed between 24 and 72 h [67]. The most common cause of failure to detect phenylketonuria is the failure to perform the test, and in 1974 this was estimated to apply to 10% of children in the United States [29]. In addition, certain other disorders, such as the mucopolysaccharidoses or disorders of the urea cycle, are not included in mass newborn screening programs.

Because of these limitations we recommend that all hospitals or clinics which routinely serve mentally retarded children or developmentally disabled children perform certain qualitative urine tests [12] for all children or clients served by the clinic. These tests are listed in table III. They are inexpensive and do not require special equipment, and will, over the course of time, identify significant disorders that would otherwise have been missed.

Clearly, these are only 'triage' tests. The more specific follow-up biochemical tests must be based upon clinical indications, and we outline some of them above. Apart from these general guidelines it seems reasonable for the physician to be particularly alert in the case of two sets of disorders: those that are most common and those for which specific treatments are available, irrespective of frequency. These two categories will form the topics of the remainder of this chapter.

The Most Common Metabolic-Genetic Disorders

Table IV lists the frequency of genetic metabolic disorders associated with mental retardation or neurological deficits. We have not listed disorders such as cystic fibrosis, which although common, 1:1,600 [20], is not

Table IV. Estimated frequency of the less uncommon metabolic disorders which may be associated with mental retardation or neurological deficits

	Frequency	Reference
Congenital hypothyroidism	1:3,500	31, 49
Phenylketonuria	1:11,000	43
Sanfilippo syndrome (MPS III; Netherlands)	1:24,000	78
Metachromatic leukodystrophy (Sweden)	1:40,000	24
Fabry's disease	1:40,000	75
Gaucher disease (Ashkenazi Jews)	1:2,500	75
Tay Sachs disease		
Ashkenazi Jews	1:5,600	54
General population	1:500,000	54
Argininosuccinic aciduria	1:60,000	75
Hunter syndrome (MPS II)		
Ashkenazi Jews	1:67,500	70
British Columbia	1:150,000	45
Galactosemia	1:75,000	75
Hurler symdrome (MPS I)	1:100,000	45
Maple syrup urine disease	1:120,000	43
Homocystinuria		
Ireland	1:40,000	75
General population	1:200,000	75

Frequency estimates are based upon results of mass screening of newborns (hypothyroidism, phenylketonuria) or on population surveys (metachromatic leukodystrophy). For the latter the results are mainly an indication of order of magnitude. Note that the frequency of these disorders may vary significantly among different population groups.

associated with mental retardation. Hypothyroidism and phenylketonuria, the two most common disorders, are detectable by mass screening of newborn infants. The disorders listed in table IV are representative of the major genetic metabolic disease categories. Congenital hypothyroidism includes a group of specific enzyme defects beyond the scope of this chapter. Initial detection is based upon mass screening of blood samples, followed by standard endocrine tests.

Phenylketonuria is the most important example of the amino acidurias, discussed in severeal excellent texts [66, 72, 75]. Disorders of amino acid metabolism are diagnosed by analysis of free amino acids in plasma and in urine [72]. The former requires 2 ml of fresh plasma, the latter 4 ml of fresh urine. If necessary they can be performed with even smaller samples.

Table V. The mucopolysaccharidoses. Clinical and laboratory findings

MPS	Name	Heredity	MR	Cloudy cornea	Urine MPS	Enzyme defect
I	Hurler	AR	+	+	DS + HS	α-L-iduronidase
II	Hunter	X-linked	+	–	DS + HS	iduronate sulfatase
III	Sanfilippo A	AR	+	–	HS	heparan sulfate sulfohydrolase
	B	AR	+	–	HS	N-acetyl-α-D-glucosaminidase
	C	AR	+	–	HS	N-acetyltransferase
	D	AR	+	–	HS	N-acetylglucosamine 6-sulfatase
IV	Morquio	AR	–	–	KS	N-acetylgalactosamine 6-sulfatase
V	Maroteaux Lamy	AR	–	+	DS	N-acetylgalactosamine 4-sulfatase
VI	Glucuronidase deficiency	AR	+	–	chondroitin sulfate	β-glucuronidase

In the study of the retarded child the most significant amino acid metabolism disorders are phenylketonuria [67], maple syrup urine disease, histidinemia, homocystinuria and the urea cycle disorders [66] including argininosuccinic aciduria (see below also). Once the newborn period has passed, the metabolic screening tests listed in table III will usually permit detection of phenylketonuria, maple syrup urine disease, histidinemia and homocystinuria. Quantitative studies of amino acids [66, 71, 72] are available in many laboratories and can be automated. We do not recommend them as routine tests, but they can and should be undertaken when there is a moderate degree of suspicion.

The Sanfilippo, Hurler and Hunter syndromes are examples of the mucopolysaccharidoses listed in table V. The Sanfilippo syndrome (MPS III) appears to be the most common of the mucopolysaccharidoses, four times as frequent as the more widely recognized Hurler syndrome (MPS I). The Sanfilippo syndrome is also pertinent to the present discussion for other reasons. Patients with this syndrome may not show the striking facial and skeletal abnormalities characteristic of the Hurler syndrome. They often present with progressive dementia and disturbed behavior [53, 78, 79] combined with moderately coarse facial features (fig. 1) and moder-

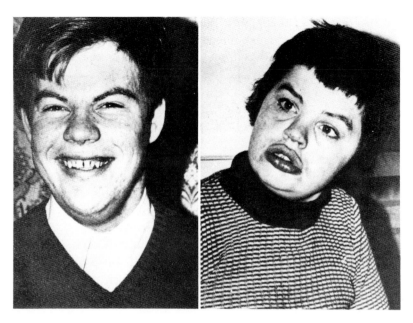

Fig. 1. Two patients with Sanfilippo syndrome, aged 24 and 27 years [from *Van de Kamp* et al., 79]. The young woman has coarsened facial features; this is not nearly as evident for the young man.

ate skeletal changes. The urine screen test for increased MPS may give a positive result, but not invariably so [53]. The most reliable test is demonstration of above normal urinary excretion of heparan sulfate: this can be achieved with a 2-ml urine sample [13]. The Sanfilippo syndrome is heterogeneous: it can be caused by four separate enzyme defects. Assays for the most common types – type A (heparan-N-sulfatase) [39] and type B (alpha-N-accetylglucosaminidase) [56] – can be performed with leukocytes or cultured skin fibroblasts. The Sanfilippo syndrome exemplifies the importance and the dilemma of specific genetic diagnosis. The disorder appears to be relatively common, particularly among clients in institutions for the mentally retarded, and it shows variability of phenotypic expression, and genetic heterogeneity (four distinct enzyme defects). The routine screening test for increased urinary MPS recommended in table III will detect some, but not all, patients. If clinical judgment indicates that this diagnosis deserves serious consideration, genetic consultation and follow-up laboratory tests [13, 39, 56] are required. While at this time there is no specific therapy, the diagnosis is of importance for prognosis, overall management plans and genetic counseling. Prenatal diagnosis is available.

Metachromatic leukodystrophy, and Fabry, Gaucher, Tay-Sachs and Niemann-Pick diseases belong to the 'lysosomal storage' disorders [36]. These are listed in figure 2. In all of these disorders there is a genetic deficiency of a specific degradative enzyme, which is normally located in the lysosome. As a consequence there is accumulation within the lysosome of the substrate of the deficient enzyme. It may take months or years before sufficient quantities of the substrate accumulate to interfere with cellular function. Probably as a result of this, the patients develop normally at first, but then show gradual and progressive loss of function.

In Tay-Sachs and in globoid leukodystrophy, the loss of function begins before the child is 6 months old; in metachromatic leukodystrophy, this does not occur until after the first year, and in Fabry's disease, symptoms do not begin before the 2nd or 3rd decade. In Tay-Sachs disease and in Sandhoff disease there is the characteristic retinal cherry red spot, and an abnormal startle response to sound. In Gaucher and in Niemann-Pick diseases, the spleen and liver are enlarged. Fabry's disease, which is a sex-linked disorder, presents with renal failure, painful extremities due to involvement of small fibers in peripheral nerves, and small red skin lesions (angiokeratoma) over the scrotum, the umbilicus and the lower abdomen.

Specific diagnosis of the lysosomal storage diseases requires enzyme assays. They are usually carried out in specialized laboratories serving a state, country or region. Specific therapy is not yet available, but research aimed to provide enzyme replacement is underway [9, 18].

Carrier detection is available for many of the disorders, and in the case of Tay-Sachs disease, effective programs have been initiated to detect Tay-Sachs carriers among Ashkenazi Jews [57] where the frequency of the carrier rate is 1:27 [23, 54]. If husband and wife are both carriers there is a 1:4 statistical chance that they will have a child with Tay-Sachs disease. Prenatal diagnosis is possible, and this is also true for all the other lysosomal storage disorders. It is cost-effective to screen for Tay-Sachs carriers among Ashkenazi Jews in the reproductive age, followed by prenatal diagnosis and abortion of fetuses shown to have the disorder [57]. In contrast, it would be prohibitively expensive to perform *routine* screening for Tay-Sachs carriers in the general population [57]. This also applies to most of the other lysosomal disorders where no special high-risk population can be identified. In the case of Gaucher disease type I, the clinical disorder is much less severe than Tay-Sachs disease, and most people would consider prenatal studies

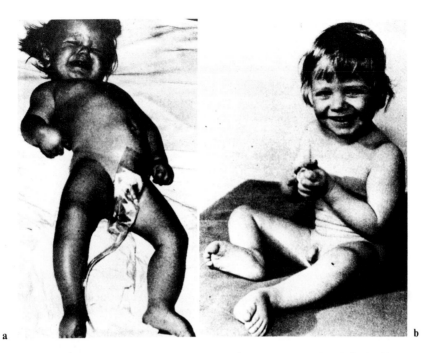

a   b

Fig. 2. a Patient with malignant phenylketonuria at age 14 months. Child had been maintained on phenylalanine-restricted diet since age 3 weeks, but was opisthotonic, spastic and had myoclonic jerks. b Same patient at 27 months following 14 months of therapy with L-dopa, carbidopa and 5-hydroxytryptophane [from *Bartholome* et al., 4].

inappropriate. Thus, for most of the lysosomal disorders other than Tay-Sachs disease, genetic counseling is reserved for families known to be at risk, that is, where an 'index case' has already occurred. This consideration highlights the importance of exact diagnosis in a person who has the disease, even in the absence of specific therapy. Without an exact enzymatic diagnosis genetic counseling cannot be offered.

Table IV shows that certain disorders are particularly common among specific ethnic groups. As already noted, Tay-Sachs disease is particularly common among Ashkenazi Jews. The same is true also for Gaucher disease type I, dysautonomia, Niemann-Pick disease A, spongy degeneration of infancy, and the autosomal recessive form of torsion dystonia [23]. Homocystinuria due to cystathionine synthase deficiency occurs most frequently in Ireland [44].

Table VI. Therapeutic strategies

---

1. Supply a missing metabolite
2. Limit intake of a precursor which may undergo toxic accumulation
3. Depletion of a toxic stored substance
4. Supply a vitamin cofactor
5. Supply a missing enzyme
6. Organ Transplantation

Disorders for Which There Are Specific Treatments

Table VI lists the therapeutic strategies now in use, and the disorders will be discussed according to this scheme.

Supply a Missing Metabolite

The most important example of this strategy is the administration of thyroid to children with congenital hypothyroidism. There is good evidence that early therapy improves prognosis in congenital hypothyroidism [34]. The capacity to detect this disorder early through newborn screening thus forms the basis for what is probably the most significant therapeutic advance in the genetic-metabolic disease category.

Treatment by supply of a missing metabolite was also successful in a child with an unusual form of phenylketonuria referred to as malignant hyperphenylalaninemia [4] (see below). It is presumed that here there is deficient synthesis of the neurotransmittors serotonin, dopamine and nor-adrenaline. In spite of dietary therapy for phenylketonuria, which had permitted maintenance of normal blood phenylalanine levels, the child was severely retarded and tetraplegic at 12 months of age, a characteristic feature of malignant hyperphenylalaninemia [16]. Because of the supposition that the neurological disability might reflect a deficit in neurotransmittors, the child was started on oral L-dopa, carbidopa and L-hydroxytryptophan, substances known to be precursors of neurotransmittors. Striking improvement was noted (fig. 3). Still more recent work suggests that similar improvements can also be achieved by the administration of vitamin cofactors [2, 16].

Another example of this type of therapeutic intervention may be in cerebrotendinous xanthomatosis, a rare autosomal recessive disorder characterized by mild mental retardation, cataracts, tendon xanthomas and pro-

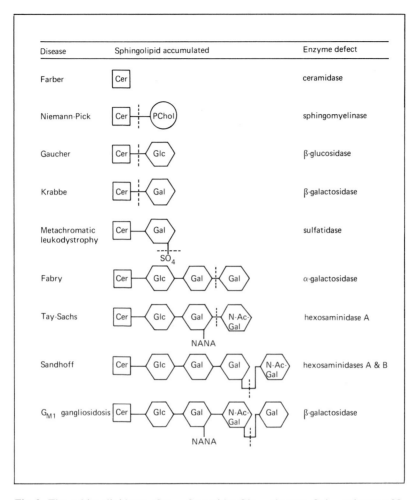

Fig. 3. The sphingolipidoses. Cer = Ceramide; Glc = glucose; Gal = galactose; N-Ac-Gal = N-acetylgalactosamine; NANA = N-acetylneuraminic acid. The dotted line indicates the location of the deficient enzyme reaction.

gressive extrapyramidal and cerebellar dysfunction. Biochemically, it is characterized by the accumulation of the sterol cholestanol, abnormal amounts of which are also present in plasma. It has been shown recently that the primary defect appears to be the deficient synthesis of certain bile acids [58]. It has also been shown that oral administration of one of these bile acids, chenodeoxycholic acid, reverses the biochemical abnormality, at least in part, probably by diminishing the abnormal overproduction of cholestanol and cholesterol which occurs in this disease [62].

Limit Intake of a Precursor Which May Undergo Toxic Accumulation

Along with the replacement therapy for hypothyroidism, described previously, the type of therapeutic intervention to be described in this section, has shown the greatest success. It has proven effective for phenylketonuria, maple syrup urine disease, galactosemia and for certain disorders of fatty acid metabolism.

Therapy of phenylketonuria is a significant public health issue: over 100 million newborn infants throughout the world have been screened for this disorder. With an incidence of 1:11,000 it is estimated that 10,000 children are now under treatment. The success of this therapeutic approach is made possible by the fact that phenylalanine is an essential amino acid, that is, it is not synthesized by man, so that dietary intake is the only source of this substance. The patient with phenylketonuria requires the same amount of phenylalanine – 200–500 mg/day for the first 5 years of life – as does the normal person. Patients with phenylketonuria differ from normal persons in that they are unable to dispose of amounts of phenylalanine in excess of this requirement. The aim of therapy is to provide a diet which contains no more than the minimum daily requirement of phenylalanine, and which nevertheless contains all other nutrients and which is palatable [1, 66, 67]. If diet is begun early, preferably within the first 60 days, the risk of severe mental retardation (which is 99% in untreated patients) is greatly decreased [82]. There is controversy about how long the diet must be maintained. While two studies reported that termination of diet at 4–5 years did not compromise follow-up IQ [30, 35], other studies indicate that in some patients the IQ scores fall after termination of therapy [81]. It is recommended that 'until the issue is resolved, it would be prudent to maintain dietary therapy of the patient with phenylketonuria as long as possible when familial and social factors permit, and then to employ a relaxed but still restricted low phenylalanine diet' [67].

Two important new issues have arisen in respect to phenylketonuria: maternal phenylketonuria and malignant phenylketonuria. 'Maternal phenylketonuria' refers to the damage incurred during fetal life, to a child born to a phenylketonuric woman. The child in almost all instances is a heterozygote for phenylketonuria, and would not be handicapped by this, were it not for the ill effects during pregnancy. Mental retardation (an IQ of less than 75) was observed in 91% of children born to mothers with a blood phenylalanine level in excess of 20 mg/dl [41]. The risk of maternal phenyl-ketonuria has been increased greatly by the very success of therapy of the phenylketonuric child. In the past the untreated profoundly retarded woman with phenylketonuria hardly ever reproduced. As a result of successful therapy, a large number of young women with phenylketonuria and normal intelligence are now considering marriage. There is hope, but no proof, that resumption of diet during pregnancy may prevent retardation in the child [41]. Resumption of diet would have to be initiated early in pregnancy, probably when pregnancy is being planned, since some of the teratogenic effects of high maternal phenylalanine levels occur during the first weeks of pregnancy. Until the efficacy of therapy is evaluated it would be most prudent for the woman with phenylketonuria not to have children.

'Malignant phenylketonuria' refers to a group of disorders in which blood phenylalanine levels are elevated – and which thus are detected by mass screening of newborns – but in which dietary restriction of phenylalanine will not prevent mental retardation or neurological deficit. These patients may have several different enzyme defects, some of which lead to a deficiency of tetrahydropterin (B-4), a cofactor required for the conversion of phenylalanine to tyrosine. Malignant phenylketonuria is estimated to be present in 2% of children with significant and persistent hyperphenylalanin-emia. Methods are being developed for their early detection [2], and there is hope that oral administration of B-4 may prove effective [16]. We have already referred to the beneficial effects of the administration of neurotransmittor precursor in one child with malignant phenylketonuria (fig. 3).

Other disorders in which success has been achieved by limiting the intake of precursor which may undergo toxic accumulation are maple syrup urine disease [74], galactosemia [37], and Refsum's disease [76]. The therapy of maple syrup urine disease differs from that of phenylketonuria in that the achievement of dietary restriction of the amino acids leucine, isoleucine and valine is more difficult than that of phenylalanine alone. Furthermore, the restriction must be maintained for life, and there may be intermittent periods of life-threatening acidosis. Nevertheless, the oldest patient, who was 15 years old at the latest report, has normal intellectual function, is performing at grade level in regular school, and has achieved normal growth and sexual maturation [50]. Varying degrees of success with dietary restriction of leucine or of isoleucine or other amino acids have also been achieved in isovaleric acidemia [44], methylmalonic acidemia [55] and propionic acidemia [10, 20]. The latter disorders may also respond dramatically to the administration of vitamin cofactors (see below).

Depletion of a Toxic Stored Substance

The most dramatic example of therapy which depletes a toxic substance, is the use of chelating agents in Wilson's disease. Wilson's disease, or hepatolenticular degeneration, is an autosomal recessive trait which is characterized by the accumulation of copper, first in the liver and later in the cornea, brain and kidney. Patients may present with cirrhosis of the liver. However, the first manifestations often relate to damage of the central nervous system, with emotional lability, dementia, school failure, tremor, dystonia or incoordination. Thus, the patient may first be referred to a clinic serving the mentally ill or mentally handicapped. A pathognomonic sign is the Kayser-Fleischer ring, a greenish ring (which contains copper) at the limbus of the cornea. This ring may be visible with the naked eye, and more definitely by examination with the slit-lamp. Other important laboratory tests are the demonstration of abnormally low serum ceruloplasmin levels and abnormally high excretion of inorganic copper in the urine [63]. Because of the distressing disability and fatal outcome of untreated Wilson's disease, and the success of therapy, failure to diagnose this condition would represent a grievous medical error. The success of therapy is illustrated by the following case history taken from a report by *Hayek* et al. [27] from Vienna.

A 14-year-old girl was seen in the University Clinic with a 6 month history of increasing difficulty with her studies, nervousness and tremor. Kayser-Fleischer ring was present, serum caeruloplasmin level reduced and urinary copper increased. During the last few months she had experienced swallowing difficulty. Speech was slow and there was difficulty in articulation. There was tremor of extremities, hypersalivation, diminished facial expression with stereotyped grin. Handwriting was impaired (fig. 4a), verbal IQ was 90, performance IQ 80, overall IQ 83. The patient had insight about her limitations and attempted to conceal the tremor. She was started on *D*-penicillamine therapy, at first 750 mg/day, later increased to 1,500 mg/day and this was continued for the next 9 years. At age 24 her handwriting was normal (fig. 4b) as was her speech and behavior, and her overall IQ was 86.

Figure 4a shows the patient's handwriting at age 14, when the diagnosis was first made, and figure 4b shows it at age 24, after 9 years of penicillamine therapy. A translation of what she wrote at age 24 is:

To the Hanusch hospital came Prof. Sternlieb from America. We drove to the hospital and I was introduced to Prof. Sternlieb. He was pleased about how well I was doing. I have continued to correspond with him, and he answers all my questions. I, of course, continue my treatment. I receive cuprimine capsules from America and I take two, three

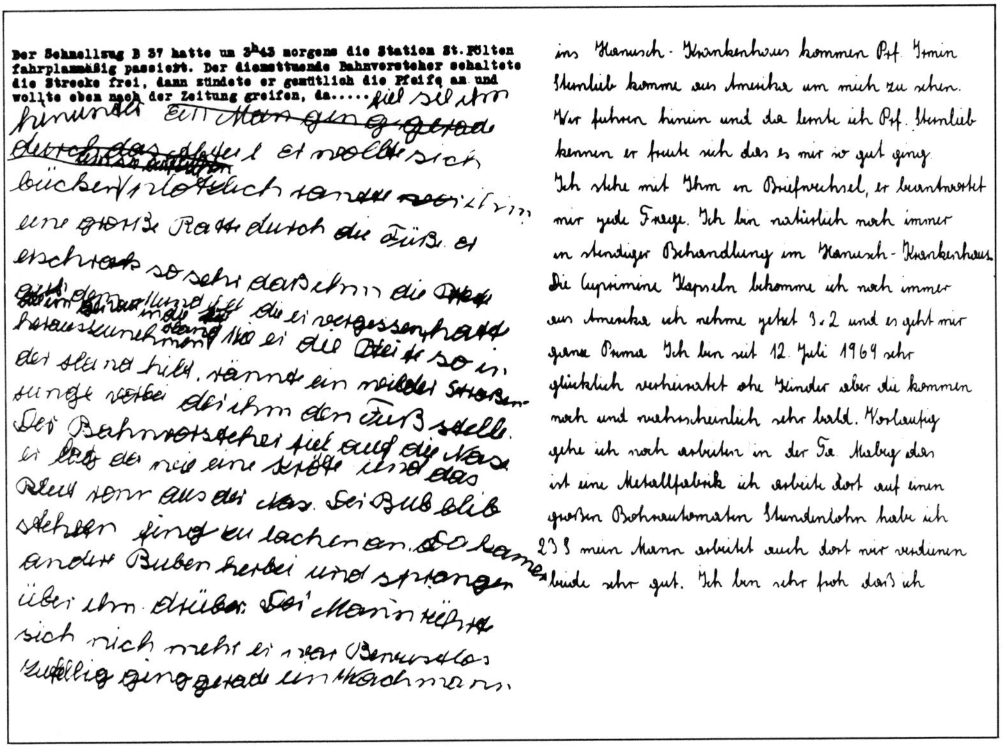

Der Schnellzug D 37 hatte um 2^h45 morgens die Station St.Pölten fahrplanmäßig passiert. Der diensttuende Bahnvorsteher schaltete die Strecke frei, dann zündete er gemütlich die Pfeife an und wollte eben nach der Zeitung greifen, da.....

[Fig. 4a: handwritten cursive text, not legibly transcribable]

[Fig. 4b: handwritten cursive text, not legibly transcribable]

Fig. 4. a Handwriting of 14 year-old-girl with Wilson's disease, at time of initial diagnosis. **b** Handwriting of same patient at age 24 years, after 9 years of penicillamine therapy. See text for translation of what she wrote at age 24 [from *Hayek* et al., 27; with permission from Springer, New York].

times daily, and feel fine. No children so far, but they will come, probably soon. At present, I work in a metal factory with automated machinery and receive 23 schillings per hour. My husband also works there, and we both receive good wages...

This history illustrates an important point: if one has specific therapy it *is* possible to reverse central nervous system damage. This applies also to other genetic metabolic disorders, and provides general encouragement for the future.

The patient did become pregnant, and delivered a normal child. At least 18 normal babies have been born by women with Wilson's disease who were maintained on penicillamine therapy during pregnancy [64]. An important new addition to the therapy of Wilson's disease, is the recent introduction by *Walshe* [80] of trienthylene tetramine 2 HCl, a new chelating agent which can be used by patients who are unable to tolerate penicillamine.

Recent work by *Batshaw and Brusilow* [5] indicates that the administration of sodium benzoate is of value for the therapy of genetic disorders of the urea cycle. These disorders include argininosuccinic aciduria, citrullinemia, ornithine transcarbamylase deficiency, hyperargininemia and other types of hyperammonemia [75]. They may manifest as mental retardation of unknown etiology, sometimes associated with abnormal hair, or more commonly by episodes of intermittent vomiting or coma. The disability is usually progressive and often fatal. Diagnosis can often be made by chromatography of amino acids in blood or urine, and by demonstrating elevated levels of blood ammonia. Specific diagnosis depends upon enzyme assays which are performed in follow-up to chromatographic studies and ammonia measurement.

The sodium benzoate therapy depends upon transformation of this substance to hippuric acid. The hippuric acid is, in turn, conjugated with glycine. This last reaction is the key therapeutic step for these disorders. Glycine excretion forms an alternate pathway for waste nitrogen excretion, and thus indirectly reduces the toxic ammonia levels. The therapeutic strategy thus involves the depletion of a toxic waste product. Other strategies for the therapy of urea cycle disorders include the administration of arginine, which acts by an analogous mechanism [11], a general reduction in protein intake, including the administration of nitrogen-free analogues of essential amino acids [77], the feeding of lactulose [73] and peritoneal dialysis.

Supply a Vitamin-Cofactor: The Vitamin-Responsive Disorders

Scriver and Rosenberg [66] have called attention to an interesting group of disorders, in which the metabolic defect can be corrected by the administration of a specific vitamin or cofactor but in doses in excess of usual daily requirement. Table VII lists some general characteristics of these disorders. Note that this concept differs sharply from the more controversial megavitamin therapy approach. For the disorders under discussion the effects are specific and verifiable, and, in each instance involve only a single substance. Recognition of these rare disorders is important: for example, a child with a vitamin-responsive form of maple syrup disease can be maintained in good health with a daily dose of 10 mg of thiamine [69] and does not require the difficult and expensive diet which is indispensable for most patients with maple syrup urine disease [50].

Table VII. General points about vitamin cofactor therapy for inborn errors of metabolism

---

1. Vitamin cofactor action is specific, and can be related to cofactor requirements of deficient enzyme reaction
2. Effective vitamin cofactor dosage may be far in excess of normal daily requirement
3. Most of the inborn errors which *may* be cofactor-responsive also have variants which are unresponsive
4. In most instances the responsive and the unresponsive forms can be distinguished only by therapeutic trial

---

The first of these disorders to be described was the pyridoxine dependency syndrome reported by *Scriver and Hutchison* [65]. They described an infant which, on a normal pyridoxine intake, grew slowly and had convulsions – but when the pyridoxine intake was raised to four to five times normal, the child got well. The activities of several pyridoxine-dependent enzymes were abnormal. Other vitamin-dependent states include methylmalonic aciduria where administration of vitamin B_{12} in a dose 1,000-fold the minimum daily requirement caused striking improvement [61] and two biotin-dependent disorders – propionyl-CoA carboxylase deficiency [3] and β-methyl-crotonylglycinuria [22]. The last three disorders all involve the metabolism of short-chain fatty acids. Such patients may present with impairment of growth and psychomotor development, intermittent metabolic acidosis and coma, and sometimes an abnormal odor. Specific diagnosis is difficult: the routine metabolic screening tests and amino acid chromatography are ususally normal. Specific diagnosis depends upon identification of the compounds by gas-liquid chromatography-mass spectometry [21, 32]. They require elaborate equipment and are performed in regional laboratories, on a referral basis. While the tests are complex, they require only 5 ml of urine. It is important for each clinical diagnostic center to establish a referral system so that these assays for organic acids can, indeed, be performed. The information provided may lead to specific and effective therapy and is essential for genetic counseling.

Enzyme Replacement and Transplant Therapy

Enzyme replacement therapy has been initiated for patients with Gaucher disease and with Fabry's disease and certain other disorders [9, 18, 19] and has formed the topic of a recent symposium [18]. At this time the practical application of such therapy is limited by the scarcity of purified enzymes, and the difficulty of targeting such large molecules to the cells and organs where they are needed, particularly the nervous system.

Bone marrow transplants have been used successfully in patients with immune deficiency states, such as adenosine deaminase deficiency [28] and the Wiscott-Aldrich syndrome [59] and in osteopetrosis [15]. In Fabry's disease, which was discussed in the previous section, renal transplantation can reverse the manifestations of kidney failure as it does in other types of renal disease. It is not yet clear, if the normal α-galactosidase contained in the donor kidney, can, in addition, help to alleviate the generalized α-galactosidase deficiency which is the basic defect in this disorder [47]. Fibro blast transplants have been used in patients with mucopolysaccharidoses. They have been well tolerated. Some biochemical improvement occurred, but clinical changes were equivocal [17]. Very recent, but still unsubstantiated reports indicate that bone marrow transplants may bring about significant improvement in patients with the Hurler syndrome [6, 30a].

Clearly, enzyme replacement, transplantation and genetic engineering are the topics of intensive investigation and hold great promise for the therapy of the disorders described in this chapter.

References

1   American Academy of Pediatrics Committee on Nutrition: Special diets for infants with inborn errors of amino acid metabolism. Pediatrics, Springfield 57: 783–791 (1976).
2   American Academy of Pediatrics Committee on Nutrition: New Developments in Hyperphenylalaninemia. Pediatrics, Springfield 65: 844–846 (1980).
3   Barnes, N.D.; Hull, D.; Balgobin, L.; Gompertz, D.: Biotin-responsive propionic acidemia. Lancet ii: 244–245 (1970).
4   Bartholome, K.; Byrd, D.J.; Kaufman, S.; Milstien, S.: Atypical phenylketonuria with normal phenylalanine hydroxylase and dihydropteridine reductase activity in vitro. Pediatrics, Springfield 59: 757–761 (1977).
5   Batshaw, M.L.; Brusilow, S.W.: Treatment of hyperammonemic coma caused by inborn errors of urea synthesis. J. Pediat. 97: 893–900 (1980).
6   Benson, P.F.: Personal communication.
7   Berry, H.K.: Screening for metabolic disorders among high risk infants and children. Hlth Lab. Sci. 14: 183–193 (1977).
8   Beutler, E.; Baluda, M.C.: A simple spot test for galactosemia. J. Lab. clin. Med, 68: 137–141 (1966).
9   Brady, R.O.; Pentchev, P.G.; Gal, A.E.: Investigations in enzyme replacement therapy in lipid storage diseases. Fed. Proc. 34: 1310–1315 (1975).
10 Brandt, I.K.; Hsia, E.; Clement, D.H.; Provence, S.A.: Propionicacidemia (ketotic hyperglycinemia): dietary treatment resulting in normal growth and development. Pediatrics, Springfield 53: 391–395 (1974).

11   Brusilow, S.; Batshaw, M.L.: Arginine therapy of argininosuccinase deficiency. Lancet *i:* 124–127 (1979).

12   Buist, N.R.M.: Set of simple side-room tests for detection of inborn errors of metabolism. Br. med. J. *ii:* 745–749 (1968).

13   Burlingame, R.W.; Thomas, G.H.; Stevens, R.L.; Schmid, K.; Moser, H.W.: Direct quantitation of glycosaminoglycans in 2 ml of urine from patients with mucopolysaccharidoses. Clin. Chem. *27:* 124–128 (1981).

14   Centerwall, W.R.: Phenylketonuria. J. Am. med. Ass. *165:* 392 (1957).

15   Coccia, P.F.; Cervenka, J.; Teitelbaum, S.L.; Kahn, A.; Clawson, C.C.; Brown, D.M.: Reversal of human osteopetrosis by bone marrow transplantation: etiologic implications. Clin. Res. *27:* 483A (1979).

16   Danks, D.: Early diagnosis of hyperphenylalaninemia due to tetrahydrobiopterin deficiency (malignant hyperphenylalaninemia). J. Pediat. *96:* 854–856.

17   Dean, M.F.; Stevens, R.L.; Muir, H.; Benson, P.F.; Button, L.R.; Anderson, R.L.; Boylston, A.; Mowbray, J.: Enzyme replacement therapy by fibroblast transplantation: long-term biochemical study in three cases of Hunter's Disease. J. clin. Invest. *63:* 138–145 (1979).

18   Desnick, R.J.: Enzyme therapy in genetic diseases. Birth Defects, Orig. Article Ser. *16/1* (1980)

19   Desnick, R.J.; Thorpe, S.R.; Fiddler, M.B.: Toward enzyme therapy for lysosomal storage diseases. Physiol. Rev. *56:* 57–99 (1970).

20   Editorial: Population screening for carriers of seemingly recessively inherited disorders. Lancet *ii:* 679–680 (1980).

21   Gates, S.C.; Dendramis, N.; Sweeley, C.C.: Automated metabolic profiling of organic acids in human urine. 1. Description of methods. Clin. Chem. *24:* 1674–1679 (1978).

22   Gompertz, D.; Draffan, G.H.; Watts, J.L.; Hull, D.: Biotin responsive β-methylcrotonylglycinuria. Lancet *ii:* 22–24 (1971).

23   Goodman, R.M.; Motulsky, A.G.: Genetic diseases among Ashkenazi jews (Raven Press, New York 1979).

24   Gustavson, K.H.; Hagberg, B.: The incidence and genetics of metachromatic leukodystrophy. Acta pediat. scand. *60:* 585–590 (1971).

25   Gustavson, K.H.; Hagberg, B.; Hagberg, G.; Stark, K.: Severe mental retardation in a Swedish county. II. Etiological and pathogenetic aspects of children born 1959–1970. Neuropädiatrie *8:* 293–304 (1977).

26   Guthrie, R.: Screening for 'inborn errors of metabolism' in the newborn infant – a multiple test program. Birth Defects, Orig. Article Ser. *4:* 92 (1968).

27   Hayek, H.W.; Knoll, E.; Widhalm, S.: Über das organische Psychosyndrom bei Morbus Wilson. Mschr. Kinderheilk. *121:* 679–683 (1973).

28   Hirschhorn, R.: Treatment of genetic diseases by allotransplantation; in Desnick, Enzyme therapy of genetic diseases. Birth Defects, Orig. Article Ser. *16/1:* 429–444 (1980).

29   Holtzman, N.A.; Meek, A.G.; Mellits, E.D.: Neonatal screening for phenylketonuria. I. Effectiveness. J. Am. med. Ass. *229:* 667–670 (1974).

30   Holtzman, N.A.; Welcher, D.W.; Mellits, E.D.: Termination of restricted diet in children with phenylketonuria: a randomized controlled study. New Engl. J. Med. *293:* 1121–1124 (1975).

30a Hobbs, J.R.; Hugh-Jones, K.; Barrett, A.J.; Byrom, N.; Chambers, D.; James, D.C.O.; Lucas, C.F.; Rogers, T.R.; Benson, P.F.; Tansley, L.R.; Patrick, A.D.; Mossman, J.; Young, E.P.: Reversal of clinical features of Hurler's disease and biochemical improvement after treatment by bone-marow transplantation. Lancet *ii:* 709–712 (1981).

31 Hulse, J.A.; Grant, D.B.; Clayton, B.E.; Lilly, P.; Jackson, D.; Spracklan, A.; Edwards, R.W.H.; Nurse, D.: Population screening for congenital hypothyroidism. Br. med. J. *280:* 675–678 (1980).

32 Jellum, E.; Stocke, O.; Eldjarn, L.: Combined use of gas chromatography, mass spectrometry and computer in diagnosis and studies of metabolic disorders. Clin. chem. *18:* 800–809 (1972).

33 Kaveggia, E.G.; Durkin, M.V.; Pendleton, E.; Opitz, J.M.: Diagnostic/genetic studies on 1224 patients with severe mental retardation; in Proc. 3rd Congr. Int. Ass. Scient. Study Mental Defic., pp. 82–93 (Polish Medical Publishers, Warsaw).

34 Klein, A.H.; Meltzer, S.; Kenny, F.M.: Improved prognosis of congenital hypothyroidism treated before 3 months. J. Pediat. *81:* 912–915 (1972).

35 Koff, E.; Kammerer, B.; Boyle, A.; Pueschel, S.M.: Intelligence and phenylketonuria: effects of diet termination. J. Pediat. *94:* 534–537 (1979).

36 Kolodny, E.H.: Current concepts in genetics: lysosomal storage diseases. New Engl. J. Med. *294:* 1217–1220 (1976).

37 Komrower, G.M.; Lee, D.H.: Long-term follow-up of galactosemia. Archs Dis. Childh. *45:* 367–373 (1970).

38 Kopelman, L.: Genetic screening in newborns; voluntary or compulsory? Perspect. Biol. Med. *22:* 83–89 (1978).

39 Kresse, H.: Mucopolysaccharidosis III A (Sanfilippo A disease): deficiency of heparin sulfamidase in skin fibroblasts and leukocytes. Biochem. biophys. Res. Commun. *54:* 1111–1118 (1973).

40 Lappe, M.; Roblin, R.O.: in Bergsma, Lappe, Roblin, Gustatson, Paul, Ethical social and legal dimensions of screening for human genetic diseases, vol. 10/6, p. 1 (National Foundation – March of Dimes, White Plains 1974).

41 Lenke, R.R.; Levy, H.L.: Maternal phenylketonuria and hyperphenylalaninemia. New Engl. J. Med. *303:* 1202–1208 (1980).

42 Levy, H.L. Personal communications.

43 Levy, H.L.: Genetic screening; in Harris, Hirschhorn, Advances in human genetics, vol. 4, pp. 1–104 (Plenum Press, New York 1973).

44 Levy, H.L.; Erickson, A.M.: Isovaleric acidemia; in Nyhan, Heritable disorders of amino acid metabolism, pp. 81–97 (Wiley, New York 1974).

45 Lowry, R.B.; Renwick, D.H.G.: The relative frequency of the Hurler and Hunter syndromes. New Engl. J. Med. *284:* 221–222 (1971).

46 Macri, J.N.; Haddon, J.E.; Weiss, R.R.: Screening for neural tube defects in the United States. A summary of the Scarborough conference. Am. J. Obstet. Gynec. *133:* 119–125 (1979).

47 Matas, A.J.; Desnick, R. J.; Najarian, I.S.; Simmons, R.L.: Clinical and experimental transplantation in enzymatic deficiency disease. Surgery Gynec. Obstet. *146:* 975–982 (1978).

48 Milunsky, A.; Annas, G.J.: Genetics and the law. II (Plenum Press, New York 1980).

49   Mitchell, M.L.; Larsen, R.; Levy, H.L.; Bennett, A.J.E.; Madoff, M.A.: Screening for congenital hypothyroidism. Results in the newborn population of New England. J. Am. med. Ass. *239:* 2348–2351 (1978).

50   Moser, H.W.: Maple syrup urine disease; in Vinken, Brayn, Handbook of clinical neurology, vol. 29: Metabolic and deficiency diseases of the nervous system. (North-Holland, Amsterdam 1977).

51   Moser, H.W.; Wolf, P.A.: The nosology of mental retardation: including the report of a survey of 1,378 mentally retarded individuals at the Walter E. Fernald State School; in Nervous system birth defects. Orig. Article Ser., vol. 7, 117–134 (Williams & Wilkins, Baltimore 1971).

52   McKusick, V.A.: Mendelian inheritance in man. Catalogs of autosomal dominant, autosomal recessive and X-linked phenotypes; 5th ed. (Johns Hopkins University Press, Baltimore 1978).

53   McKusick, V.A.; Neufeld, E.F.: The mucopolysaccharide stroage diseases: in Stanbury, The metabolic basis of inherited disease; 5th ed. (McGraw-Hill, New York, in press).

54   Neel, J.V.: History and the Tay-Sachs allele; in Goodman, Motulsky, Genetic diseases among Ashkenazi jews, pp. 285–299 (Raven Press, New York 1979).

55   Nyhan, W.L.; Fawcett, N.; Anda, T.; Rennert, O.M.; Julius, R.L.: Response to dietary therapy in B_{12} unresponsive methylmalonic acidemia. Pediatrics, Springfield *51:* 539–548 (1973).

56   O'Brien, J.S.: Sanfilippo syndrome. Profound deficiency of alpha-acetylglucosaminidase activity in organs and skin fibroblasts from type B patients. Proc. natn. Acad. Sci. USA *69:* 1720–1722 (1972).

57   O'Brien, J.S.: Tay-Sachs disease: from enzyme to prevention. Fed. Proc. *32:* 191–199 (1973).

58   Oftebro, H.; Bjorkhem, I.; Skrede, S.; Schreiner, A.; Pedersen, J.I.: Cerebrotendinous xanthomatosis. A defect in mitochondrial 26-hydroxylation required for normal biosynthesis of cholic acid. J. clin. Invest. *65:* 1418–1430 (1980).

59   Parkman, R.; Rappeport, J.; Geha, R.; Belli, J.; Cassady, R.; Levey, R.; Nathan, D.G.; Rosen, F.S.: Complete correction of the Wiskott-Aldrich syndrome by allogenic bone-marrow transplantation. New Engl J. Med. *298:* 921–927 (1978).

60   Rapin, I.: Progressive genetic-metabolic disorders of the central nervous system in children. Pediat. Ann. *5:* 313–349 (1976).

61   Rosenberg, L.E.; Lilljequist, A.C.; Hsia, Y.E.: Methylmalonic aciduria: metabolic block localization and vitamin B_{12} dependency. Science *162:* 805–807 (1968).

62   Salen, G.; Meriwether, T.W.; Nicolau, G.: Chenodeoxycholic acid inhibits increased cholesterol and cholestanol synthesis in patients with cerebrotendinous xanthomatosis. Biochem. Med. *14:* 57–74 (1975).

63   Sass-Kortsak, A.; Bearn, A.G.: Hereditary disorders of copper metabolism, in Stanbury, Wyngaarden, Fredrickson, The metabolic basis of inherited disease; 4th ed., pp. 1098–1126 (McGraw Hall New York 1978).

64   Scheinberg, H.; Sternlieb, I.; Pregnancy in penicillamine-treated patients with Wilson's disease. New Engl. J. Med. *293:* 1300–1302 (1975).

65   Scriver, C.R.; Hutchison, J.H.: Vitamin B_6 deficiency syndrome in human infancy: biochemical and clinical observations. Pediatrics, Springfield *31:* 240–250 (1963).

66   Scriver, C.R.; Rosenberg, L.E.: Amino acid metabolism and its disorders (Saunders,
      Philadelphia 1973).
67   Scriver, C.R.; Clow, C.L.: Phenylketonuria: epitome of human biochemical genetics.
      New Engl. J. Med. *303:* 1336–1342, 1394–1400 (1980).
68   Scriver, C.R.; Feingold, M.; Mamunes, P.; Nadler, H.L.: Screening for congenital
      metabolic disorders in the newborn infant: congenital deficiency of thyroid hormone
      and hyperphenylalaninemia. Pediatrics, Springfield *60:* 389–404 (1977).
69   Scriver, C.R.; Mackenzie, S.; Clow, C.L.; Delvin, E.: Thiamine responsive maple
      syrup urine disease. Lancet *i:* 310–312 (1971).
70   Schaap, T.; Bach, G.: Incidence of mucopolysaccharidoses in Israel: is Hunter disease
      a 'Jewish disease'? Hum. Genet. *56:* 221 (1971).
71   Schmidt, L.: The biochemical detection of metabolic disease: screening tests and a
      systematic approach to screening; in Nyhan, Heritable disorders of amino acid
      metabolism. Patterns of clinical expression and genetic variation (Wiley, New York
      1974).
72   Shih, V.E.: Laboratory techniques for the detection of hereditary metabolic disorders
      (CRC Press, Cleveland 1973).
73   Simmons, F.; Goldstein, H.; Boyle, T.D.: A controlled clinical trial of lactulose in
      hepatic encephalopathy. Gastroenterology *59:* 827–832 (1970).
74   Snyderman, S.E.; Norton, P.; Roitman, E.; Holt, L.E., Jr.: Maple syrup urine disease,
      with particular reference to diet therapy. Pediatrics, Springfield *34:* 454–472
      (1964).
75   Stanbury, J.B.; Wyngaarden, J.B.; Fredrickson, D.S.: The metabolic basis of inherited
      disease; 4th ed. (McGraw-Hill, New York 1978).
76   Steinberg, D.; Mize, C.E.; Herndon, J.H., Jr.; Fales, H.M.; Engee, W.K.; Vroom,
      F.Q.: Phytanic acid in patients with Refsum's syndrome and response to dietary
      treatment. Archs intern. Med. *125:* 75–87 (1970).
77   Thoene, J.; Batshaw, M.; Spector, E.; Kulovich, S.; Brusilow, S.; Walser, M.; Nyhan,
      W.: Neonatal citrullinemia: treatment with keto-analogs of essential amino acids. J.
      Pediat. *90:* 218–224 (1977).
78   Van de Kamp, J.J.P.: The Sanfilippo syndrome: a clinical and genetical study of 75
      patients in the Netherlands; thesis (Pasmans, The Hague 1979).
79   Van de Kamp, J.J.P.; van Pelt, J.F.; Liem, K.O.; Giesberts, A.H.; Niepoth, L.T.M.;
      Staallman, C.R.: Clinical variability in Sanfilippo B disease: a report on six patients
      in two related sibships. Clin. Gen. *10:* 279–284 (1976).
80   Walshe, J.M.: The management of Wilson's disease with trienthylene tetramine
      2 HCL (Trien HCl); in Papadatos, Bartsocas, The management of genetic disorders
      (Liss, New York 1979).
81   Williamson, M.; Koch, R.; Berlow, S.: Diet discontinuation in phenylketonuria. Pedi-
      atrics, Springfield *63:* 823–824 (1979).
82   Wrona, R.M.: A clinical epidemiological study of hyperphenylalaninemia. Am. J.
      publ. Hlth *69:* 673–679 (1979).

2 Genetics of Mental Retardation
Mark W. Steele

If one defines mental retardation as a consistent IQ score of less than 70 on standard intelligence tests, then approximately 3% of the population in the US may be identified as mentally retarded at some time during their lifetime. Etiological classification of mental retardation has been complicated by problems of definition and ascertainment. At least 5% of mental retardation can be attributed solely to environmental (nonhereditary) factors. Simple Mendelian traits and chromosomal abnormalities can account for another 20% of the mentally retarded, and multifactorial polygenic traits (such as neural tube defect) can account for another 10% of the mentally retarded. The etiology for the remaining 65% of the mentally retarded is still quite controversial. Most affected individuals in this last group are categorized as familial or subcultural retardates. If one accepts that the etiology here also may be multifactorial, then clearly the etiology of over 90% of the mentally retarded may be related in part to some heritable (genetic) factors [6, 9]. The diagnosis and classification of mental retardation may be found on pages 70 and 124 of this textbook.

Multifactorial Mental Retardation

The term 'multifactorial' refers to an interaction of environmental and polygenic factors. Respecting the genetic component at least two and usually more genetic loci are involved. For most multifactorial traits the crucial environmental factors are not known. Several birth defects represent multifactorial traits and some, such as neural tube defects, are often associated with mental retardation. The environmental factors in such situations must be in utero, but their exact nature remains a mystery.

Neural tube defects include anencephaly, spina bifida cystica (often with secondary hydrocephalus) and isolated congenital hydrocephalus. The three are simply different manifestations of the same multifactorial trait. The overall incidence of neural tube defects in the United States is approximately 1/350–1/750 live births with higher frequencies in Caucasians of Welsh, Scottish and English ancestry and lower frequency in Blacks [5]. If a normal couple have a child with a neural tube defect, the recurrent risk for another is 5%. This risk increases to 13% when a second affected sib is born. For a couple with one affected child in which one parent also had a neural tube defect, the recurrent risk for another affected child is again 13%. One cannot predict in advance the severity of a neural tube defect in a subsequent affected child. However, if a child is affected the risk of anencephaly is 47%, spina bifida cystica (with or without secondary hydrocephalus) is 47% and hydrocephalus is 6%. Anencephaly is not compatible with postnatal life for more than a few hours. Among those with spina bifida cystica or isolated hydrocephalus at least one half of the survivors will have some degree of mental retardation even after surgical treatment.

It is important to differentiate multifactorial hydrocephalus in newborns from congenital X-linked recessive hydrocephalus. The latter is a single-genic trait found only in males and is a consequence of stenosis of the Sylvian aqueduct. The hydrocephaly at birth is usually more severe than with the multifactorial type and a 'cortical' thumb is often found. In about one half of instances X-linked hydrocephalus does not become clinically apparent until the 2nd or 3rd month of life. With surgical treatment, 80% of children with X-linked hydrocephalus have normal intelligence or are educable retardates. The recurrent risk (the risk after the birth of one affected child) is 50% for each male newborn. Female newborns should be unaffected although the chance of each normal female newborn carrying the X-linked gene is 50%. Congenital hydrocephalus can also result from atresia of the foramina of Luschka and Magendie. This is an autosomal recessive trait. The prognosis is similar to that for the X-linked variety of hydrocephalus. The recurrent risk is 25% with each newborn.

About 90% of clinically significant neural tube defects can be diagnosed in the fetus prenatally. This is done by a combination of sonography and assay for alpha-fetoproteins in amniotic fluid obtained by amniocentesis at 15 weeks' gestation. Recently it has been observed that alpha-fetoproteins may be significantly elevated in the peripheral blood of pregnant women carrying a fetus with an open neural tube defect. This blood test is now done routinely at 16 weeks' gestation in Britain where the incidence of neural tube defects is 1/200 live births [5]. However, the frequency of false-positive and negative results may still be too high for routine application of

Table I. Hypothetical model for multifactorial mental retardation (MR)

Matings[b]		Each parent		Most negative child	Most negative		Relative risk for MR child
mother	father	algebraic sum	IQ		algebraic sum	IQ	
a 2 alleles (+, −)[a]; each negative allele at different gene locus; IQ average if algebraic sum of all alleles is 36							
39+, 1−	× 39+, 1−	38	superior	38+, 2−	36	average	0
38+, 2−	× 38+, 2−	36	average	36+, 4−	32	MR	1 (4−)[c]
37+, 3−	× 37+, 3−	34	inferior	34+, 6−	28	MR	3 (4, 5 or 6−)
36+, 4−	× 36+, 4−	32	MR	32+, 8−	24	MR	5 (4, 5, 6, 7 or 8−)
b 3 alleles (+, 0, −)[a]; each +, −, or (0) allele at different locus; IQ average if algebraic sum of all +, 0, and − alleles is 32 and < 4 (−) alleles							
38+, 2−	× 38+, 2−	36	average	36+, 4−	32	MR	1 (4−)
36+, 4 (0)	× 36+, 4 (0)	36	average	32+, 8 (0)	32	average	0
38, 2−	× 36+, 4 (0)	36	average	34+, 2−, 4 (0)	32	average	0

Assume: 20 genetic loci; total of 40 alleles; 4 or more negative (−) alleles = MR.
[a] A + allele = superior IQ; a negative allele equals inferior IQ; a (0) allele equals average (90–110) IQ.
[b] Couple have no children.
[c] The numbers in parentheses are the possibilities for negative alleles in MR children.

this prenatal screening test to the lower-risk general population of the United States.

Another condition associated with mental retardation is 'congenital cerebral encephalopathy'. This is a nonspecific term to describe microcephaly of unknown and heterogeneous etiology. It includes nongenetic fetal insults such as prenatal infection with cytomegalic or herpes viruses, toxoplasmosis, or other infectious agents; large amount of radiation to the maternal pelvic area early in gestation, and also maternal ingestion early in pregnancy of alcohol (over 2 oz/day) or drugs such as Aminopterin, warfarin, trimethadione and hydantoin [10, 17]. Some cases represent in utero fetal cerebral vascular accidents and these often are associated with porencephaly. Some cases represent autosomal recessive inheritance with a 25% recurrent risk but many cases simply represent multifactorial type inheritance. Therefore, in those instances where an environmental etiology or

Table II. Some empiric risks for mental retardation [9, 13]

Parents, IQ	Children	Risk, %	Relative risk
Normal × normal	none	0.5[a]	1
Normal × normal	retarded[b]	6[a]	12
Normal × retarded	retarded	20[c]	40
Retarded × retarded	retarded	42[c]	84
Normal × normal sib of retardate	none	2.5[c]	5
Normal × normal sib of retardate	retarded	13[c]	26
Retarded × normal sib of retardate	none	24[c]	48

[a] ~ 60% diagnosed as 'familial'.
[b] One or more.
[c] ~ 85% diagnosed as 'familial'.

porencephaly can be ruled out, a recurrent risk for a couple who had an affected child lies somewhere between 6 and 25% [17]. Serial fetal sonography from 13 to 18 weeks of pregnancy might be helpful in the prenatal diagnosis of this condition.

The individuals termed familial or subcultural retardates usually are normal except for mild (educable) mental retardation and are most often found within the lower economic strata of society. The etiology of this retardation is more physiological than pathological; that is, it probably represents nothing more than the bottom tail of the normal distribution curve for intelligence in the general population. This, then, implies that the normal variation of intelligence in the general population is itself a consequence of multifactorial factors. The environmental part of these multifactorial factors includes pre- and postnatal nutrition and postnatal psychosocial-economic circumstances. The evidence for polygenic factors comes mainly from numerous twin and sib studies correlating IQs with biological and nonbiological relationships [2]. Other evidence for polygenic factors in the variation of intelligence comes from studies of adopted children showing correlates with their biological rather than their foster parents. A hypothetical model to illustrate how polygenic factors may produce familial mental retardation is given in table I. The model predicts that a couples' risk for a familial retarded child is inversely proportional to parental intelligence and increases with the birth of affected offspring. Actual (empiric) risks (table II) for a couple having a familial retardate follow these predictions. Particularly note that the risk for a familial retardate is increased for a normal person who has a retarded sib. This datum strongly supports the influence of polygenic factors in the etiology of familial mental retardation, for such a normal person leaves his retarded sib at home when he marries and takes only his genes into the marriage.

Simple Mendelian Traits

Simple Mendelian traits account for about 15% of the mentally retarded and include the inborn errors of metabolism, syndromes of congenital anomalies, certain cranial anomalies, and neuronal degenerative diseases. Mental retardation in most of these conditions is in the severe-to-moderate range and is usually associated with other severe congenital morphological and physiological anomalies. Affected individuals rarely reproduce. (For details on inborn errors of metabolism associated with mental retardation, see page 5 in this textbook.)

There are more than 180 well-known syndromes of congenital anomalies. These are recognizable patterns of childhood malformations constituting a group of medical entities which have in common only the presence at birth of at least two different primary developmental anomalies and which individually often are rare in occurrence, genetic in etiology, variable and overlapping in quality and quantity of expression, difficult to diagnose or treat, grim in overall prognosis, and poorly understood [1, 12]. About 80% of these are inherited as simple Mendelian traits. Those which are inherited as autosomal recessive or X-linked recessive traits are more likely to be associated with mental retardation than those inherited as autosomal dominant traits. A list of the essential syndromes associated with mental retardation can be found on pages 9 and 190, 191 in this textbook.

Chromosomal Disorders

About 5% of mental retardation result from a chromosomal abnormality, the most common of which is mongolism or Down's syndrome (DS) with an overall incidence of 1/900 live births. This represents about one third of all DS conceived, the rest having aborted spontaneously early in gestation [16]. 95% of DS children have an extra chromosome 21 (trisomy

21). This results from a maternal meiotic error in two thirds of instances and a paternal meiotic error in one third of instances. Since maternal meiotic errors increase with age, the risk of a couple having a DS child does likewise. The risk probably does not increase with paternal age. Approximate maternal risks for trisomy 21 DS in a live-born infant are as follows [15]:

Maternal age	Risk/live births
Under 20	1/1,550
20–24	1/1,550
25–29	1/1,050
30–34	1/700
35–39	1/250
40–42	1/85
over 42	1/40

If a couple already have a DS child with trisomy 21, then the risk for a second affected child is at least 1%. About 1% of DS infants are mosaics; that is, they have trisomy 21 in some cells and normal chromosomes in others [15]. The mechanism for this is a mitotic error occurring after fertilization has taken place. The recurrent risk for another DS child should be only slightly greater than that for the general population. The degree of mental retardation is not correlated to the percentage of chromosomally normal versus abnormal cells, but intelligence is somewhat higher in mosaics compared to non-mosaics. Other physical stigmata of DS, however, are the same in mosaics as in non-mosaics.

The remaining 4% of DS infants result from centric fusion type translocation between the long arms of a chromosome 21 and the long arms of either a D or G group chromosome. Of these, approximately 65% are chromosomal accidents restricted to that particular conception. The risk of this chromosomal accident happening again to an at-risk couple is slightly higher than that for the general population. The remaining third of such mongols inherit their translocation from one of their parents who is a balanced translocation carrier. If the father is the balanced translocation carrier, the risk at each conception of his having DS children is less than 2% [15]. Of his other offspring about one half would be chromosomally normal and one half would be balanced translocation carriers like himself. The latter in turn would produce children like their father, etc. ... If the mother is the balanced translocation carrier, about 10% of her offspring would have DS; and of the remaining offspring about one half would be chromosomally normal and the remaining one half would be balanced translocation carriers like herself. If a parent carries a 21/21 translocation, all offspring will have DS. The clinical stigmata and degree of mental retardation in translocation DS are no different from those of trisomy 21 DS.

Although virtually all mongols are mentally retarded, the degree of mental retardation varies over a broad range. Removal of mongols from the parental home inevitably depresses intellectual development significantly [4]. Consequently, institutionalization of mongols is contraindicated unless family circumstances allow no other option. Males with DS cannot reproduce. Female mongols are fertile. If a female (trisomy 21) mongol is impregnated, the theoretical risk of a child with DS is 50%, of a normal child is 50%. However, since two thirds of DS fetuses abort spontaneously, normal children should be more common than DS among the live-born offspring.

Rarer autosomal chromosomal abnormalities are 13(D_1) trisomy, 18(E) trisomy, 5p– (cri-du-chat), and 4p– syndromes. These abnormalities are all associated with profound mental retardation and are usually incompatible with long postnatal life. Another rare chromosomal syndrome is the cat's eye syndrome which is associated with an extra small acrocentric chromosome (most likely a delection of one half of the long arms of a chromosome 22). Other stigmata of this syndrome are coloboma of the iris, ear anomalies, and anal atresia. About one half of affected individuals are mentally retarded while the remaining one half have normal intelligence. About 50% of the offspring of affected individuals are expected to inherit the condition.

Other more common chromosomal abnormalities associated with mental retardation are those involving the sex chromosomes (either the X or the Y). About 1/1,000 females chromosomally are 47,XXX while about 1/1,000 males are 47,XXY. About 25% of such male and females are mildly retarded. 47,XXY (Klinefelter's syndrome) males are invariably sterile. 47,XXX females are fertile, and, interestingly, rarely produce XXX daughters or XXY sons; that is, their offspring are usually chromosomally normal. If an individual has more than one extra X chromosome, moderate to severe mental retardation is usually present along with various other congenital anomalies. About 1/1,000 newborn males chromosomally are 47,XYY. They are usually fertile (producing normal children) and quite tall.

About 5% of XYY males are mildly mentally retarded while 95% are normal. XYY males are not overly aggressive or psychopathic. About 1/10,000 females chromosomally are 45,XO (Turner's syndrome). They are sterile and usually have normal intelligence. A chromosomally normal genocopy of Turner's syndrome is Noonan's syndrome. The latter affects both males and females, results from an abnormal autosomal dominant gene and has an incidence of about 1/1,000 live births. Most cases are sporadic, presumably the result of a new mutation. About 50% of cases demonstrate moderate to severe mental retardation. Finally, about 1/1,300 male and 1/3,000 female newborns have some other abnormality of the sex chromosomes which may or may not be associated with mental retardation.

Because meiotic chromosomal errors increase with maternal age, the risk of a couple having an abnormal child due to a chromosomal abnormality also increases with maternal age. This is seen in the risks for DS, but also applies to other chromosomal conditions where there is an increase over 46 in the number of chromosomes present. The risk for monosomic conditions, such as 45,XO (Turner's syndrome), and structural chromosomal rearrangements is not maternally age-dependent. Chromosomal abnormalities of any type do not appear to increase with paternal age. The risk of a white couple having a live-born child with a chromosomal abnormality is about 1/200 for maternal age < 35; 1/140 for maternal ages 35–39, and > 1/100 for maternal age over 40. The risks for black couples may be lower [8].

There is almost an infinite number of chromosomal rearrangements and gene mutations possible, and when these occur usually a newborn is born with congenital abnormalities some of which are inherited from a carrier parent while some are spontaneous genetic accidents. Microcephaly, mental retardation and multiple congenital anomalies are often found. About 10% of the unclassifiable mentally retarded (with microcephaly and multiple congenital anomalies) have been found to have unique chromosomal abnormalities [3]. Although the incidence of mental retardation in individuals with inherited balanced structural rearrangements of autosomal chromosomes is not greater than in the general population, mental retardation is found with increased frequency when such chromosomal rearrangements occur de novo (not inherited from a carrier parent) [3].

Recently it has been shown that a significant proportion of undifferentiated mentally retarded males, particularly with macro-orchidism, demonstrate a morphological abnormality of their X-chromosome called a 'fragile site' when their cells are cultured in special growth medium. It has been estimated that possibly 1/1,100 live-born males have a 'fragile site' X-chromosome. This chromosomal marker can be demonstrated in carrier mothers, which could become helpful in genetic counseling. Prenatal diagnosis of affected males also may become possible. However, unfortunately the correlation between this chromosomal marker and mental retardation is not absolute. Males with a 'fragile site' X-chromosome rarely can have normal intelligence, and many instances of X-linked mental retardation do not demonstrate an X-chromosome with a 'fragile site' [18]. Consequently, one must be still cautious in applying this technique to genetic counseling.

Recent advances in clinical cytogenetics, somatic cell, and biochemical genetics have been of great help in diagnosing the etiology of mental retardation, and elucidating the mode of inheritance and recurrent risk in individual cases. Of particular help has been the ability to diagnose defective fetuses prenatally early in gestation. Prenatal diagnosis in most instances is accomplished through a combination of sonography and transabdominal amniocentesis at 15–16 weeks' gestation. Cultured amniotic fluid cells (which are derived from the fetus) can be analyzed biochemically or cytogenetically as required. Reliable information is obtained in over 95% of instances. There is no evidence that sonography is harmful to the mother or fetus. The risk of transabdominal amniocentesis inducing an abortion lies between 0.5 and 1.5% depending upon the data from various US, Canadian, and British studies [14]. The risk of this procedure otherwise harming the mother or fetus is so small that it can be ignored. Nevertheless, because there is some risk of inducing an abortion, prenatal diagnosis by transabdominal amniocentesis should be considered primarily in those instances where the chance of benefit is at least equal to that of harm. Consequently, prenatal techniques such as fetoscopy (which are useful for visualizing the fetus and obtaining fetal blood samples for biochemical or chromosomal analysis) must still be considered experimental, for the risk of inducing an abortion by fetoscopy lies between 4 and 8%.

Prenatal diagnosis by transabdominal amniocentesis to detect fetal chromosomal abnormalities should be considered when: the mother is 35 years old or more; a child with a chromosomal abnormality has been born to the couple; a parent is a known carrier of a balanced or unbalanced chromosomal abnormality.

In addition to chromosomal disorders, numerous simple Mendelian traits associated with mental retardation can be diagnosed by appropriate analysis of cultured fetal amniotic cells obtained by amniocentesis (see pages 2, 7, 10 of this textbook).

Impact of Genetic Counseling

The impact of genetic counseling on the incidence of mental retardation has been quite limited. Numerous studies on the effects of genetic counseling indicate that less than a quarter of those counseled change their precounseling reproductive intents but, of those who do, not all avoid high risks or chance low risks [11]. This behavior apparently results primarily from poorly understood psychological influences rather than from the level of intelligence or education. In America, less than 20% of older women (> 35 years) avail themselves of prenatal diagnosis for fetal chromosomal abnormalities. A recent study in Atlanta, Georgia, suggests that intense educational efforts for the professional and lay communities or even free care is unlikely to increase the utilization rate of prenatal diagnosis by older women past 25% [7]. This suggests to me that the people *in general* do not want prevention of genetic disease, rather they want treatment of genetic disease; and, be that right or wrong, it may be futile for geneticists to insist otherwise. If genetic counseling is to have more impact on reducing the incidence of mental retardation, there will have to be much more psychological research in this area to complement the rapid scientific advances in medical genetics.

References

1   Bergsma, D. (ed.): Birth defects compendium; 2nd ed. (Liss, New York 1979).
2   Bouchchard, T.J., Jr.; McGue, M.: Family studies of intelligence: a review. Science *212:* 1055–1059 (1981).
3   Breg, W.R., Jr.: Euploid structural rearrangements in the mentally retarded; in Hook, Porter, Population cytogenetics, pp. 99–101 (Academic Press, New York 1977).
4   Cornwell, A.; Birch, H.: Psychological and social development in home-reared children with Down's syndrome (mongolism). Am. J. mental Defic. *74:* 341–350 (1968).
5   Milunsky, A.: Prenatal diagnosis of neural tube defects; in Milunsky, Genetic disorders and the fetus, pp. 379–430 (Plenum Press, New York 1979).
6   Milunsky, A.: The causes and prevalance of mental retardation; in Milunsky, The prevention of genetic disease and mental retardation, pp. 19–50 (Saunders, Philadelphia 1975).
7   Oakley, G.P., Jr.; Brantley, K.; Chen, A.T.H.; Fernhoff, P.M.; Goldberg, M.F.; Priest, J.H.; Trusler, S.: A community approach to prenatal diagnosis; in Hook, Porter, Service and education in medical genetics, pp. 163–182 (Academic Press, New York 1979).
8   Patil, S.R.; Lubs, H.A.; Kimberling, W.J.; Brown, J.; Cohen, M.; Gerald, P.; Hecht, F.; Moorhead, P.; Myrianthopoulos, N.; Summit, R.L.: Chromosomal abnormalities

ascertained in a collaborative survey of 4,342 seven- and eight-year-old children: frequency phenotype and epidemiology; in Hook, Porter, Population cytogenetics, pp. 103–131 (Academic Press, New York 1977).

9   Reed, E.W.; Reed, S.C.: Mental retardation: a family study, pp. 1–82 (Saunders, Philadelphia 1965).

10 Smith, D.W.: Recognizable patterns of human malformations; 2nd ed., pp. 336–347 (Saunders, Philadelphia 1976).

11 Steele, M.W.: Lessons from Tay-Sachs programme. Lancet *ii:* 914 (1980).

12 Steele, M.W.: Syndromes of congenital anomalies; in Kelley, Practice of pediatrics, vol. 1, pp. 1–40, chapter 91 (Harper & Row, London 1976).

13 Stern, C.: Principles of human genetics; 3rd ed., pp. 696–715 (Freeman, San Francisco 1973).

14 Editorial: The risk of amniocentesis. Lancet *ii:* 1287–1288 (1978).

15 Thompson, J.S.; Thompson, M.W.: Genetics in medicine; 3rd ed., pp. 142–180 (Saunders, Philadelphia 1980).

16 Uchida, I.A.: Maternal radiation and trisomy 21; in Hook, Porter, Population cytogenetics, pp. 285–299 (Academic Press, New York 1977).

17 Warkany, J.: Congenital malformations, pp. 237–244 (Yearbook Medical Publishers, Chicago 1971).

18 Editorial: X-linked mental retardation. Lancet *i:* 1086–1087 (1981).

3 Mental Retardation: Some Pathological Considerations

John J. Kepes

While it is impossible to discuss all the aspects of pathology of mental retardation in one brief chapter, it is safe to say that normal mental development and function requires a brain which, to a great extent, is anatomically and functionally intact. The proviso 'to a great extent' is being applied here, because the brain is not a homogeneous organ and it is certainly possible to suffer anatomical damage to some isolated areas in the brain that would not affect mentation. This of course is true for the developed brain also. There are so-called 'silent' areas in the brain, particularly in the non-dominant hemisphere, where an acquired lesion such as a stroke may not result in any detectable functional deficit. In addition lesions, like a small infarct in the internal capsule, may cause problems for the motor system, but will not likely affect the mental abilities of the patient. Similarly, in the developing brain injuries may take place that have either no detectable effect on central nervous system activities or cause a type of deficit that does not involve higher mental functions.

In general, however, there is a limit as to how extensive an injury or malformation the developing brain will tolerate before its normal mental development will suffer. Any discussion of normal mental function must of course take into consideration a person's age, since at birth our central nervous system has not yet completed its anatomic and functional development, and 'normal' mental activity for a given age is determined by comparing the level of that individual's mental function to that of a large number of presumably normal other individuals of the same age. Another difficulty in the attempted delineation and definition of 'pathology of mental retardation' is related to the fact that the brain is not only the anatomic center of higher mental functions, but is a vital organ in every other sense of the word as well. It is very questionable, indeed, whether developmental abnormalities or destructive processes in the brain, that are of such severe nature as to interfere with the brain's basic function (regulation of respiration, of vasomotor control, etc.) thereby endangering the patient's very life, should be included in this discussion. True, they often will, among others, interfere with normal mental development, but in the presence of an abnormality or disease that is likely to lead to the patient's demise within a few weeks or months, the problems of retarded or regressive mentation, although saddening for the parents, usually come to be regarded as of secondary importance. This is true not only of malformations incompatible with life to begin with, such as anencephaly (fig. 1), but also genetic diseases manifesting themselves in extrauterine life, such as infantile Gaucher's disease or Tay-Sachs disease, or for that matter other acquired diseases, e.g. a devastating bout of viral encephalitis or bacterial meningitis with fatal complications.

Other patients, with brain defects not serious enough to place their very life in jeopardy, nevertheless may become blind, deaf, or disabled by spastic diplegia, choreoathetosis, or hard-to-control seizures because of these defects. It is true, however, that many disease entities exist that may occur with various degrees of severity and whereas the most severe forms will lead to the patient's demise or serious physical disabilities, the milder forms of the same will cause 'only' mental retardation. This is also true for developmental abnormalities. The spectrum of holoprosencephaly serves as a good example. Cyclops monsters representing the most severe form of this abnormality are either deadborn or die shortly after birth, whereas milder forms of the same problem may cause only mental retardation. A similarly wide spectrum of effects exists also with various forms of physical birth trauma, perinatal anoxia, congenital hydrocephalus, kernicterus, and infectious diseases of the central nervous system, to name just a few.

Finally, there are disease entities like the neuronal storage diseases with a relatively slow but progressive course (some forms of mucopolysaccharidosis and the later forms of neuronal lipofuscinosis come to mind) that will eventually cause the patient's demise, but the course of the disease is sufficiently protracted to be measured in years and even decades, and the problems of institutionalization and training, to the degree possible in such cases, become matters of concern.

The above considerations, I believe, sufficiently explain why it is difficult to define the proper territory for 'pathology of mental retardation'.

As to etiology, the list of causes, events, and episodes that may lead to cerebral maldevelopment and brain damage is almost endless and includes genetic, environmental, physical, toxic, nutritional, metabolic, and infectious factors that cover the entire spectrum of human pathology, and it is definitely beyond the scope of a short chapter to consider in detail the pathologic changes created by all of them [1].

Fortunately, there exist excellent special textbooks dealing with this matter, outstanding among them are 'Pathology of Mental Retardation' by *Crome and Stern* [2] and 'Developmental Neuropathology' by *Friede* [3]. The reader is advised to review these books for detailed information on the subject. The purpose of this chapter can only be to outline the *basic principles* governing the development of cerebral lesions in the immature brain, lesions that in their cumulative effects will lead to the clinically observable forms of mental retardation. An attempt will be made to illustrate some of the more important types of malformations and cerebral injuries that result in diminished mental capacity of a growing individual.

General Classification of Causes of Mental Retardation

One way of classifying the causes of mental retardation is to separate 'true development malformations' of the brain from 'acquired destructive lesions'. In the first category, one may include the problems of certain normal developmental steps not having taken place or having done so in an abnormal way. In the second category one would list noxious events and episodes that destroyed brain tissue which had already been formed in a normal fashion. Even this seemingly simple classification has to contend with many instances of overlap due to the fact that changes in both categories may be caused by the same agent. For example, cytomegalovirus infection of the fetal brain may interfere with normal developmental organization of the cortex and lead to micropolygyria on the one hand, [4] while it will often cause necrosis and calcification in nearby brain tissue that has already been properly formed [5], on the other.

Another problem that patients with certain developmental as well as acquired brain lesions must face is possible anoxic tissue damage to the brain as a result of repeated epileptic seizures. Among the developmental anomalies, micropolygyria, cortical and subcortical heterotopias, Sturge-Weber syndrome, and tuberous sclerosis are particularly likely to cause seizures; among the acquired lesions, meningocortical scars of previous infections, anoxia-induced scarring of the cortex in ulegyria (sclerotic microgyria) and cerebral hemiatrophy play an important role in predisposing to epileptic seizures.

Developmental Anomalies (Malformations) of the Brain

It is helpful to consider the fact that development of the central nervous system takes place at three levels, or modes that can be listed as (1) gross organogenesis, (2) histogenesis, and (3) cytogenesis. Naturally, these three modes of development are closely interrelated and interdependent. For a detailed review of normal steps of embryonal, fetal and postnatal development of the central nervous system, the reader is referred to textbooks of embryology, but a brief review may be appropriate for this chapter.

The brain and spinal cord develop from the germinal layer called ectoderm. Its main product is the integument, but since the nervous system (both central and peripheral) is also derived from this germinal layer, the latter is frequently referred to as 'neuroectoderm'. The first visible event taking place in neurogenesis is the formation of a *neural plate* in the posterior midline of the embryo which soon develops a depression along its long axis turning in the process into a *neural groove*. Eventually, starting in the future cervical region and extending both in a cranial and a caudal direction, the lips of the neural groove will close to form the *neural tube*. Partial or total failure of this closure leads to various degrees of spina bifida or rachischisis, the more severe forms being incompatible with life. Since the upper and lower ends of the tube are the last to become closed, lumbosacral and posterior occipital defects are among the most common anomalies of failure of closure (dysraphism). The degree of closure defect varies from a small dimple in the lumbar area with an underlying defect in the vertebral arch (spina bifida occulta) to protrusion of a meningeal sac through the defect (meningocele) and to spinal cord and brain tissue forming contents of the meningeal sac (meningomyelocele (fig. 2) and meningoencephalocele (fig. 3), respectively) [6–8]. Of these, encephaloceles represent perhaps the most direct danger to the tissues of the cerebrum, but lumbar meningomyeloceles, in addition to serving as ports of entry to an often fatal meningeal infection, are also frequently associated with debilitating hydrocephalus. Usually in the latter cases at the cervical-occipital junction, one or another form of the Arnold-Chiari malformation may be found [9, 10]. The downward displacement of the cerebellar tonsils and associated 'buckling' of the medulla oblongata serve to obstruct the foramen magnum and contribute to the hydrocephalus. While the lumbar meningomyelocele is not directly responsible for the Arnold-Chiari malformation (this earlier notion has been successfully dispelled by pertinent animal experiments [11]) it is often present as an associated anomaly.

Anencephaly [12, 13] formerly thought of as a primary failure of development of the cerebral hemispheres, is now believed to be yet another form of a failure in closure [14, 15]. According to this theory, in the absence of the protective calvaria, the already formed cerebral hemispheres degenerate and become destroyed through exposure (fig. 1).

A further step in the gross pathogenesis of the brain is the development of the primitive cerebral vesicles: prosencephalon or forebrain, mesencephalon or midbrain and rhombencephalon or hindbrain. These vesicles become evident by the time the neural tube is completely closed. The prosencephalon further differentiates into telencephalon (the future cerebral hemispheres and basal ganglia, having for their cavities the lateral ventricles) and diencephalon (thalamus, hypothalamus, optic vesicle nerves, and tracts with the third ventricle as cavity). Throughout the development of the brain the mesencephalon with its aqueduct undergoes the least changes, whereas the rhombencephalon, which has for its cavity the fourth ventricle, divides into metencephalon (future pons and cerebellum) and myelencephalon (medulla oblongata).

A further important developmental step is the division of the telencephalon into two hemispheres. Failure of this to happen will result in holoprosencephaly, also called telencephalon impar [16–19]. In its most severe form this anomaly affects the entire facial development including the formation of the eyes (cyclops deformity; fig. 4). In milder forms the anteroposterior diameter of the head is shortened, the eyes are closely placed, and the nose is deformed (fig. 5). In all forms of holoprosencephaly there is absence or incomplete development of the sagittal interhemispheric fissure (fig. 6), creating direct communication between the gray matters of the two hemispheres (fig. 7), and in addition in these brains the lateral ventricles form a single cavity. In many instances the olfactory portions of the frontal lobe are absent (arhinencephaly). A mild degree of holoprosencephaly is compatible with life, but is usually accompanied by mental retardation of varying severity.

The corpus callosum, the great commissural fiber bundle connecting the two cerebral hemispheres, develops between the 3rd and 5th fetal months. Partial or total agenesis of this structure (fig. 8) is often associated with other malformations, but even by itself may be responsible for mental retardation and seizures [20, 21]. Other less common failures of gross morphogenesis include the Dandy-Walker malformation [22–24], where the cerebellar vermis is absent and the roof of the greatly enlarged fourth ventricle is formed by fibrous membrane (fig. 9). Absence of the septum pellu-

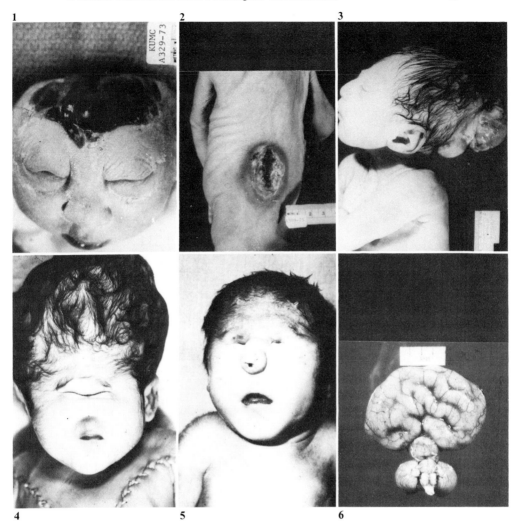

Fig. 1. Anencephalic monster. The calvaria is missing, and the exposed hemispheres degenerated into a highly vascular mushy mass.

Fig. 2. Lumbar meningomyelocele after rupture of the sac.

Fig. 3. Occipital meningoencephalocele.

Fig. 4. Cyclops monster with single eye in midline and undeveloped nose.

Fig. 5. A somewhat milder form of holoprosencephaly. Eyes are close, the nose is represented by proboscis with single nostril.

Fig. 6. Holoprosencephaly: the interhemispheric fissure is absent and frontal gyri are continuous from one side to the other.

cidum [25] and/or of the fornices, cystic enlargement of the cavum of the septum pellucidum and a host of other variations of developmental disorders also occur in some patients [26, 27].

Effect of Cranial Osseous Development on the Brain

Apart from partial failure of cranial bone development leaving portions of the cerebral surface exposed and vulnerable, the most important abnormalities to consider are related to premature closure of sutures. Many variants exist which cannot be discussed in this short review, but what they all have in common is moderate to severe interference with the normal growth and expansion of the brain. Many of these osseous anomalies are associated with some degree of mental retardation (fig. 10) [28]. Fortunately, various modes of linear craniectomies exist that can 'open up' the sutures and alleviate the pressure on the brain.

Disturbed Histogenesis and Mental Retardation

The original source of nerve cells and glial cells (except for microglia) in the brain and spinal cord is the neural tube or canal. In the beginning the lining of this canal (and its cranial extension, the cerebral vesicles) is a layer of columnar cells called the medullary epithelium. In the developing embryo and fetus a feverish mitotic activity takes place in that layer, followed by centrifugal migration of the cells derived from the medullary epithelium. In the case of the brain, migrating neuroblasts will settle in the area of the basal ganglia, and successive waves will carry others to the surface of the hemispheres, the site of the future cerebral cortex. Recent studies have demonstrated that matrix cells play an important role in providing a scaf-

---

Fig. 7. Full mount section of brain with holoprosencephaly, from a patient who was only moderately retarded. The interhemispheric fissure is incompletely formed. Single lateral ventricle with horizontally lying caudate nuclei developed. Weil-Weigert myelin stain.

Fig. 8. Agenesis of the corpus callosum.

Fig. 9. Dandy-Walker malformation with absence of cerebellar vermis and greatly enlarged fourth ventricle. The patient also had generalized hydrocephalus.

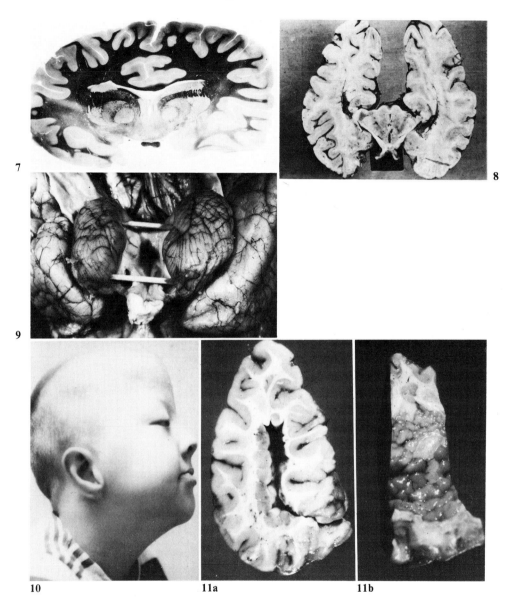

Fig. 10. Pointed head with shortened anteroposterior diameter in a patient with acro-cephalosyndactylism (Apert's disease).

Fig. 11. Gray matter heterotopias surrounding the lateral ventricle, a result of arrested migration of neuroblasts. a Coronal section of occipital lobe. b Protruding gray matter islands as viewed from the ventricular surface.

folding for the migrating neurons, helping them to reach the surface of the brain [29]. Particularly large masses of neurons migrate in the 12th week of gestation.

Abnormalities of migration (due to genetic causes or to interruption by noxious events in intrauterine life) will cause migratory arrest, either quite close to the outskirts of the ventricles [30] or at any point en route to the future cortex. The cells will usually undergo individual development to mature neurons in the place, where they got bogged down in the migratory arrest and thus become heterotopic islands of gray matter. Large numbers of such heterotopic neurons possibly will make their absence felt in the cortex, but more importantly these ectopic nerve cell islands often become the starting foci for epileptic seizures (fig. 11).

At the completion of normal neuronal migration, the cortical neurons first form a thick undifferentiated layer of cells, and at that point the cortical surface is still quite smooth. The principal fissures (Sylvian, central and parietooccipital) are next in developing, these to be followed by the formation of the various cortical gyri and sulci as we know them from normal neuroanatomy. The insula remains exposed until fairly late in fetal life, until it becomes overgrown by other parts of the cerebral cortex [8]. One of the characteristics of the brain in Down's disease is that, mostly due to poor development of the first temporal gyrus, a part of the insula will remain uncovered by opercular cortex, even in postnatal life (fig. 28).

In some individuals gyral development never takes place, and the smooth surface of the brain is maintained into postnatal life [31]. This condition is known as *agyria* or, because of the smoothness of the surface, *lissencephaly* [32] (fig. 12). In these brains the undifferentiated cortex forms a very thick layer. Children with this anomaly are usually severely retarded, mentally. A less severe failure of gyral development results in the presence of a few coarse convolutions (*pachygyria;* fig. 13).

In *micropolygyria* [33–35] (or polymicrogyria) the alteration of the cortex may be focal or extensive. The former sometimes represents merely an incidental finding at autopsy, but the latter is conducive to severe neurological problems, epileptic seizures and mental retardation. Morocco leather-like appearance with very shallow depressions between small ridges and elevated areas characterize this abnormality (fig. 14). The depressions are not true sulci; the undulating gray matter is fused, and the cortex characteristically consists of only four instead of the more common six layers. This abnormality of intracortical organization dates to near the 5th and before the 6th months of gestation.

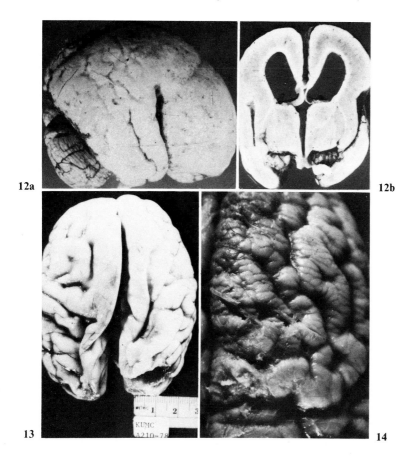

Fig. 12. Agyria (lissencephaly). **a** View of convexity: only the Sylvian fissure and the first temporal sulcus are normally formed. Note the normal cerebellar surface. **b** Coronal section of the same brain shows large ventricles, thin periventricular white matter, and a wide band of unstructured cortical gray matter (4-year-old severely retarded girl).

Fig. 13. Pachygyria in a 4-week-old infant, born at term. Only a few major gyri have formed.

Fig. 14. Micropolygyria. The surface of the brain resembles Morocco leather. Sulci are very shallow. Unlike sclerotic microgyria or ulegyria, brains with micropolygyria have normal consistency on palpation, since there is usually no gliosis present.

Disturbed Cytogenesis and Mental Retardation

The cells that migrate through the hemispheres to populate the cerebral cortex are primitive neuroblasts. Having arrived at their destination, the mantle layer of the brain, and having arranged themselves in an ordered fashion to form the normal layers of the cortex microscopically, and the gyri and sulci of gross topography, they also must undergo individual maturation in order to become fully functional cortical neurons. This entails enlargement of the cell bodies (perikarya) to their ultimate size (different from layer to layer and from region to region) and the sprouting of processes. The axons will extend to shorter or longer distances depending on the role of the neuron, while the growth of dendrites will make interconnections, synapses, and circuits possible. With the development of rich dendritic expansions, the perikarya will be more separated from each other spatially, and on ordinary cell stains (e.g., hematoxylin and eosin, Nissl, etc.) a given area of the cortex will appear less populated than it was in the developing fetus or the newborn. Failure of adequate development of dendrites and synapses will prohibit interaction between neurons and may be the sole morphological change appreciable in some forms of mental retardation [36], as has been suggested for example for congenital hypothyroidism or cretinism [37].

An additional and very important final event in neuronal development is the myelinization of axons by the oligodendroglial cells. Although some parts, particularly the phylogenetically older fiber tracts of the brain and spinal cord, are completely myelinated at the time of birth, many others are not [38, 39], and it takes several years of postnatal life for myelinization to become completed. Insufficient production of developing myelin may be due to metabolic problems, such as those present in phenylketonuria (phenylpyruvic oligophrenia) [40–42] and many other diseases. These include disturbances of amino acid metabolism, e.g. hyperprolinemia, tyrosinemia, hyperpipecolactemia, branch chain ketonuria (maple syrup urine disease), hyperglycinemia, homocystinuria, and others [43]. As to profound *intrinsic* abnormalities of neuronal cytogenesis, one has to cite the neuronal changes of tuberous sclerosis. In this disease the migration of neuroblasts to the cortex has duly taken place, but the neurons in the pathognomonic 'tubers' are not only in spatial disarray, they also show evidence of dysplastic changes: processes sprouting from abnormal locations and extending in the wrong directions, nuclear abnormalities, including binucleated cells, and others. As an indication that the cytological problems start at a very early phase of development, it has been suggested that in the brains of these patients some mixed forms between glial and neuronal cells exist which would place the date of the onset of cellular maldevelopment to the time when neuroblasts and spongioblasts (primitive glial cells) were not yet distinct from each other [44].

Destructive Lesions of Already Formed Portions of the Central Nervous System

Mental retardation may result from destruction of brain tissue during intrauterine or postnatal developmental phases. Unlike true malformations in the strict sense, these latter changes affect structures that had already formed, although even in this situation secondary malformations may result from these events. For example, hemorrhagic necrosis of a cerebellar hemisphere in the fetus may result in faulty development of the contralateral inferior olive, even though there was no necrotic change in the olive itself. In most instances, however, the functional consequences of the tissue destruction relate to the loss of neuronal population in the affected area itself.

Among the causes of neuronal loss are harmful influences that may be *prenatal, perinatal,* or *postnatal.* The long list of *prenatal* factors includes malnutrition of the mother, exposure to ionizing radiation, infectious diseases which may affect the fetus transplacentally (e.g., syphilis, rubella, cytomegalovirus infection, toxoplasmosis, etc.). Toxic substances such as alcohol and certain drugs ingested or used by the mother, perfusion problems of the placenta (e.g., partial detachment, placental fibrosis, etc.) represent other very important factors to consider [45]. *During the birth process* the prolongation of the actual delivery with accompanying hypoxia of the brain [46], and interference with cerebral blood supply through pressure on the umbilical cord or the carotid arteries in the neck, must be considered. Also during the process of birth, physical trauma, e.g., undue degree of molding of the head or forceps injury may result in subarachnoid and/or subdural hemorrhages [47, 48].

Hypoxia with accompanying hypotension (shock) is thought to be instrumental in the development of hemorrhagic necrosis in a very fragile vulnerable area, the subependymal matrix layer of the ventricular walls, particularly in the region of the heads of the caudate nuclei bordering the lateral ventricles. Some infants develop fatal intraventricular hemorrhages from these lesions [49, 50] (fig. 15), others survive with residual tissue damage [51, 52]. In an occasional infant suffering from such bleeding, organizing hemorrhage in the aqueduct may become one of the causes of aqueductal stenosis and secondary hydrocephalus (fig. 16). Perinatal anoxia also affects the cortex (particularly in the so-called watershed areas and more so in the perisulcal than in the crown portion of the gyri) and the basal ganglia. White matter destruction is most prominent in the periventricular areas [53–62] and in other instances in the subcortical zones.

In the immediate *postnatal* state infants with severe Rh or ABO incompatibility may suffer toxic necrosis of neurons that become imbibed with unconjugated bilirubin which in turn was derived from hemolyzing red blood cells and gained access to the nerve cells, particularly those of the brain stem and basal ganglia, through the still immature, therefore, penetrable blood-brain barrier [63, 64].

Cases of bacterial meningitis acquired through aspiration of coliform organisms in the birth canal or through infection in the nursery (these days most commonly in the form of *Streptococcus bovis* infection) account for another group of early postnatal injuries. Bacterial meningitis may not only lead to brain damage [65–67], but, if incompletely treated, will often result in leptomeningeal adhesions with subsequent communicating or noncommunicating forms of obstructive hydrocephalus that will have secondary deleterious pressure effect on the brain [68] (fig. 17). Bacterial meningitis, including tuberculosis meningitis, may also cause vasculitis with secondary obstruction in meningeal blood vessels, and that in turn may lead to infarcts of the brain parenchyma [69].

Morphologic Manifestations of Injury to the Developing Brain

For the clinical appraisal of brain tissue damage and its role in the causation of mental retardation, it would seem that the most important item to consider would be the *loss of nerve cells and their processes* because this is the factor that is ultimately responsible for the functional deficit. Instead, classical descriptions in neuropathology place great emphasis on morphological changes that occur *after* the neurons have been destroyed by whatever noxious agent or event claimed them. After neuronal destruction the appearance of an affected area will, to a great extent, depend on somewhat extraneous factors, e.g., to what extent were tissue elements other than neurons (e.g., glia, mesenchymal tissues) affected by the harmful influences?

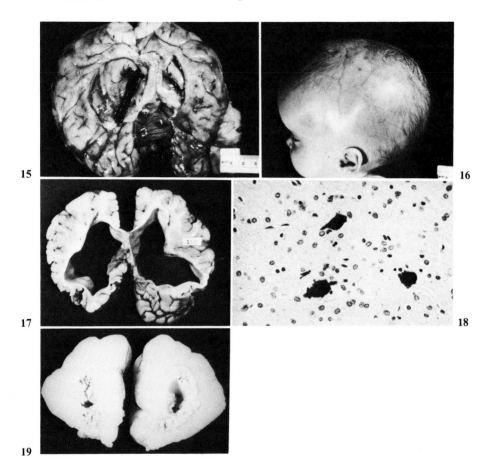

Fig. 15. Hemorrhage in the lateral ventricle, a frequent complication of perinatal asphyxia and hemorrhagic necrosis of periventricular 'matrix layer'.

Fig. 16. A complication of intraventricular hemorrhage: blood clot obstructed the aqueduct, resulting in secondary obstructive hydrocephalus.

Fig. 17. Healed bacterial meningitis caused by *Haemophilus influenzae* in a 5-month-old infant. Fibrous meningeal adhesions caused marked hydrocephalus.

Fig. 18. A result of perinatal asphyxia: necrotic neurons in the thalamus have become calcified and ferruginated (mineralized).

Fig. 19. Newborn infant with extensive cytomegalovirus disease: periventricular necrosis and calcification in frontal lobes.

Since neurons themselves do not regenerate, this will determine to what extent shall nonneuronal repair occur in the damaged territory? The neurons themselves, after they became necrotic, will usually disappear altogether from the area, although sometimes they become mineralized (calcified and ferruginated) before macrophage action can remove them from the scene, and then, like trunks of a petrified forest, they will persist indefinitely in the areas of the tissue damage (fig. 18). Calcification can involve much more than individual necrotic neurons, since entire territories often become calcified in tissue destruction caused by toxoplasmosis [70] and by cytomegalovirus infection (fig. 19).

Repair by astrocytic gliosis, when present, will result in glial scars, sometimes dense and *solid* as in the cortex in cases of sclerotic microgyria (ulegyria; fig. 20) [71] sometimes *spongy* with microcystic areas intermingled with more solid strands of gliosis. At times the atrophy and gliosis involve one hemisphere asymetrically (hemiatrophy; fig. 21) [72]. In cases of severe tissue damage, particularly if occurring at the time of glial immaturity, sometimes there is very little gliosis to replace the tissue loss, the result being cystic cavitation. This may be present in the form of single or multiple, small or large cysts. The largest ones nowadays are sometimes loosely referred to as 'porencephalic cysts' (fig. 22), whereas in the past only malformations resulting in open connections between ventricular and subarachnoid space were considered as being true examples of porencephaly [73, 74].

Subcortical multilocular cavitation is often listed among the typical gross morphological findings of 'cerebral birth injury' (usually of a hypoxic nature) (fig. 23). In the most severe cases only the walls of the dilated ventricles and the subpial outermost layers of the cortex remain, with the rest of the brain being transformed into a sponge-like substance created by a multitude of thin-walled cysts (hydranencephaly) [74].

Marbled state ('status marmoratus') [75–78] is an interesting morphological consequence of the fact that oligodendroglial cells may be in the process of forming myelin at the time when the tissue damage occurs in the developing brain. In such cases the glial scar that results from the tissue loss may be heavily endowed with myelin which in this instance has lost its chance to be wrapped around axons, but its presence nevertheless provides a marbled appearance to the affected areas – most commonly the basal ganglia (fig. 24) but often also the cortex – that is best seen on appropriate myelin stains. Needless to say that in these instances too the most important problem is the loss of the nervous parenchyma, not the type of scar

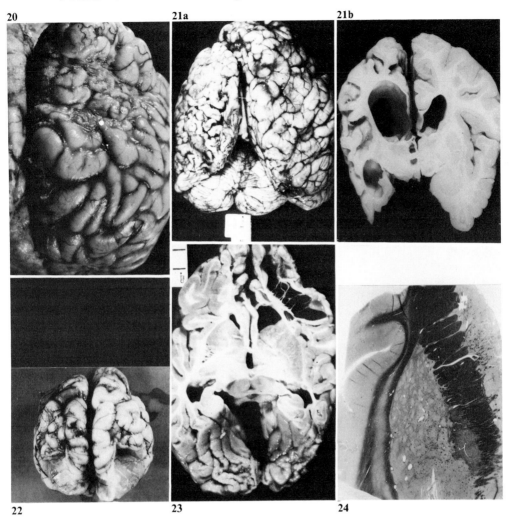

Fig. 20. Ulegyria (sclerotic microgyria). The shrunken, gliotic gyri are predominantly seen in 'watershed zones'. There was underlying subcortical cyst formation present.

Fig. 21. Left hemiatrophy with scarring and shrinkage of convolutions. **a** Superior view. **b** Coronal section showing compensatory dilatation of the left ventricle.

Fig. 22. Poorly developed brain with pachygyria and symmetrical large porencephalic cysts.

Fig. 23. Anoxic perinatal brain injury: note sclerotic microgyria of occipitotemporal convolutions and large subcortical cyst of the right frontal lobe with glial strands making a feeble attempt to bridge cyst cavity.

Fig. 24. Basal ganglia in status marmoratus. Note specks of irregular myelin deposits in the head of caudate nucleus and in putamen. Weil-Weigert myelin stain.

(even though a myelinated one in this instance), that develop in the affected area. It is possible, nevertheless, that fibrous gliosis in an area of previous tissue damage will be of some future clinical significance as in the case of temporal lobe epilepsy where 'incisural scarring', believed to have developed secondary to a form of birth injury, e.g., transient uncal herniation, is considered to be instrumental in provoking temporal lobe epilepsy in later life. Indeed, the formation of glial scars *anywhere* in the brain, whether secondary to pre-, peri- or postnatal injuries of the brain may be an aggravating factor for the patient's condition because of epileptic seizures with their often-associated episodes of anoxia. These in themselves are likely to further impair the integrity of the brain parenchyma, particularly that of the cerebral cortex.

Viral Infections

Subacute Sclerosing Panencephalitis

This is a tragic 'slow motion' form of measles encephalitis of young children and adolescents involving both gray and white matter (hence the term 'panencephalitis') and usually leading to the patient's demise in a matter of a few months or years. The problem faced, therefore, is more of a relentlessly progressive fatal disease than one of mental retardation, but since some of the patients do live for a number of years and since behavioral problems (often first detected at school) and gradually diminishing mental capacity play an important role in the symptomatology of this condition, it deserves to be included in this discussion. The entity was first described by *Dawson* [79] in 1933 as 'subacute inclusion body encephalitis'. White matter changes have been emphasized, and the term *subacute sclerosing leukoencephalitis* was given to this entity by *van Bogaert* [80]. The multifocal aggregates of inflammatory cells were highlighted by the term 'panecenphalitis nodosa' by *Pette and Döring* [81]. Gradually it became recognized that these terms in reality described one and the same disease, the subacute to chronic form of measles encephalitis. The protracted nature of the 'conflict' between virus and defensive forces of the brain is believed by some to be due to a defective character of the measles virus strains involved, and by others to altered defense mechanisms of the host. The disease occurs in individuals who either have had exposure to or, less commonly, have been vaccinated against measles. The infection brings about the presence of intracytoplasmic and intranuclear inclusion bodies in nerve

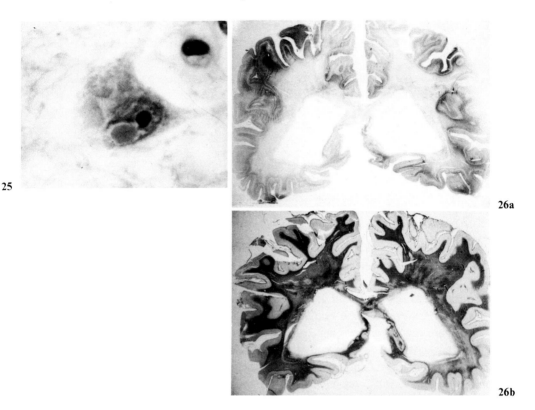

25

26a

26b

Fig. 25. Cortical neuron in subacute sclerosing panencephalitis. Viral inclusion bodies are present in both cytoplasm and nuclei.

Fig. 26. Full-mount coronal sections of brain with long-standing subacute sclerosing panencephalitis. **a** Almost total disappearance of hemispheric myelin. Weil-Weigert myelin stain **b** Holzer stain for glial fibers shows dense gliosis replacing lost myelin.

cells (fig. 25) and glial cells that are not greatly different from inclusions seen in other organs, e.g., giant cell pneumonia of measles. Unlike conventional viral encephalitides, the protracted course of this disease allows much destruction of myelin (probably due in great part to viral damage to oligodendrocytes) and the development of widespread fibrous gliosis, hence the term 'sclerosing' encephalitis. In the end there will be much tissue loss with demyelination, gliotic shrinkage of the parenchyma, and secondary dilatation of the ventricles (fig. 26). Microscopically, inflammatory changes usually persist to the end with perivascular lymphocytic cuffing and micro-glial nodules. The measles virus can be visualized with the immunofluores-cence technique and electron microscopy. By light microscopy, the charac-teristic intracytoplasmic and intranuclear inclusions originally described and beautifully illustrated in *Dawson's* original paper [79] allow the diagno-sis to be made.

Rubella Encephalitis

Maternal infection with rubella virus during the first trimester of preg-nancy has been known for a long time to lead to various congenital malfor-mations in the fetus, most commonly some forms of congenital heart dis-ease. Sometimes psychomotor retardation is seen in children of such preg-nancies which may be slight to moderate and not infrequently associated with microcephaly. In addition to these developmental defects, rubella virus may cause a persistent chronic infection in such babies which eventu-ally disappears during postnatal life. This condition, which may involve the liver, spleen, lungs, and myocardium and may also cause meningoencephal-itis, is known as the congenital rubella syndrome. The process may be quiescent for as long as 13 months after birth. Surviving infants show microcephaly, intracranial calcification, severe mental retardation, sei-zures, deafness, and focal neurological defects, according to *Friede* [82]. Cerebral lesions consist of chronic meningitis and foci of necrosis in the nervous parenchyma. Vascular mineralization is part of the rubellar vascu-lopathy and the characteristic presence of PAS-positive material in the ves-sel walls is thought to be helpful in making this diagnosis [83–85].

Cytomegalovirus Infection and the Brain

Cytomegalovirus is believed to reach the developing fetus through transplacental infection in mothers with viremia due to this agent. As pointed out in the introduction, this is one of the conditions in which developmental arrest and destruction of already developed tissues may be observed side by side. The former is often manifested by micropolygyria [4], the latter by necrosis of brain tissue leading to extensive secondary calcification frequently involving periventricular tissues [5] (see figure 17). This change may be visualized by plain films of the skull in the newborn.

Toxoplasmosis

The causative agent is a protozoon, *Toxoplasma gondii,* first discov-ered in a North African rodent, the gondi. Cats appear to be the principal host of the disease and play an important role in the infestation of other species, including humans [70]. In adults the infection is often of a mild nature, manifested by lymphadenopathy and low fever, but without more serious effects, except in immunosuppressed individuals where toxoplasmosis may have a stormy course, including a devastating form of necrotizing encephalitis [70]. Cerebral toxoplasmosis in newborns is an important source of brain damage. Infestation occurs transplacentally, and the organisms produce necrotizing changes in the brain with secondary calcification. *Frenkel* [70] emphasizes the frequency with which the walls of the ventricles and that of the aqueduct are affected by the disease, leading to secondary obstruction and hydrocephalus with accumulation of the toxoplasma antigen in the stagnating cerebrospinal fluid proximal to the occlusion. This will result in particularly severe damage in the area surrounding the third and lateral ventricles. Chorioretinitis is a common and diagnostically helpful associated finding in neonatal toxoplasmosis.

Relationship between Small Brain Size and Mental Retardation

Microcephaly, Micrencephaly
The first term means a small head, the second a small brain. The two are often closely interrelated since a cranium that is small because of abnormal osseous development (e.g., premature closure of cranial sutures) will simply not allow the brain to grow and expand; indeed, it will cause pressure on the developing brain. A reverse relationship also exists since it is the growing brain that stimulates the enlargement of the cranium. If, for example, a brain suffers extensive damage during the birth process and becomes arrested in its growth as a consequence, the head circumference will also stagnate at its perinatal level. Damage to the brain, however, will only prevent the further growth of the cranium, it will not cause it to become smaller, so if the destructive process of the brain eventually leads to scarring and shrinkage of the cerebrum, this may lead to the finding of a shriveled-up brain in a cranium with a larger capacity.

Attempts have been made to differentiate between 'true' or 'primary' microencephaly and acquired of 'secondary' micrencephaly. In the first, the brain is proportionately developed with no evident focal area of atrophy or hypoplasia, only its total weight and size are below what is considered to be normal. Such true micrencephaly is sometimes inherited and familial [27]. True micrencephaly would have to be distinguished from 'secondary forms' where degeneration and scarring were responsible for the diminished size of the brain. The distinction between the two forms is not always easy, suffice to say that the secondary form is much more common. For the pathologist the most valuable clue for the secondary character of micrencephaly is either obvious external deformities of the gyral and sulcal pattern, or the more insidious but equally important diffuse presence of fibrous gliosis throughout the white matter of an otherwise misleadingly normally proportioned small brain ('gliotic encephalopathy').

Morphological Changes of the Brain in Down's Disease

The genetic and chromosomal characteristics and the facial (fig. 27) and general somatic features of this entity are discussed elsewhere in this book. It would also exceed the proposed confines of this chapter to discuss the possible relationships between the chromosomal abnormalities of somatic cells and the biochemical alterations (deviations from normal standards) found in patients suffering from this condition [86].

The gross morphological changes of the brain can be summarized as usually consisting of a moderate degree of symmetrical micrencephaly with a fairly proportionate development of the cerebral hemispheres, but smallness of the frontal lobes is often noted. The anterior-posterior diameter of the brain is usually shortened and the occipital lobes, rather than showing the normal 'slope', may end abruptly in a more vertical plane. This configuration and the smallness of the frontal lobe are also related to the *shortened anterior-posterior diameter of the head as a whole* in these individuals. The convolutional pattern appears somewhat 'simplified', and a rather constant feature is the underdevelopment of the first temporal gyrus on both sides [87]. This gyrus plays a role in covering the insular cortex, and its hypoplasia together with smallness of other components of the operculum will result in the insula being exposed to the examining eye. Finally, the cerebellum and to some extent the brain stem are proportionately smaller compared to the cerebrum than is seen in normal individuals. (fig. 28).

Patients with Down's disease often also suffer from extraneural congenital malformations that can bring about secondary harmful effects to the brain. Those individuals having one form or another of congenital heart disease are liable to develop thromboembolic phenomena of the brain, sometimes resulting in devastatingly large and even fatal infarcts. These patients will also suffer from the consequences of acute and chronic anoxia

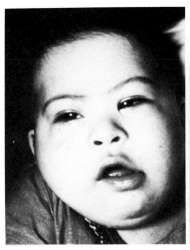
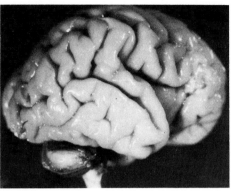

27

28

Fig. 27. Typical facial features of an infant with Down's disease.
Fig. 28. Brain in Down's disease. Convolutions appear 'simplified', the insula is exposed, the first temporal gyrus and the cerebellum are hypoplastic.

and/or of chronic passive congestion of the brain. Nutritional deficiencies often also affecting the brain are complications of congenital malformations involving the gastrointestinal tract (e.g., duodenal atresia). In this disease there is also a higher than normal incidence of leukemia [88]. This, however, usually represents more danger to survival than to mental functions. The patients with Down's disease, if free from associated extraneural, somatic abnormalities, usually follow a limited but otherwise undisturbed mental developmental pattern with various training schools and programs engaged in providing a slot for these individuals in a society where they can function according to their limited abilities. The latter usually reach a plateau that is determined by the anatomic limitations of the individual's brain [89]. There is, however, a group among these patients who, usually some time during the third decade of their life, develop definite signs of *mental regression.* In the cortices of these individuals neurons show neurofibrillary tangles indistinguishable from those seen in Alzheimer's disease. It is these structural alterations that are believed to be the cause of the clinically observed mental deterioration [90, 91].

Storage Diseases and Mental Retardation

As pointed out earlier, there are many organic diseases involving the central nervous system that are life threatening and eventually fatal so that impairment of the patient's mental functions is not the physician's primary concern. Many storage diseases fit this category, but some others allow the patient to live long enough to necessitate special concern for mental capacities of the individual. In storage diseases there is usually a congenital, genetically determined absence of a certain enzyme in the intermediate catabolic metabolism of cells, causing an abnormal accumulation of the substance the missing enzyme was supposed to break down. The nervous system may be spared, moderately or severely involved, either as the principal victim or in association with other involved organs. Examples of this spectrum include adult Gaucher's disease or glucocerebrosidase insufficiency, an abnormality involving mostly the reticuloendothelial system (bone marrow and spleen) with sparing of the brain. In the *infantile* form of the disease, however, the central nervous system is severely involved and affected nerve cells soon disintegrate, and the patient dies early. In Tay-Sachs disease (GM2 gangliosidosis) the malfunction of involved neurons of the CNS and the retina stand in the clinical foreground. The patients usually die before 3 years of age. In generalized gangliosidoses and in Niemann-Pick's disease, visceral (e.g. hepatic) damage also plays a part in the clinical picture. In Pompe's disease (glycogenosis type II or infantile acid maltase) deficiency neurons store abnormal amounts of glycogen, but massive cardiac involvement in the disease may overshadow other problems leading to death by congestive heart failure. The absence of galacto-cerebrosidase in Krabbe's globoid cell distrophy causes a profound change in myelin metabolism, leading to white matter destruction and death, usually before the second year of life. In neuronal storage diseases the accumulation of abnormal amounts of a catabolite in a neuron causes damage by crowding out the functioning portions of the perikaryon, but the same material may also cause disruption of synaptic structures and thus further impair the function of the brain.

In terms of institutionalized children with mental retardation secondary to neuronal storage diseases, the slower evolving forms of neuronal lipofuscinosis, e.g. the juvenile Vogt-Spielmeyer form, play an important part (although in these cases a more generalized lysosomal dysfunction, rather than the absence of a single enzyme, seems to play a causative role). Abnormal collections of autofluorescent lipofuscin in neurons characterize

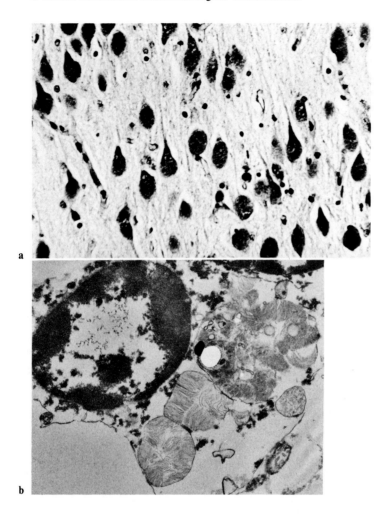

Fig. 29. a Characteristic appearance of cortical neurons in neuronal storage disease (in this instance Hunter type of mucopolysaccharidosis). The material stored in the perikaryon lends the cells a 'pregnant' appearance. PAS. b Same case. Electron micrograph of K cerebellar granule cell shows characteristic membrane-bound striated ('zebra') bodies often seen in gargoylism.

these entities and under the electron microscope the stored membranous debris assumes the shape of 'curvilinear bodies' in the younger patients and 'fingerprint-like inclusions' in the older ones.

In the various forms of gargoylism (mucopolysaccharidoses) there is accumulation of mucopolysaccharides in the viscera and bones (the latter explaining problems of the skeletal system and of growth) whereas the nerve cells contain much lipid debris as well, often in the shape of membrane-bound multilinear 'zebra bodies' (fig. 29). Particularly with the milder forms of the disease (e.g. Hunter's syndrome) patients may live for many years in institutions for the mentally retarded. One special feature of the mucopolysaccharidoses, as distinct from other neuronal storage diseases, is the eventual development of obstructive hydrocephalus secondary to fibrous thickening of the leptomeninges: apparently a response to the deposition of mucopolysaccharides in the meninges.

Dysplastic States and Phacomatoses

Of the five principal forms of phacomatoses (neurofibromatosis, neurocutaneous melanosis, von Hippel-Lindau disease, Sturge-Weber disease, and tuberous sclerosis), the first three, while creating potentially very serious problems for the central nervous system, particularly in the form of neoplasia, seldom are the cause of mental retardation (except in the rare form of diffuse gliomatosis in von Recklinghausen's disease).

Patients with encephalo-trigeminal angiomatosis (Sturge-Weber disease) have malformed, angiomatous blood vessels in the meninges, usually overlying the parietooccipital convexity on the same side of the facial skin hemangiomata. The underlying cortex often shows gliosis and extensive calcification [92]. These patients are subject to repeated epileptic seizures and to mental retardation.

In tuberous sclerosis, an autosomal recessively inherited condition, again, mental retardation and epileptic seizures occur in the same patient. As mentioned before, a profound multifocal dysplasia of the brain is present in these individuals with giant misshapen neurons and astrocytes clustered in cortical 'tubers' (fig. 30) (likely sources of seizures) and groups of subependymal large astrocytes forming the characteristic 'candle guttering' of the ventricles. Although the cortical tubers play an important role in the clinical manifestations of mental retardation and seizures, true neoplasms (giant cell astrocytomas) if and when they develop, usually start their growth from the subependymal astrocytic nodules.

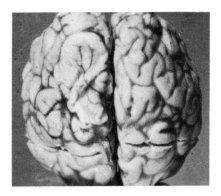

Fig. 30. Brain in tuberous sclerosis. Note the pale, grossly deformed and protuberant area in the left parasagittal cortex. This area was very firm on palpation and contained, in addition to poorly organized cortex and dysplastic neurons, heavy fibrous gliosis and calcification.

References

1   Ch'eng, L.Y.: Mental retardation – a question and suggestion about classification. J. Kans. med. Soc. *67:* 310–316 (1966).
2   Crome, L.; Stern, J.: Pathology of mental retardation; 2nd ed. (Churchill-Livingstone, Edinburgh 1972).
3   Friede, R.L.: Developmental neuropathology (Springer, New York 1975).
4   Crome, L.; France, N.E.: Microgyria and cytomegalic inclusion disease in infancy. J. clin. Path. *12:* 427–434 (1959).
5   Haymaker, W.; Girdany, B.R.; Stephen, J.; Lillie, R.D.; Fetterman, G.H.: Cerebral involvement with advanced periventricular calcification in generalized cytomegalic inclusion disease in the newborn. J. Neuropath. exp. Neurol. *13:* 562–586 (1954).
6   Holmes, L.B.; Driscoll, S.G.; Atkins, L.: Etiologic heterogeneity of neural-tube defects. New Engl. J. Med. *294:* 365–369 (1976).
7   Padget, D.H.: Neuroschisis and human embryonic development. New evidence on anencephaly, spina bifida and diverse mammalian defects. J. Neuropath. exp. Neurol. *29:* 192–216 (1970).
8   Dorovini-Zis, K.; Dolman, C.L.: Gestational development of brain. Archs Pathol. Lab. Med. *101:* 192–195 (1977).
9   De Reuck, J.; Eecken, H. van der: Transitional forms of Arnold-Chiari and Dandy-Walker malformations. J. Neurol. *210:* 135–141 (1975).
10 De Barros, M.C.; Farias, W.; Ataide, L.; Lins, S.: Basilar impression and Arnold-Chiari malformation. A study of 66 cases. J. Neurol. Neurosurg. Psychiat. *31:* 596–605 (1968).

11   Goldstein, F.; Kepes, J.J.: The role of traction in the development of the Arnold-Chiari malformation. An experimental study. J. Neuropath. exp. Neurol. *25:* 654–666 (1966).

12   Nichols, J.: Anencephaly. Geographic incidence, etiology and hormonal relations of the pituitary and adrenal cortex; in Bajusz, an introduction to clinical neuroendocrinology, pp. 273–298 (Karger, Basel 1967).

13   Sarraf Chirazi, M.T.: L'anencéphalie. Etude épidemiologique. Annls Pédiat. *23:* 737–740 (1976).

14   Friede, R.L.: Anencephaly; in Developmental neuropathology, pp. 230–236 (Springer, New York 1975).

15   Hamilton, W.J.; Mossman, H.W.: Human embryology, p. 488. (Williams & Wilkins, Baltimore 1972).

16   Goldberg, B.; Foster, D.B.; Segerson, J.A.; Baumeister, J.: Congenital brain malformations in the mentally retarded. Bull. Menninger Clin. *27:* 275–290 (1963).

17   Jellinger, K.; Gross, H.: Congenital telencephalic midline defects. Neuropädiatrie *4:* 446–452 (1973).

18   Gross, H.; Jellinger, K.: Morphologische Aspekte zerebraler Missbildungen. Häufigkeit und diagnostische Probleme im Rahmen kindlicher Hirnschäden. Wien. Z. NervHeilk. *27:* 9–37 (1969).

19   Khodadad, G.; Putschar, W.G.J.: The cerebral arteries in cyclopia and arrhinencephaly. An arteriographic and anatomical study. Acta anat. *72:* 12–24 (1969).

20   Loeser, J.D.; Alvord, E.C.: Clinicopathological correlations in agenesis of the corpus callosum. Neurology *18:* 745–756 (1968).

21   Barth, P.G.; Stam, F.C.; Harten, J.J. v.d.: Tuberous sclerosis and dysplasia of the corpus callosum. Report of their combined occurrence in a newborn. Acta neuropath. *42:* 63–64 (1978).

22   D'Agostino, A.N.; Kernohan, J.W.; Brown, J.R.: Dandy-Walker syndrome. J. Neuropath. exp. Neurol. *22:* 45–471 (1963).

23   Hart, M.N.; Malamud, N.; Ellis, W.G.: The Dandy-Walker syndrome: a clinicopathologic study based on 28 cases. Neurology *22:* 771–780 (1972).

24   Raimondi, A.J.; Samuelson, G.; Yarzagaray, L.; Norton, T.: Atresia of the foramina of Luschka and Magendie: the Dandy-Walker cyst. J. Neurosurg. *31:* 202–216 (1969).

25   Dolgopol, V.B.: Absence of the septum pellucidum as the only anomaly in the brain. Archs Neurol. Psychiat. Chicago *40:* 1244–1248 (1938).

26   Kepes, J.J.; Clough, C.; Villanueva, A.: Congenital fusion of the thalami (atresia of the third ventricle) and associated anomalies in a 6 month old infant. Acta neuropath. *13:* 97–104 (1969).

27   Norman, R.M.; revised by Urich, H.: Malformations of the nervous system, perinatal damage and related conditions in early life; in Greenfield, Neuropathology, chapter 10, pp. 385–391 (Edward Arnold, London 1976).

28   Palacios, E.; Schimke, R.N.: Craniosynostosis-syndactylism. Am. J. Roentg. Rad. Ther. nucl. Med. *106:* 144–155 (1969).

29   Ikuta, F.; Ohama, E.; Yamazaki, K.; Takeda, S.; Egawa, S.; Ichikawa, T.: Morphology in migrating glial cells in normal development, neoplasia and other disorders; in Zimmerman, Progress in neuropathology, vol. 4 (Raven Press, New York 1979).

30   Bergeron, R.T.: Pneumographic demonstration of subependymal heterotopic cortical gray matter in children. Am. J. Roent. Rad. Ther. nucl. Med. *101:* 168–177 (1967).
31   Chi, J.G.; Dooling, E.C.; Gilles, F.H.: Gyral development of the human brain. Ann. Neurol. *1:* 86–93 (1977).
32   Jellinger, K.; Rett, A.: Agyria-Pachygyria (lissencephaly syndrome). Neuropädiatrie *7:* 66–91 (1976).
33   Williams, R.S.: The cellular pathology of microgyria. A Golgi analysis. Acta neuropath. *36:* 269–283 (1976).
34   Levine, D.N.; Fisher, M.A.; Caviness, V.S.: Porencephaly with microgyria: a pathologic study. Acta neuropath. *29:* 99–113 (1974).
35   Leon, G.A. de; Grover, W.D.; Morinigo Mestre, G.: Cerebellar microgyria. Acta neuropath. *35:* 81–85 (1976).
36   Huttenlocher, P.R.: Dendritic development in neocortex of children with mental defect and infantile spasms. Neurology *24:* 203–210 (1974).
37   Crome, L.; Stern, J.: Pathology of mental retardation; 2nd ed., p. 53 (Churchill-Livingstone, Edinburgh 1972).
38   Riggs, H.E.; Rorke, L.B.: Myelination of the brain in the newborn (Lippincott, Philadelphia 1969).
39   Gilles, F.H.: Myelination in the neonatal brain. Human Pathol. *7:* 244–248 (1976).
40   Malamud, N.: Neuropathology of phenylketonuria. J. Neuropath. exp. Neurol. *25:* 254–268 (1966).
41   Oteruelo, F.T.; Partington, M.W.; Haust, M.D.: Ultrastructure of phenylketonuric (PKU) brains. Fed. Proc. *29:* 290 (1970).
42   Oteruelo, F.T.: 'PKU bodies' characteristic inclusions in the brain in phenylketonuria. Acta neuropath. *36:* 295–305 (1976).
43   Erdohazi, M.; Barnes, N.D.; Robinson, M.J.; Lake, B.D.: Cerebral malformation associated with metabolic disorder. A report of 2 cases. Acta neuropath. *36:* 315–325 (1976).
44   Bender, B.L.; Yunis, E.J.: Central nervous system pathology of tuberous sclerosis in children. Ultrastruct. Path. *1:* 287–299 (1980).
45   Brann, A.W., Jr.; Myers, R.E.: Central nervous system findings in the newborn monkey following severe in utero partial asphyxia. Neurology *25:* 327–328 (1975).
46   Jakab, I.: The role of neonatal anoxia and its prevention. Acta paedopsychiat. *32:* 329–338 (1965).
47   Towbin, A.: Spinal cord and brain stem injury at birth. Archs Path. *77:* 620–632 (1964).
48   Takagi, T.; Nagai, R.; Wakabayashi, S.; Mizawa, I.; Hajashi, K.: Extradural hemorrhage in the newborn as a result of birth trauma. Child's Brain *4:* 306–318 (1978).
49   Leech, R.W.; Kohnen, P.: Subependymal and intraventricular hemorrhages in the newborn. Am. J. Path. *77:* 465–476 (1974).
50   Donat, J.F.; Okazaki, H.; Kleinberg, F.; Reagan, T.J.: Intraventricular hemorrhages in full-term and premature infants. Mayo Clin. Proc. *53:* 437–331 (1978).
51   Courville, C.B.: Birth and brain damage. An investigation into the problems of antenatal and paranatal anoxia and allied disorders and their relation to the many lesion complexes residual thereto (Courville, Pasadena 1971).
52   Towbin, A.: Mental retardation due to germinal matrix infarction. Science *164:* 156–161 (1969).

53 Banker, B.Q.; Laroche, J.C.: Periventricular leukomalacia in infancy. Archs Neurol. 7: 386–410 (1962).

54 Gilles, F.H.; Murphy, S.F.: Perinatal telencephalic leucoencephalopathy. J. Neurol. Neurosurg. Psychiat. 32: 404–413 (1969).

55 Towbin, A.: Central nervous system damage in the human fetus and newborn infant. Mechanical and hypoxic injury incurred in the fatal neonatal period. Am. J. Dis. Child. 119: 529–542 (1970).

56 Leviton, A.; Gilles, F.H.: Morphologic correlates of age at death of infants with perinatal telencephalic leukoencephalopathy. Am. J. Path. 65: 303–309 (1971).

57 Towbin, A.: Organic causes of minimal brain dysfunction. Perinatal origin of minimal cerebral lesions. J. Am. med. Ass. 217: 1207–1214 (1971).

58 De Reuck, J.; Chattha, A.S.; Richardson, E.P.: Pathogenesis and evolution of periventricular leukomalacia in infancy. Archs Neurol. 27: 229–236 (1972).

59 Armstrong, D.; Norman, M.G.: Periventricular leucomalacia in neonates: complications and sequelae. Archs Dis. Childh. 49: 367–375 (1974).

60 Schneider, H.; Schachinger, H.; Dicht, R.: Telencephalic leukoencephalopathy in premature infants dying after prolonged artificial respiration. Report on 6 cases. Neuropädiatrie 6: 347–362 (1975).

61 Volpe, J.J.: Perinatal hypoxic-ischemic brain injury. Symp. on Pediat. Neurol. Pediat. Clins N. Am. 23: 383–396 (1976).

62 Marriage, K.J.; Davies, P.A.: Neurological sequelae in children surviving mechanical ventilation in the neonatal period. Archs Dis. Childh. 52: 176–182 (1977).

63 Stern, L.; Denton, R.L.: Kernicterus in small premature infants. Pediatrics 35: 483–485 (1965).

64 Blanc, W.A.; Johnson, L.: Studies on kernicterus. J. Neuropath. exp. Neurol. 18: 165–187 (1959).

65 Lademan, A.: Postneonatally acquired cerebral palsy. A study of the etiology, clinical findings and prognosis in 170 cases. Acta neur. scand. 57: suppl. 68 (1978).

66 Fitzhardinge, P.M.; Kazemi, M.; Ramsay, M.; Stern, L.: Long-term sequelae of neonatal meningitis. Devl. Med. Child Neur. 16: 3–10 (1974).

67 Berman, P.H.; Banker, B.Q.: Neonatal meningitis. A clinical and patholgocial study of 29 cases. Pediatrics 38: 6–24 (1966).

68 Crosby, R.M.N.; Mosberg, W.H.; Smith, G.W.: Intrauterine meningitis as a cause for hydrocephalus. J. Pediat. 52: 94–101 (1958).

69 Friede, R.L.: Cerebral infarcts complicating neonatal meningitis. Acute and residual lesions. Acta neuropath. 23: 245–253 (1973).

70 Frenkel, J.K.: Toxoplasmosis. Curr. Top. Pathol. 54: 28–75 (1971).

71 Norman, R.M.: Atrophic sclerosis of the cerebral cortex associated with birth injury. Archs Dis. Childh. 19: 11–121 (1944).

72 Crome, L.: Congenital hemiatrophy of the brain. Archs Dis. Childh. 26: 608–615 (1951).

73 Heschl, R.: Gehirndefekt und Hydrocephalus. Wschr. prakt. Heilk. 72: 102–104 (1861), cit. by Friede; in Developmental Neuropathology, p. 108 (Springer, New York 1975).

74 Lindenberg, R.; Swanson, P.D.: 'Infantile hydranencephaly' – a report of five cases of infarction of both hemispheres in infancy. Brain 90: 839–850 (1967).

75 Bielschowsky, M.: Über den Status marmoratus des Striatums und atypische Mark-fasergeflechte der Hirnrinde. J. Psychol. Neurol., Lpz. *31:* 121–151 (1924).

76 Löwenberg, K.; Malamud, W.: Status marmoratus. Etiology and manner of develop-ment. Archs Neurol. Psychiat. *29:* 104–124 (1933).

77 Carpenter, M.B.: Status marmoratus of the thalamus and striatum (associated with athetosis and dystonia). Neurology *5:* 139–146 (1955).

78 Borit, A.; Herndon, R.M.: The fine structure of plaques fibromyeliniques in ulegyria and in status marmoratus. Acta neuropath. *14:* 304–311 (1970).

79 Dawson, J.R.: Cellular inclusions in cerebral lesions of lethargic encephalitis. Am. J. Path. *9:* 7–15 (1933).

80 Bogaert, L. van: Une leuco-encéphalite sclerosante subaigue. J. Neurol. Neurosurg. Psychiat. *8:* 101–120 (1945).

81 Pette, H.; Döring, G.: Panencephalitis nodosa. Cit. by Nieberg and Blumberg; in Minckler, Viral encephalitides, pathology of the nervous system, vol. III. p. 2308 (McGraw Hill, New York 1972).

82 Friede, R.L.: Developmental neuropathology, pp. 154–156 (Springer, New York 1975).

83 Naeye, R.L.; Blanc, W.: Pathogenesis of congenital rubella. J. Am. med. Ass. *194:* 1277–1283 (1965).

84 Monif, G.R.G.; Sever, J.L.: Chronic infection of the central nervous system with rubella virus. Neurology *16:* 11–112 (1966).

85 Rorke, L.; Spiro, A.: Cerebral lesions in congenital rubella syndrome. J. Pediat. *70:* 243–255 (1967).

86 Friede, R.L.: Dysplasias in chromosome disorders. Down's syndrome (mongolism); in Developmental neuropathology, pp. 351–353 (Springer, New York 1975).

87 Colon, E.J.: The structure of the cerebral cortex in Down's syndrome. A quantitative analysis. Neuropädiatrie *3:* 362–376 (1972).

88 Krivit, W.; Good, R.A.: Simultaneous occurrence of mongolism and leukemia. Report of a nationwide survey. Am. J. Dis. Child. *94:* 289–293 (1953).

89 McGowen, C.H.: Prolonged survival in a patient with Down's syndrome. J. Am. med. Ass. *237:* 673–675 (1977).

90 Jervis, G.A.: Early senile dementia in mongoloid idiocy. Am. J. Psychiat. *105:* 102–106 (1948).

91 Solitare, G.B.; Lamarche, J.B.: Alzheimer's disease and senile dementia as seen in mongoloids: Neuropathological observations. Amer. J. ment. Defic. *70:* 840–848 (1966).

92 Krabbe, K.H.: Facial and meningeal angiomatosis associated with calcifications of brain cortex: clinical and anatomo-pathologic contribution. Archs Neurol. Psychiat. Chicago *32:* 737–755 (1934).

Diagnostic and Treatment Procedures

4 Diagnosis and Differential Diagnosis of Mental Retardation

Irene Jakab

Mental retardation is not a disease. It is a disability which must be differentiated from other conditions manifested in similar symptoms. Furthermore, the basic mental retardation itself must be differentiated from conditions associated with it, whether or not they have a causal relationship with each other.

About 1% of the population meets the criteria of retardation at any given time and it is twice as common in males as in females [DSM III, 1980]. The etiological and the detailed symptomatological differential diagnosis is essential in order to establish the prognosis and to assist in planning the strategies of intervention for habilitation, education or treatment. The details of the diagnostic evaluation are the building blocks of the treatment plan.

Diagnostic Criteria

The presence of the following three diagnostic criteria must be established in order to arrive at a working diagnosis of mental retardation: (A) subaverage intellectual functioning (IQ under 70); (B) deficits in adaptive behavior, and (C) age of onset under 18 years.

These criteria have been accepted both by the American Association of Mental Deficiency [*Grossman,* 1973] and by the American Psychiatric Association. They are listed in the third edition of the Diagnostic and Statistical Manual of Mental Disorders [DSM III, 1980]. Mental retardation may be listed on axis I in the diagnostic process of multiaxial evaluation. A graphic representation of the three basic criteria will be used for building up the differential diagnostic speculations related to each of the three components of the definition of mental retardation. Figure 1 illustrates the definition of mental retardation. The graphic representation of the diagnostic criteria may be conceived as a mobile structure. The fixed criteria (C) is the

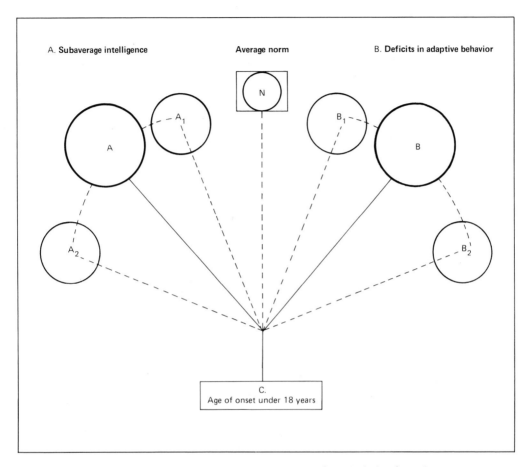

Fig. 1. Diagnosis of mental retardation. Variations of the deviation from the norms (N) on the diagnostic mobile. Distance from N: (1) A = B, even developmental delay of intellect and behavior; (2) A > B, greater intellectual deficit and less behavioral problems; (3) B > A, more behavior problems and less intellectual deficit.

age of onset, which must be under 18 years. From here the structure may tilt in any direction, either by keeping the angle between the arms A and B constant, or by moving either arm independently closer to or away from the midline which represents the average norms of intelligence and behavioral adaptation.

Of the above represented three criteria, A and B must be present simultaneously assuming a flexible upper margin of IQ between 65 and 75.

(A) Criteria of Low Intellectual Functioning (IQ under 70)

The demarcation line of IQ 70 between 'normal' and subnormal intelligence is based on the Gaussian distribution curve of the intelligence levels in the general population, as measured by standardized tests. Therefore, the criteria of a given individual's subaverage intellectual functioning at an IQ of 70, or under, is an arbitrary, but essentially objectively measurable entity. (A list of psychological tests is presented by *Shapiro* in this volume.) The most frequently used IQ tests, the Standford-Binet-LM, the WISC and the WAIS are each composed of several subtests measuring different elements of the intellectual functioning. A detailed analysis of their subtests is provided by *Sattler* [1974]. Several authors have designed specific evaluation forms [*Ozer*, 1980; *Feldman*, 1980; *Agranowitz and McKeown*, 1964]. *Walls* et al. [1977] list a large number of tests including the sources of ordering them. *Freeman* et al. [1981] give a checklist of 67 objectively defined behaviors.

For differential diagnostic purposes the intelligence profile representing the scores on each subtest of a given test allows a more refined assessment which may indicate specific deficiencies requiring further neuropsychological investigation. As a criteria for mental retardation the IQ under 70 is less rigidly applied in the new diagnostic manual [DSM III, 1980] than in previous editions. Some flexibility in diagnosis pertains to the cases of mild mental retardation with an IQ margin between 65 and 75, allowing the clinical decisions to be based on the presence or absence of deficits in the adpative behavior. This means that a person with an IQ as low as 65 without deficiencies in adaptive behavior will not be classified mentally retarded while another one with deficiencies in adaptive behavior and with an IQ up to 75 would be diagnosed as mentally retarded.

Based on the severity of the intellectual deficit, four subtypes of retardation are established. Mild: IQ 50–70; moderate: IQ 35–49; severe: IQ 20–34; profound: IQ below 20.

(B) Criteria of Deficits in the Adaptive Behavior

The ability to meet the social-behavioral criteria, is judged in the context of the subject's own environment. This is a relative (subjective) measure which may designate the same person as retarded in one environment (school) and not in another, where the demands of 'normality' are different (home). Developmental norms are considered when defining age-appropriate behavioral criteria for children.

The testing for social adaptive functions may help by determining the social quotient (SQ) relevant in the context of the subject's age and the population used for standardization of the test. A useful list of behavioral assessment tools, including bibliographical data on 28 tests, was compiled by the Pennsylvania Office of Mental Retardation [1976].

(C) Criteria of the Age of Onset

The age of onset as being under 18 years must be confirmed either by the age at the time of the referral itself or by history in a person with a low IQ and adaptive deficits in order to establish the diagnosis of mental retardation.

Diagnostic Methods

The established diagnosis of mental retardation itself does not provide any guidelines as to the prognosis, nor any help in designing methods of intervention. Therefore detailed differential diagnostic guidelines are provided below, based on one hand on the presenting symptoms, on the other hand on the etiology of the retardation and of the associated conditions.

Symptom-Related Differential Diagnosis

General Remarks

The methods of symptom-related differential diagnostic workup include the developmental history, clinical examination, observation and testing. Clusters of symptoms may be characteristic of diseases other than mental retardation. These may either cause secondary retardation, or be associated with, but not causally related to the primary retardation.

Low IQ and associated deficiencies in adaptive behavior may be caused by a general and even-level developmental delay of both intellectual and emotional maturity (A_1 and B_1 in fig. 2). In these cases of uncomplicated retardation the IQ tests reveal no substantial differences in performance versus verbal IQ, both being lower than normal, producing an intelligence profile of rather even level on all subtests. The neuropsychological testing reveals no specific cortical function deficits. In children within the given level of the achieved mental age all functions are essentially on the same level. The behavioral adaptation is characterized by emotional immaturity, but it is not grossly deviant, rather the child acts like one of younger

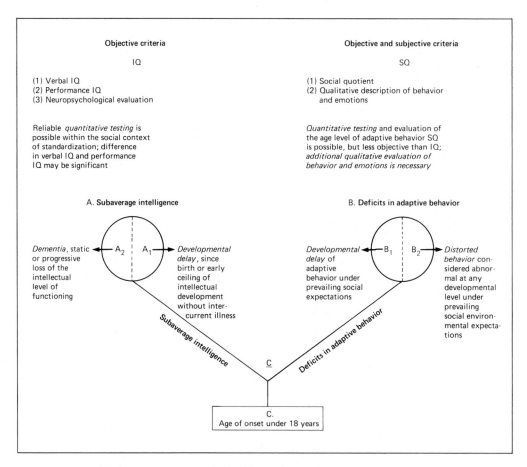

Fig. 2. Mental retardation. Symptom-related differential diagnosis.

age. At most he/she may be on a slightly 'different timetable emotionally and intellectually' [*Pearson, 1968*].

The sequence of appearance of symptoms is of differential diagnostic importance. Repeated testing may show a relatively constant IQ and the possible progression of the behavioral maladaptation (A₁ and B₂ in fig. 2). In this case the question of the occurrence of an unrelated psychiatric illness must become the focus of the differential diagnosis. The quality of the behavioral adaptation of a retarded person may be distorted and considered to be abnormal at any developmental level, for example stereotype movement patterns, severe aggression, self-abuse, attention deficit disorder, hyperactivity, hallucinations, delusions, autistic withdrawal, etc. (B_2 in fig. 2). An appropriate psychiatric diagnosis will be added to the diagnosis of mental retardation in these cases.

For detailed differential diagnosis of emotional problems and illustrative case presentations, the reader is referred to the chapter on 'Psychiatric Disorders in Mental Retardation' [this volume].

Retardation may be caused or aggravated by physical illness at an early age with loss of specific functions and/or dementia (A_2 in fig. 2, and organic mental disorders in fig. 3). If dementia is suspected, a detailed history must complete the present evaluation in order to confirm the type of the dementia as either being static or progressive. In the static organic mental disorder, on repeated testing, the IQ subtests will reveal each time essentially the same deficits and uneven achievements (splinter skills). The progressive dementing processes, on the other hand, lead to increasingly more severe deficits – ending in death in many cases, within a short time.

The arrest of maturation or the destruction of already developed parts of the brain are manifested in the alterations of its functions.

In diffuse organic brain damage, those functions which are acquired phylogenetically and ontogenetically the latest (i.e., the highest functions) are the ones which get lost first, or are prevented from developing at all. The developmentally oriented differential diagnostic technique provides the clue to the assessment of the general cerebral functions affected by diffuse brain damage (fig. 4).

The destruction of nervous tissue can manifest itself in: (1) loss of function related to the destroyed area; (2) impairment of higher functions in which the lost basic function plays an important role; and (3) abnormal or exaggerated function as a result of release of nervous mechanisms by destruction of higher centers.

Any damaging agent which affects the brain could cause either an organic lesion of a circumscribed nature (forceps pressure, shot or stab wound, abscess, embolism, thrombosis, tumor, etc.) or it could affect the whole brain diffusely (genetic, metabolic disorders, inflammation, intoxication, anoxia, contusion, sclerotic vascular diseases, etc.). These two types of lesions in many cases are not that distinguished but often the diffuse damage is associated with destruction of important centers and vice versa.

In diffuse lesions the amount of the brain substance lost or impaired in its function will be grossly paralleled by the amount of functional impairment; animal experiences [*Lashley,* 1943] and neurological cases [*Hecaen and*

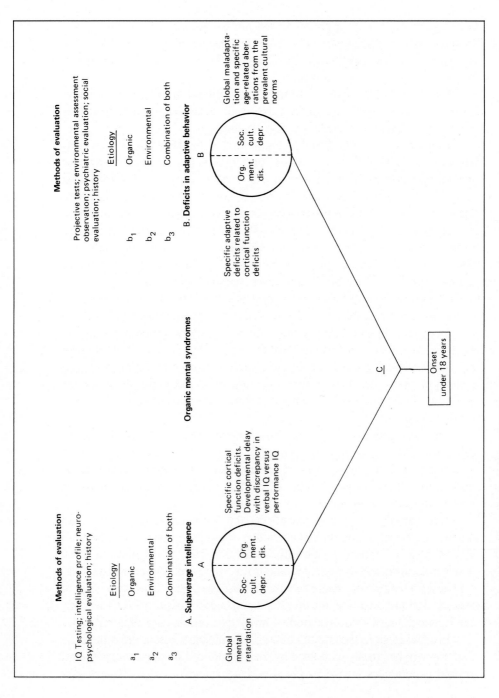

Fig. 3. Mental retardation. Etiological differential diagnosis.

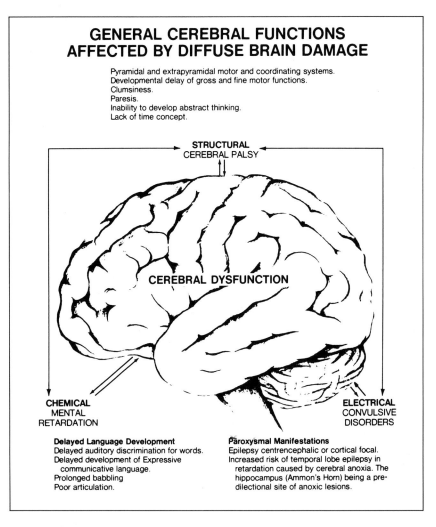

GENERAL CEREBRAL FUNCTIONS AFFECTED BY DIFFUSE BRAIN DAMAGE

Pyramidal and extrapyramidal motor and coordinating systems.
Developmental delay of gross and fine motor functions.
Clumsiness.
Paresis.
Inability to develop abstract thinking.
Lack of time concept.

STRUCTURAL
CEREBRAL PALSY

CEREBRAL DYSFUNCTION

CHEMICAL
MENTAL
RETARDATION

ELECTRICAL
CONVULSIVE
DISORDERS

Delayed Language Development
Delayed auditory discrimination for words.
Delayed development of Expressive
  communicative language.
Prolonged babbling
Poor articulation.

Paroxysmal Manifestations
Epilepsy centrencephalic or cortical focal.
Increased risk of temporal lobe epilepsy in
  retardation caused by cerebral anoxia. The
  hippocampus (Ammon's Horn) being a pre-
  dilectional site of anoxic lesions.

Fig. 4

Angelergues, 1963] give evidence to this assumption. The results are different in the cases of anatomical destruction of the more differentiated 'centers'. A loss of ½ ounce of brain substance of the calcarine fissure will give a more obvious impairment than the removal of about half of a prefrontal area.

In localized lesions the neuropsychological testing needs to be done with special care for the following functions: conceptual thinking, speech,

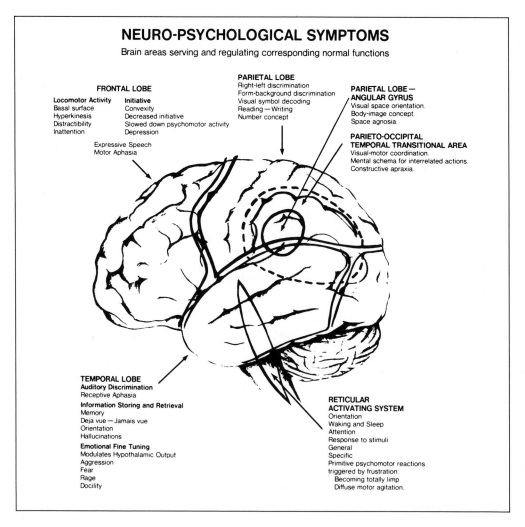

Fig. 5

symbol-understanding, reading, writing, understanding of space-relations and the ability to manipulate objects purposefully. Figure 5 represents the cortical mapping of these functions. Recently, substantial differences have been recorded in the level of initiative for conversational speech following frontal lesions depending on the side of the lesion [*Kolb and Taylor,* 1981].

The psychiatric implications of brain damage in children were described by *Eisenberg* [1957].

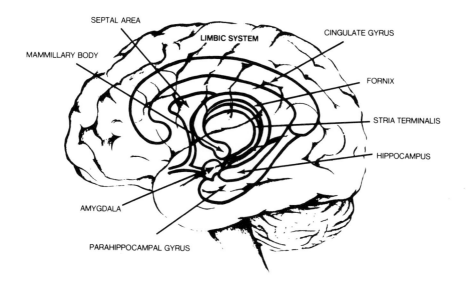

PSYCHIATRIC SYMPTOMS

Assumed correlations:
  with anatomical cortical and subcortical areas and with complex interdependent
  regulating systems.

SEPTAL AREA

LIMBIC SYSTEM

CINGULATE GYRUS

MAMMILLARY BODY

FORNIX

STRIA TERMINALIS

HIPPOCAMPUS

AMYGDALA

PARAHIPPOCAMPAL GYRUS

Motivation—interpersonal relations.
Egocentric thinking.
Idiosyncratic, distorted psychotic speech.
Lack of play skills and lack of interest in toys.
Lack of eye contact or active avoidance of eye contact.
Inability or refusal to interact with adults or children.

Emotional lability and ambivalence.
Low frustration tolerance.
Uncontrollable aggressive impulses.
Psychotic anxiety.
Self injury.
Hallucinations. Delusions. Bizarre posturing.

Fig. 6

In order to understand all possible ramifications of organic brain damage, including the occurrence of psychotic states, it is equally important to assess the phases of ego-development regarding the level of emotional stabil-
ity and the range of emotional flexibility in the adaptive behavior (fig. 6).

In the multiaxial diagnosis, identified clinical entities should be listed
on axis I, in addition to the mental retardation, or on axis II if they meet the
criteria of special developmental disorders. Underlying neurological condi-

tions should be listed on axis III (these may well represent the etiological background of the retardation). In cases of multiple diagnoses on the same axis, the condition requiring major attention will be marked 'principal diagnosis'. Behavioral symptoms which are not part of another disease will be recorded on the fifth digit of the principal diagnosis.

Assessment of the Functions of the Brain and Signs of Organic Brain Damage

The procedure of identifying signs of organic brain damage includes the following methods of evaluation: (1) clinical neurological examination, and if necessary, genetic-metabolic laboratory procedures, EEG, cerebral blood flow recordings, CAT scan, evoked potential studies, etc.; (2) psychological testing and neuropsychological evaluation.

(1) Guidelines to the Neurological Examination

To detect discrete neurological signs in cases of organic brain disorder not manifested in gross cerebral palsy or other clear-cut neurological syndrome on standard clinical neurological examination, the evaluation of the higher integrative functions of praxis, gnosis and language is necessary. For details of the standard neurological examination, see the Pediatric Neurology section [this volume]. Some neurological signs easily overlooked during the evaluation of retarded persons are listed below.

Cranial Nerves

Olfactory Nerve. Bilateral hyposmia or anosmia, of which the patient might be unaware, may be the only detectable permanent sign of past head injury. Retarded persons may not complain of lack of smell, therefore, testing whenever feasible should be performed. Unilateral hyposmia or anosmia usually signals focal lesions affecting the olfactory nerve or the temporal lobe. In the latter case hallucinations can also develop and be misdiagnosed as psychogenic, while the hyposmia itself may remain unknown, unless tested.

Optic Nerve. In diffuse brain damage, visual field defects may be found quite often due to the widely spread-out visual pathways. Children with good central vision but reduced visual fields may be misdiagnosed as alexic (learning-disabled) when they cannot read the large letters written by the teacher on the black-board – and the larger they are the less they can be perceived through a pinpoint central visual field, even if visual acuity for central vision is normal. Observers should be alerted by these children's method of compensating through 'macula transport'. This is a phenomenon of moving the head, for following the outline of letters to be read when the visual field is substantially narrowed. In other cases, before assuming non-compliance, one should remember that the use of only one-half of a sheet of paper when writing or drawing can reveal hemianopsia or parietal inattention manifested in neglecting one-half of the visual field. This can be further clarified if one of two stimuli applied simultaneously to the visual fields, or to other sensory areas (touch, pain), is suppressed.

Substantial discrepancy between the visual acuity of the two eyes, or monocular vision may lead to problems in depth perception. This in turn could cause clumsiness in eye-hand coordination and make the person's walking appear clumsy or even ataxic.

Shapiro [1972] shows the importance of the organization of visual perception in the development of the total child, while *Tarnopol* [1971] points out the importance of disorders of vision and hearing in learning disorders.

Extraocular Nerves. Their lesion may cause deviation of one eye and, if it is severe, ambliopia may result. The oculomotor reaction time reflects the degree of cerebral dysfunction by decreased latency in Alzheimer's disease [*Pirozzolo and Hansh,* 1981]. This technique may be useful in the diagnosis of retarded brain-damaged subjects, especially in Down's syndrome patients who have a higher incidence of Alzheimer's disease than the average population.

The abducens nerve has the longest trajectory on the base of the skull and therefore, is the most vulnerable during head injury, especially during delivery. In some cases the lesion is minimal and does not lead to visible strabismus, although on examination it is revealed by horizontal nystagmus at extreme lateral gaze in the direction of the weakened muscle innervation. Early detection of visual deficit is important, since it may prevent the loss of vision in one eye. *Kurzberg and Vaugham* [1981] report differential findings on evoked potential in high risk infants as early as at 40 weeks of age.

Facial Nerve. Nuclear or supranuclear paresis of the facial nerve of different extent can be found in retardates with cerebral palsy. In other cases, however, a thalamic lesion may interfere with spontaneous emotional smiling in spite of intact voluntary facial innervation. This may give the impression of emotional dullness, causing a person to appear more retarded than in reality, when actually only the physiological pathway of the expression, but not the feeling itself, is suppressed [*Watson* et al., 1981]. Myoclonic jerks and choreiform movements which often involve the facial muscles might be misinterpreted as tics or grimacing. *Blumberg* et al. [1981] have described a case of myoclonus in Down's syndrome. *Bender* [1961] called attention to the importance of the evaluation of subcortical mechanisms as a 'possible approach to the pathophysiology of manneristic and clowning movements of schizophrenics.' Her observations are also quite relevant to the differential diagnosis of behavioral disturbances of retarded children who frequently have organic brain disorders, and who are also prone to stereotype behavior.

Acoustic and Vestibular Nerves. Audiological testing may help in differentiating hearing deficit from retardation, attention deficit syndrome, sensory aphasia, and infantile autism. In adult retardates, the social-interpersonal isolation caused by hearing deficit may be confused with depression. Impaired vestibular function may explain the 'clumsy gait' of some retarded persons.

Locomotor System
Hypertonia and hypotonia are both frequent in retardates. Slight muscle tone changes can be proven by 'shaking' the relaxed arm and leg of the patient and observing the extent of the passive movements made by the hand or foot. Hyperextensibility in the joints of the

fingers may indicate lesions of the thalamus with or without pronounced athetoid movements ('thalamus hand'). Muscle rigidity and weakness may appear as clumsiness, Barré's sign is useful to detect slight weakness. It can be examined on the arms in standing, sitting or prone positions – on the legs it can be examined in prone position by having the patient raise both legs from the hip with straight knees, and (just like the weaker extended arm) the weaker leg will sink. Some retarded children, who may not cooperate with standard examination of muscle strength, may be willing to lie down and raise their legs for this test.

Lately, since the use of psychotropic drugs is frequent in the treatment of retarded persons [*Breuning*, 1981], one should carefully watch retarded patients to avoid misdiagnosing tardive dyskinesia or other drug side effects by ascribing them to manneristic oddities of the retarded person. Protruding tongue, fidgeting, smacking lip movements or occasional choreiform jerking, as well as rigidity and mask-like face should be investigated through good observation and history from reliable relatives or staff about the onset of these manifestations. If connections with drug taking is established, appropriate therapeutic measures must be initiated.

Cerebellar Signs

These signs should be looked for carefully in cases of perinatal anoxia, which frequently leads to damage of the Purkinje cells in the cerebellar cortex. Tremor, ataxia and dysdiadochokinesis, in slightly affected cases, may appear as clumsiness. The presence of rebound phenomenon or other cerebellar signs such as nystagmus, hypotonia or Romberg's sign will help confirm the diagnosis.

Reflexes

The absence, hyper- or hypoactivity, of reflexes (especially if asymmetrical) and the appearance of pathological reflexes as well as the persistence of infantile reflex behavior signal organic damage or delay in maturation of the central nervous system.

The following reflexes are normally found in infancy [*Ford*, 1946]: sucking reflex until the age of 1 year; grasping reflex from the first weeks to the age of 4 months; grasping reflex of the foot until 2 years; Moro's reflex until the age of 5 months; Babinski's sign until the age of 1 year; otolith righting reflex appears after the 2nd month and persists throughout life; for this, children have to be examined with blind-folded eyes; Landau reflex, between 1 and 2 years of age; tonic neck reflex, until the age of 3 years (this reflex is usually incomplete in normal infants). Righting reflexes are employed in rising from dorsal recumbent position. Young children arise as do quadrupeds. This quadrupedal stage corresponds to the crawling period, and may persist for a long time in retarded children. *Ford* [1946] uses some lovely terms to characterize the psychomotor development stages of infants and children. 'Eighteenth month. . .the children should walk well, use two or three words and understand much of what is said. Should now be badly spoiled and cry for whatever is desired.' 'Fifth year . . .tonic neck reflexes should be absent. Galvanic irritability of muscles and nerves of adult standard. The child should now be into mischief almost all day.'

Sensory System

Pathological signs to be considered here are not in the realm of elementary sensations, but in the pathology of combined sensations: two points discrimination, graphesthesia, stereognosis, and higher visual and auditory integrative functions. The testing of higher sensory functions will involve the clinical examination of the psychological function of 'recognizing' and 'naming' objects; of coordinating visual and auditory stimuli, and the assessing of visual-motor coordination. Even in the nonverbal tests the understanding of verbal instructions is often needed. In conditioned reflex experiments the function of 'recognizing' can be examined separately from that of 'naming'. Evoked potential studies are useful in differentiating hearing deficit, aphasia and infantile autism. More refined studies of brain electrical activity mapping (BEAM) [*Duffy,* 1981] may help in the identification of functional learning deficit versus global developmental delay. Based on the dynamic spaciotemporal electrical patterns, *Gevins* et al. [1981], clearly distinguished two visual-motor tasks during cognition.

In the clinical observation of young infants, *Brazelton and Heidelise* [1979] found that they achieve homeostatic control over stimuli by reaching out for, or shutting out, individual stimuli.

The following two cases show the need for extended clinical observation, beyond the routine neurological examination, in order to interpret correctly some behavioral symptoms related to organic causes.

Case sample: Illustration of the difficulties of a retarded woman, caused by inadequate depth perception:

Case 1. Mary (all names in case vignettes in this paper are fictitious to protect the anonymity of the patients) is a middle-aged, mildly retarded woman living in the community and commuting to a mental health clinic for supportive social casework. The social worker was puzzled by the client's behavior who would come to her office without any difficulty, but when leaving she had frequently asked to be escorted and leaned on the social worker for support until she reached the exit door. A case of 'exaggerated dependency' was suspected. Inspection of the premises by the social worker, revealed the following conditions: the distance from the main entrance of the clinic to the social worker's office was a carpeted surface (no problem of walking), while the distance to the back door exit, for the pick-up by bus, was a tile-surfaced corridor in alternating black and white tiles (where the client required physical support to walk the distance to the door). For persons with impaired depth perception the dark surfaces seem to recede while the white squares may appear as elevated surfaces, thus giving the impression of unevenness and causing insecurity in placing each step. This case of 'exaggerated dependency' was solved by advising the client to use the carpeted corridor to the front entrance each time and then walk to the bus on the sidewalk.

Case sample: The 'eye-poking' (self-abusive) behavior of a retarded child signaling discomfort caused by occasional double vision due to eye muscle weakness:

Case 2. Roland, a 9½–year-old Caucasian boy, born after 7 months' gestation, was admitted to the John Merck Program in 1980 (a program for emotionally disturbed-retarded children, at the University of Pittsburgh, Department of Psychiatry). Past history:

Roland had grand mal and myoclonic seizures since the age of 5 months. He was severely retarded in all psychomotor milestones and had repeated ear infections. After 5 years of special education, Roland was still nonverbal and only partially toilet trained. Seizures were under control with medication. Complaints at admission: loud screaming, whining with a hissing sound (when demands were placed on him in school or at home), self-abusive behaviors such as head-banging, beating his head and face with objects, biting his palm and fingers. ('He also presses hard on his right eyeball.') Standard neurological examination revealed scaphocephaly and high-arched palate. (This explains the hissing quality of his whining.) No metabolic genetic disorder was detected. Repeated and lengthy observation of the child's spontaneous behavior revealed that the 'eye-poking' was indeed restricted to the right eyeball. For instance, Roland focused straight ahead on a distant object for a short time, his left eye remained in the midline while his right eye turned slowly inward, revealing the weakness of the right abducens innervation. This was followed each time by his pushing with his index finger the right corner of his right eye. This maneuver brought the right eyeball back into the midline, obviously alleviating the distressing experience of double vision, of which this retarded nonverbal child was unable to complain. *His apparently self-abusive symptom of 'eye-poking' was actually an adaptive maneuver counteracting the right abducens paresis.* His other symptoms were considered to be signs of emotional disturbance and were treated successfully with behavioral therapy, milieu therapy and tranquilizers (Milieu therapy is described in the chapter on Psychiatric Disorders in Mental Retardation [this volume]).

A word of caution is in order here: in similar cases, the 'eye-poking' behavior could be suppressed by behavior modification. However, the double vision will reoccur and without 'pushing the eyeball' back to parallel position it may lead to physiological suppression of the vision in the deviant eye, ending in amblyopia. Similar cases, therefore, should have an ophthalmological evaluation for latent strabismus.

(2) Psychological Testing and Neuropsychological Evaluation

On intelligence tests a substantial discrepancy between the performance IQ and the verbal IQ helps identify organic brain damage, if the performance IQ is at least by 15 points lower than the verbal IQ. 'The common outcome of early hydrocephalus is an uneven growth of intelligence in childhood, with nonverbal intelligence developing less well than verbal intelligence' [*Dennis* et al., 1970]. On the contrary, in low IQ caused by psychosis, or noncompliant behavioral disorder, the verbal IQ is usually lower than the performance IQ. An erratic intelligence profile where some subtests measuring similar functions are solved at a developmentally higher level than others, within the same testing period, indicates the likelihood of emotional disturbance. It is especially revealing if at repeated testing, some of the previously passed items are failed and vice versa. The narrative description of a patient's behavior during testing should further clarify the diagnosis. (For a systematic and detailed description of psychological evaluation see *Yando* [this volume].)

In the differential diagnosis of organic brain syndromes in mental retardation, testing is best done with selected tests assessing special cortical functions. These tests will detect uneven maturational levels on different categories of intelligence subtests and on the neuropsychological evaluation of cortical functions. This will help differentiate the mental retardation caused by general intellectual developmental delay from specific developmental disabilities.

It is indeed the most challenging task to differentiate, through detailed neuropsychological evaluation, the etiology of the retardation when the global IQ values may provide no clues to distinguish cases of cultural deprivation from cases where the retardation is due to a mosaic of several cortical deficits. Sociocultural retardation is often aggravated by malnutrition. In these cases, organic brain damage may be superimposed on the social neglect. The importance of the first 3 years is crucial in this respect [*Maggio,* 1971].

The discrepancies in test findings led to polemics in the literature regarding the developmental theory [*Kahmi,* 1981; *Ross,* 1968] versus the difference (defect) theories [*Balla and Zigler,* 1971; *Das,* 1972; *Detlerman,* 1979; *Deutsch and Schumer,* 1970; *Dutton,* 1975; *Greenspan,* 1979; *Humphreys and Parsons,* 1979; *Luria,* 1970, 1973; *Milgram,* 1971; *Reed,* 1971; *Spitz,* 1979; *Winters,* 1977; *Zigler,* 1969].

Communication disorders, being quite frequent in childhood (*Richardson and Normanly* [1965] found 52% in a sample of 800 cases), require special attention in differentiating aphasia from the disorders caused by emotional disturbance which at times may be induced by the aphasia itself [*Mapelli* et al., 1981]. *Ramsay-Graeme* [1980] found that multilinguals show less rigidity in using learning sources to acquire a new language than those speaking a single language. This phenomenon was related to the emotional aspect of the motivation to learn. Rigidity in using available language sources may play a role in the language delay of retarded children. Language delay (not aphasia) of Down's syndrome children is found to be due to deficits in vocal imitation skills [*Mahoney* et al., 1981]. Other perceptual dysfunctions may lead to emotional problems in adolescents unless diagnosed and treated early [*Reiser,* 1981]. For children over 6 years of age the Wechsler-Bellevue intelligence scale for children (WISC), and for adults the Wechsler adult intelligence scale (WAIS) are useful in detecting organic mental disorders. In organic cases the digit-symbol and block design subtests show low scores on these tests, while the vocabulary, the information and the comprehension subtests yield relatively higher scores.

Special tests useful in the differential diagnosis of developmental arrest and dementia, both in children and in older retardates, are listed below.

The *Reitan* battery for logical memory, memory span and associate learning.

The *Wechsler* memory scale (information, orientation, mental control tests of abstraction or concept formation).

The *Goldstein-Scheerer* sorting test with quantitative scoring by Rapaport measures adequacy, conceptual level and concept span.

The *Halstead* category test and the tactual performance test, based on the biological concept of intelligence are very useful in detecting organic brain damage.

In organic lesions a tendency of concrete thinking will interfere with the solving of the Goldstein-Scheerer, and Halstead tests. The *Reitan* battery and the *Bender* gestalt test are both excellent indicators of organicity. Intelligence tests are revealing of the underlying cause of the failure only if the scores are not all too low in a battery. Failing essentially all subtests might be caused by several disorders including any of the following entities: advanced organic brain disorder, severe mental retardation, catatonic or hysterical stupor, and delusional behavior [*Jakab,* 1950]. In such cases, the examiner must rely on the history of former achievements and on behavioral observations, before making a diagnosis.

Projective tests are especially useful in the cases of adolescents, and adults, functioning in the mild range of retardation, where organicity versus emotional disturbance is in question.

Rorschach test. One of the most reliable single indicators of organicity is the lowering of the (form) F+% under 70 [*Piotrowski,* 1937], especially if this is not paralleled by low scores on vocabulary and information tests. Such discrepancies have been seen in lobotomized patients whose intelligence test performance showed improvement as compared to the level measured shortly before lobotomy, while at the same time the F+% was lower after lobotomy [*Jakab,* 1957]. In these patients, the use of the full capacity of their intelligence was previously impaired by the psychotic symptoms causing the low preoperative scores. The lowering of the F+ percentage after lobotomy was a sign of organicity revealing their inability to integrate the details of nonspecific stimuli, in spite of an increased IQ as compared to their performance before the lobotomy.

Thematic apperception test (TAT) and the *Children's apperception test* (CAT). Concrete answers and simplicity characterizes the stories given by brain-damaged persons similarly to those of retarded persons. *Sarason* [1959] found that in the stories of mentally retarded children aggression, loneliness and a desire for affection is prevalent. These facts, however, seem to be signs of reaction to the environmental deprivation and are not diagnostic of the retardation itself.

Affectivity

Emotional instability can be observed and recorded in the test situation. It may be revealed in restlessness or in a tendency to joke inappropriately (moria of the frontal-lobe-damaged patients). In other cases the lack of initiative can lower the score beyond the actual capabilities of the patient. The role of lesion site and side in the affective behavior of patients with localized cortical excisions was demonstrated by *Kolb and Taylor* [1981].

Brain-damaged children may either show regression from a former level of functioning or remain developmentally delayed by lack of achieving higher intellectual functions. The pathological course of the physiological developmental phases was found also in cases of brain tumors by *Corboz* [1958]. In these children, primitive drives and instincts dominate the egocentric personality. The tolerance for anxiety is lowered in traumatic brain damage and anxiety is easily provoked either by overprotection, or by too demanding parents and through loss of contact of the brain-damaged child with children of the same age [*Laux*, 1965].

(3) Assessment of Special Developmental Disabilities Frequently Associated with Mental Retardation: Aphasias, Alexia, Agraphia, Acalculia, Agnosias and Constructive Apraxia

The definition, cortical localization and testing (methods of neuropsychological evaluation) of these symptoms are listed in tables I–V and their cortical localization is presented in figure 5.

These symptoms reveal the pathology of the highest intellectual functions of speech, symbol-understanding, integrative visual-motor functions and space-orientation. The intellectual development of retarded patients with diffuse brain damage may never reach the level of abstract thinking and symbol-understanding. In some cases, however, in addition to generalized developmental delay one or more of the specialized cortical functions may be critically impaired. *Proper recognition and differential diagnosis in such cases may lead to habilitation with substantial improvement, by using the same methods as for nonretarded learning-disabled children.*

If the remedial methods are successfully alleviating the special developmental disability, the general level of functioning of the retarded person will be improved substantially. The improvement can lead to an accelerated increase of the IQ (see cases 3 and 4).

The higher psychological functions of speech, concept formation, abstraction, symbol-understanding and goal-directed motor activity are all liable to show impairment in diffuse brain damage, and would then be manifested in low scores on most tests measuring the functions beyond the level of abstract concept formation. *Pruyser* [1979] gives a most lucid description of abstract concept formation as it hinges on the capacity to establish identity between various visual stimulus configurations. This author also demonstrates how the language remains specific in concretism without attaining global concept formation. There are also physiological variations at different ages in the cognitive development of the infant and the child, as it was masterfully described by *Piaget* [1952].

Table I. Tabulation of specific developmental disorders frequently associated with general developmental delay

Definition	Localization	Testing
Aphasias		
Motor, or expressive aphasia: the inability to produce meaningful words and sentences without impairment of vocalization	dominant hemisphere, frontal lobe (Broca center); third frontal gyrus and/or operculum	spontaneous speech (in mother tongue and other languages spoken by the patient) and repetition of words spoken by others; automatic speech patterns representing rote memory: the days of the week, a prayer, the national anthem, etc.
Sensory, or receptive aphasia: the inability to understand speech without hearing impairment	dominant hemisphere; temporal lobe (Wernicke center); first temporal gyrus	auditory decoding and speech understanding; following commands, pointing to objects named by the examiner; repeating words spoken by the examiner
Amnestic aphasia: the inability to name persons or objects, while recognizing people and using objects appropriately; inability to remember numbers; both the encoding and the retrieval may be affected	diffuse-cortical lesions; observed also in most frontal lesions and the lesion of the mamillary bodies	standardized memory tests; object naming; word pair learning; clinical memory evaluation for recent and long past events; orientation in time, space and for person; assessment of concomitant confabulation.

Table II. Tabulation of specific developmental disorders frequently associated with general developmental delay

Definition	Localization	Testing
Alexia		
The inability to read, or spell out written material, to recognize letters or words and to understand the meaning of written words and sentences	dominant hemisphere, parietal lobe, cortical area; for alexia due to general space agnosia (in spite of intact parietal lobe), see localization of spacial agnosia	reading individual letters, words, and sentences
Agraphia		
The inability to write letters and words; making directional errors in the writing of letters; the inability to copy letters or words	dominant hemisphere, parietal lobe, cortex; for agraphia due to constructive apraxia (inspite of intact parietal lobe), see localization of constructive apraxia; the inability to copy is lost only in bilateral lesions	spontaneous writing, writing upon dictation (requires auditory decoding also); copying: letters, words, sentences (printed and cursive writing to be tested each); the examiner must keep in mind that both alexia and agraphia can be combined with aphasia

Table III. Tabulation of specific developmental disorders frequently associated with general developmental delay

Definition	Localization	Testing
Acalculia		
The lack of number concept; inability to do mathematical operations (add, substract, multiply, divide); inability to read (decode) multi-digit numbers or to write them upon dictation;	dominant hemisphere, parietal lobe, cortical area; inability to read and write multi-digit numbers may be due to space agnosia or to constructive apraxia; for localization, see space agnosia and constructive apraxia	recognizing written, single- and multi-digit numbers; operations with numbers; mental calculation and using paper and pencil for mathematical operations should be tested separately – the latter requires ability to write (may be impaired in agraphia) – while mental operations with numbers are still possible; assembling numbers using three-dimensional blocks showing numbers on their surface or being shaped like numbers may be impaired in-spite of intact number concept in space agnosia and in constructive apraxia

Table IV. Tabulation of specific developmental disorders frequently associated with general developmental delay

Definition	Localization	Testing
Agnosias and asymbolia		
The inability to recognize: objects, symbols, relations of concrete objects, pictures or schematic representations without	visual agnosia: dominant hemisphere; angular gyrus, parieto-temporo-occipital cortical transitional area lesions of either	orientation on the own body orientation in the concrete space, finding one's way in the home, on the street, etc.; recognizing figures, shapes, and their spacial relationships; recognition of pictures of geometrical figures, hu-

Definition	Localization	Testing
impairment of the elementary sensory organs (tactile, visual or auditory agnosia, asymbolia); body image disturbances (somatoagnosias, autotopagnosia); inability to recognize, name, and point to one's own body parts	hemisphere, or sub-cortical lesions of the same areas on the nondominant side; autotopagnosia: white matter nondominant hemisphere with corpus callosum lesion	man figures, face, hand, orientation on a map; persons suffering from severe visual agnosia, are also alexic; the meaning of the letters and words as a distinct gestalt is missing; some patients with space agnosia are oriented in the actual space and disoriented on the map or unable to sort out the gestalt of a picture assembly test

Table V. Tabulation of specific developmental disorders frequently associated with general developmental delay

Definition	Localization	Testing
Constructive apraxia		
The inability to perform purposeful movements or movement sequences in assembling objects or movement patterns representing a symbolical meaning, without impairment or ataxia of the locomotor system	the transitional parieto-temporo-occipital areas of either hemisphere; caused mostly by cortical lesions of the dominant hemisphere and subcortical lesions of the nondominant hemisphere	manikin assembly; block design; picture arranging; form board with open eyes and with closed eyes; draw a person; copy the picture of a stick figure; draw a map; building blocks, towers, bridges; assemble words and numbers from block letters and block numbers; puzzles, stick-figure making; purposeful practical movement series: folding and placing a letter in an envelope, hammering a nail; use of the telephone; opening and closing doors; switching on and off of the light; symbolical gestures, (as if) movements: waving good-bye, clapping hands, drinking from a cup, combing one's hair, pulling a rope, grinding coffee

In the case samples cited in this chapter, the higher psychological functions are assessed based on the medical model of evaluation. The medical model of neuropsychological evaluation is not culture bound [*Mercer and Ysseldyke*, 1977]. *Ross* [1968] criticizes the medical diagnostic model, quoting *Reitan* [1962] about the label of 'brain damage' as not being a meaningful entity. *Ross* is perfectly correct in pointing out the lack of meaning of a diagnosis of 'brain damage' which is not further qualified. Such diagnosis, however, becomes meaningful, both in a retarded and in a nonretarded person, if the localization can be substantiated by further diagnostic procedures. The perceptual disturbances and eye-hand coordination deficits will require different rehabilitation methods, depending on the cortical localization of the underlaying brain dysfunction. A rather pessimistic attitude is evident when *Ross* states, by paraphrasing *Gallagher's* [1957] opinion, that an educator gains far more information from the fact that a child is perceptually disturbed than from the fact that he is brain injured. Of course, *Ross's* pessimism is not justified any more in the light of the tremendous advances in the new technology of evoked potential studies which can provide refined information on the dynamic patterns of the cortical processing of mental operations [*Gevins* et al., 1981] and in the light of other refined neurophysiological methods [*Denes and Caviezel*, 1981; *Rossi, and Rossadina*, 1967; *Sipress-Goodwin* et al., 1981]. These latter methods are not yet in common clinical practice. Nonetheless, cortical localization of different brain dysfunctions can be achieved even presently with less sophisticated neuropsychological testing. This knowledge should be used in the planning of the remediation.

Diagnostic guidelines for the recognition of cortical function deficits in retardates are listed below.

Aphasias. The inability to produce speech (expressive, motor aphasia), and the inability to understand speech (receptive, sensory aphasia) are frequent complications of mental retardation. For the definition, localization and testing of aphasias see table I and figure 5.

Recent research in aphasia focuses on the role of the right hemisphere in motor aphasia [*Assal* et al., 1981; *Denes and Caviezel*, 1981]. A more refined localization of motor aphasia within the third frontal gyrus and the Rolandic operculum is attempted by *Tonkonogy and Goodglass* [1981].

Amnestic aphasia may be caused in adult retardates by degenerative diseases. It is known that Alzheimer's disease is more frequent and is manifested at relatively younger ages in Down syndrome patients than in the general population. [*Crapper* et al., 1975; *Dalton* et al., 1974; *Ellis* et al., 1974; *Heston and Mastri,* 1977; *Malamud,* 1957; *Olson and Shaw,* 1969]. The difference between the remote memory patterns in amnesic and in demented patients has been documented also [*Albert* et al., 1981].

Case sample: Differential diagnosis of expressive aphasia, mental retardation, and severe behavioral disturbance:

Case 3. Peter is a 10-year-old Caucasian boy who has a younger retarded brother. Peter was admitted to the John Merck Program in 1975 for treatment of the following symptoms: almost continuous screaming in extremely shrill, high-pitched voice; negativism; self-abuse and aggression have also been noted when the child felt frustrated. Past history includes: metatarsus varus; feeding problems with poor sucking; and an inguinal hernia, operated in infancy. Previous to his admission to the John Merck Program, many individuals who dealt with Peter believed him to be severely retarded, primarily because of his apparent lack of communication ability. On previous testing before admission, at the age of 9.5, Peter obtained an MA of 1:9 (IQ 25) on the Bayley scales of infant development. At admission, the clinical neurological evaluation revealed several minor anomalies: metatarsus varus; height in the 20th percentile; weight in the 25th percentile; Peter's teeth were discolored and ground down by bruxism. He had no gag reflex. Muscle hypotonia and hyperreflexia were also found. Psychiatric evaluation showed withdrawal, anxiety, negativism with intolerable screaming, apparently not influenced by any environmental measure. At admission he obtained an MA of 2:3 on the Peabody picture vocabulary test. At that time, the psychologist noted that Peter took little notice of test demands, made little eye contact, and tantrumed in the face of difficult tasks. Similarly, the testing in February 1976 produced extremely anxious reactions in Peter, and he hurled the testing equipment across the room. On repeated testing, the psychological profile revealed failure on the subtests requiring a verbal answer and those requiring fine motor coordination. However, because of noncompliance and continuous screaming it was difficult to assess his level of comprehension and his performance IQ. A dramatic turning point in the differential diagnosis came about when he wrote spontaneously a word on the blackboard, as an answer to the teacher's question (addressed to another child) about the name of a TV cartoon character.

We realized at that point that Peter suffered from expressive (Broca) aphasia with essentially intact internal speech and adequate receptive language. *His screaming and most other symptoms developed secondary to the frustration of being unable to communicate.* It is indeed not rare among aphasic children to become psychotic, or at least severely emotionally disturbed [*Agranowitz and McKeown,* 1964; *Jakab,* 1972]. Peter's potential level of functioning assessed later on the Binet L-M, administered in a nonstandardized way through written instruction, indicated strengths in the areas of conceptualization at the 3- to 4-year level (comparison of sizes, integrating split forms) and abstract representation (copying a circle and vertical line), both of which involve a visual component. His strengths continued to be primarily conceptual, as he could express a considerable range of needs through writing, and could understand much that was communicated to him.

Tests administered at discharge: Arthur adaptation of the Leiter international scale for children; Stanford-Binet L-M; Vineland social maturity scale; CA: 12:3. Test results: Leiter scale: MA = 4:10; IQ = 45 (moderate range of retardation); basal = 3.0; ceiling = 5.0;

Binet L-M: MA = 3–4 years (estimate through nonstandardized administration); Vineland social age equivalent = 6:0.

Strengths were noted in the areas of visual conceptual and representational skills, whereas weaknesses were found in the expressive language and fine motor areas. Peter's ability to control his anxiety has significantly improved, increasing his test performance (and documented IQ) to its present stable level.

In Peter's case, assuming the presence of intact subcortical pathways between the Broca area of internal speech and the reading-writing center of the parietal lobe, intensive educational efforts were instituted in order to teach him to communicate through reading and writing. Many times one could witness Peter suddenly calming down in the middle of a temper tantrum when his teacher produced a written clarification related to the apparently frustrating situation. Peter achieved second-grade-level reading. Naturally, this was not the only treatment method in dealing with Peter's complex symptomatology. Multimodality treatment brought about substantial improvement. After a short unsuccessful trial on Ritalin and on tranquilizers, no medication was prescribed. A specially designed behavioral program has successfully decreased the screaming behavior (this aspect of Peter's treatment is presented in fig. 7). Of course, the long-standing severe emotional disturbance of this retarded and aphasic youngster did not have a favorable prognosis in spite of the intensive therapeutic interventions. Peter was discharged in a nonpsychotic state to a residential facility for further total communication training and special education. As compared to his earlier IQ of 25, Peter's discharge psychological evaluation showed a substantially increased IQ of 45 (9/20/77) at a chronological age of 12.3.

The so-called critical age for learning to communicate has been missed, unfortunately, by not detecting and remedying Peter's aphasia before he was admitted to the John Merck Program at 9½ years of age.

The method of rehabilitation by substituting written communication for the missing expressive verbal communication is possible only in those patients with congenital aphasia whose intellectual developmental level reached a mental age of 6–7 years, this being the required developmental level of maturity for understanding abstract symbols (individual letters) and composite gestalts (words).

Based on this case (and on similar cases from the author's practice), it is strongly recommended to attempt teaching reading and writing to nonverbal retarded children whose mental age is at least on the 6- to 7-year level. Through correct differential diagnosis and therapeutic trial, the practitioner may save a retarded aphasic youngster from a lifelong frustration due to the inability to communicate.

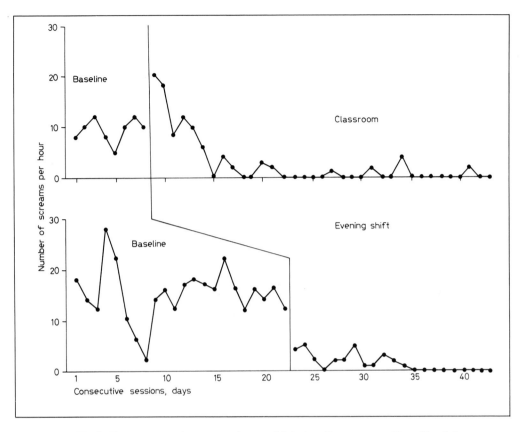

Fig. 7. Program to reduce screaming, multiple baseline across settings (the John Merck Program, staff psychologist *E. Shapiro,* PhD). Case 3: Peter, aphasic child, severely retarded at admission. Program consisted of getting close to the child face to face and looking at him sternly until the screaming stopped.

Case sample: In the following case the differential diagnosis of retardation due to sociocultural deprivation versus aphasia and early infantile autism was based on the absence of specific neurological or neuropsychological signs of organic brain damage and on proof of social cultural deprivation.

Case 4. Lila, a 9-year-old, severely retarded black girl was admitted to the John Merck Program because of extremely withdrawn, anxious behavior and language disorder.
    History: Uneventful neonatal history. She was toilet trained. She was reared in a household with her mother, who suffered from schizophrenia and was frequently hospital-

ized. When at home, the mother lived 'upstairs', while the grandmother who lived 'down-stairs' shared her room with Lila. The family was on welfare. The grandmother watched TV from the earliest morning show to the latest night show and Lila stayed up until the end of the last show, long past midnight. There was practically no conversation between her and her grandmother. Lila started repeating TV ads in a singsong voice. She missed school most of the time, and when in class, the teacher found her 'unreachable'. Her intellectual level was estimated at IQ 25.

Present status: This child repeated the words of long TV commercials endlessly (delayed echolalia), but did not use verbal or gestural language to communicate. Lila showed a high level of stranger anxiety. She was restless, negativistic and did not tolerate classroom setting. Lila often fell asleep during daytime.

Differential diagnosis: Developmental delay secondary to organic brain damage was ruled out by history and by neurological examination and EEG. Sociocultural deprivation was confirmed by history and home visit. In the differential diagnostic evaluation, the echolalia was considered as a 'positive proof of language readiness', instead of a sign of brain damage. Essentially, this child's only language source was the television. The items most frequently heard (the commercials) have formed her bank of accumulated auditory verbal memory.

Treatment consisted of integrating Lila as an inpatient into small group recreational activities and language therapy progressing from total communication (gestures and words) to vocal language. Lila's high level of stranger anxiety has subsided. She was able, before her discharge, to participate in group activities, also outside of her classroom. For example, she was choosen to perform in the children's Christmas pageant and she even enjoyed a brief solo dance in front of a large audience of parents and staff.

Lila was discharged in an improved state to a foster home. As she became 'socialized' and learned communicative verbal language (as opposed to the former delayed echolalia), Lila also showed accelerated intellectual growth with a measured IQ of 68 at discharge as compared to her admission IQ of 25.

Alexia and Agraphia in Mental Retardation. For definition, localization and testing, see table II and figure 5.

At the early stages of learning how to read and write, normal young children frequently have difficulties in sounding out certain letters within words, or using them appropriately when attempting to write. The most common errors are reversals in directionality in the perception (reading) and/or in the production (writing) of the following letters: right-left reversals: b - d and p - g; up-down reservsals: b - p and d - g. In more extensive directionality confusion all four of these letters will be interchanged at random. Up-down reversal is also frequent with the letters W, M and u, n.

These errors will be overcome quickly by nonretarded children, as they learn reading. Developmentally delayed children may continue to make the same directionality mistakes for a longer time.

In parietal lobe lesions the alexia and agraphia will be persistent, both in otherwise normal children and in retarded children, while they advance in other educational tasks according to their maturational level.

The most efficient remediation of directionality errors is achieved by practicing to read and write each variation repeating these letters in pairs by emphasizing the differences in the position of their long stem. Examples: right-left pairs: d - b and g - p. Up-down pairs: d - g and b - p.

This is far more efficient than having the child write each letter separately 'a hundred times'.

Agraphia without alexia may be caused by constructive apraxia as part of a global inability to conceive and to write symbols, including letters in their planned sequences according to the mental schema required for writing meaningful words. These patients are equally unable to assemble a written word like 'TABLE' by using block letters. Even if the elements (block letters) are provided, this requires the cognitive analysis of the written word and resynthesis of the elements (block letters) in the proper spacial sequence.

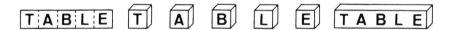

To reproduce the same word in a vertical direction, using the block letters, requires an additional mental operation of sequencing. The 'bottom letter' must be placed first. Otherwise, due to the force of gravity the other letters would not stay suspended in mid-air while the subject is trying to assemble randomly this gestalt.

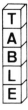

Case sample: Differential diagnosis of congenital alexia and agraphia versus developmental delay and attention deficit disorder with hyperactivity:

Case 5. Bobby is a 9-year-old child functioning on the 5.9-year mental age level. He had no signs of organicity. His mother is mildly retarded, his father is albino and quite paranoid, one of his brothers is not retarded, another younger brother is albino, blind and retarded. No other genetic anomaly was detected. The home environment was chaotic. Bobby was admitted to the John Merck Program in 1975 for oppositional behavior, anxiety states and hyperactivity. Educational testing revealed that he could identify individual letters and could also recognize individual words which he previously learned to identify – 'like a picture' (gestalt reading), such as his name and the names of other children in his classroom. Nonetheless, he was unable to recognize, read (sound out) and understand the meaning of new words. The gestalt composed of a specific sequence of letters (a word) had no meaning for him, unless it was related to the rote memory of that gestalt. The concept of letters as symbols, to be used in different combinations to become words with specific meanings is acquired at a mental age above 6 years. Thus, Bobby, whose mental age was below 6, was unable to read new words by decoding the specific constellation of letters in a given word. His learning was also hindered by attention-deficit disorder.

Bobby's attention improved with Ritalin treatment (20 mg/day). The most successful method of teaching him to 'read' was by the gestalt method of providing him with a site vocabulary by accumulating a data bank of paired picture-word items, where he later could identify the words as a gestalt even without the picture.

Bobby had no specific localized cortical deficit. His reading problem was caused by generalized developmental delay in abstract concept formation and symbol-understanding.

Alexia and agraphia may be only part of the symptoms in more extensive parietal lobe damage. A frequent combination of cortical-function deficits is the simultaneous presence of acalculia, finger agnosia, right-left discrimination deficit (Gerstmann syndrome). The localizational value of the Gerstmann syndrome is questioned by *Heimburger* et al. [1964]. In determining whether or not the reading-writing deficit is part of a more extensive parietal lobe lesion the differential diagnosis will rest on additional neuropsychological testing for finger agnosia and acalculia. A normal 6-year-old child does not have finger agnosia, or right-left discrimination deficits related to his/her own body axis. Similarly, a 9-year-old retarded child, whose general developmental delay is around 6 years of MA, will be able to perform well on right-left directionality tests. Also, retarded children, once they have learned the names of each of their fingers, should not fail the finger agnosia test. When the examiner points to a finger, without touching it, they should be able to name it. The finger agnosia test is a visual test not aided by touching the finger, or by allowing the subject to move the finger to which the examiner is pointing.

Retarded children with a parietal lobe lesion will confuse the names of their fingers in this visual-gnostic test, even after repeated attempts. They may be able to name each finger correctly if the finger in question is touched, or if they are allowed to move it, i.e., when another channel of tactile or proprioceptive information is added to the visual perception.

In some cases, alexia may be a consequence of more generalized space agnosia (asymbolia) due to lesions in the cortex of the parieto-occipital transitional areas and of the angular gyrus of the dominant hemisphere, or to the lesions of the subcortical white matter of the same areas in the non-dominant hemisphere. In the left-handed persons the cerebral lateralization of functions may be less predictable. Observations of left-handed writing posture may predict cerebral language laterality according to *Volpe* et al. [1981].

Case sample: Differential diagnosis of a case of alexia and agraphia caused by space agnosia and constructive apraxia, versus global mental retardation:

Case 6. Ronald was a 10-year-old, retarded emotionally disturbed Caucasian boy, functioning at a mental age of 7 years and on several subtests of the Stanford-Binet L-M test over 7 years. He was unable to learn reading or writing by conventional educational methods. He was enrolled in 1973 in the diagnostic classroom of the Community Evaluation and Rehabilitation Center (CERC) in Waltham, Mass. (Director: *R. Flynn,* MD). An example of Ronald's reading difficulty is the following. The written word FATHER was learned, recognized and 'read' correctly by Ronald. However, if the same word was spelled FA*HT*ER, where one letter is transposed, it was perceived as an 'unknown word' by Ronald. His global retardation was complicated by alexia due to space agnosia. Without these specific developmental disabilities, Ronald (whose intellectual level was above the concrete thinking phase) should have been able to 'read' the word spelled FAHTER and recognize that it has a spelling error, or even read it by mentally correcting the spelling error without becoming conscious of its presence. This mechanism is responsible for reading past typographical errors, many times without noticing them.

Ronald learned to write when the teacher first provided him with little squares for each letter of a word (fig. 8). Past this phase, Ronald learned to write into spaces separated by vertical lines to indicate the end of each word and the beginning of the next one. Finally, he learned to write between the lines of his writing pad. Ronald's reading was more successful when he was allowed to cover up the lines above and below the line he was reading. This helped him to focus his attention to a small space.

Alexia and agraphia may be caused by suppression of the differences of gestalts with a predominant similarity of one of their elements. This phenomenon of mental suppression of the differences among gestalts with a predominant similarity of one of their components was described in congenital agraphia and alexia by *Ranschburgh* as early as in 1927. This disorder may lead to perceptual deficiencies similar to those seen in parietal lobe lesions or in space agnosia, and constructive apraxia.

In these cases, besides impaired directionality concept, the details within a single gestalt (a letter) are not perceived as distinct elements of that gestalt. For example, the letters b - d, p - g are essentially *composed of a circular detail 'o' and a vertical line attached to it in different locations:* either on the right or on the left of the circular detail, and extending either upwards or downwards. This is especially confusing when these letters are part of a word surrounded by other letters. The mental suppression of the linear details of letters may be caused by the predominant similarity of their circular component which is in itself a 'gestalt' (a circle).

Suppression of the differences applies also to certain printed capital letters. For example, the letters P, R, B, D are often confused, because the basic D-like shape as the common element monopolizes the attention of the reader to the detriment of the 'insignificant' linear details which determine the differences of those letters. If one covers the bottom half of these letters, it becomes more evident that the remaining visible top half is not sufficient anymore to distinguish them from each other:

P R B D

The remedial efforts should emphasize the differences between these letters and the basic D shape, by using comparative pairing:

D - - - P, D - - - R, D - - - B, P - - - R

Acalculia. The inability to acquire number concepts and to perform simple mathematical operations in mental calculations or by working on paper with pencil indicates parietal lobe lesion, if the general developmental age is above the MA of 7 years (table III, fig. 5).

In developmental delay, the concrete level of thinking will interfere with reading and writing (using letters as symbols in specific groupings to form words with meaning), as well as with the correct reading and writing of

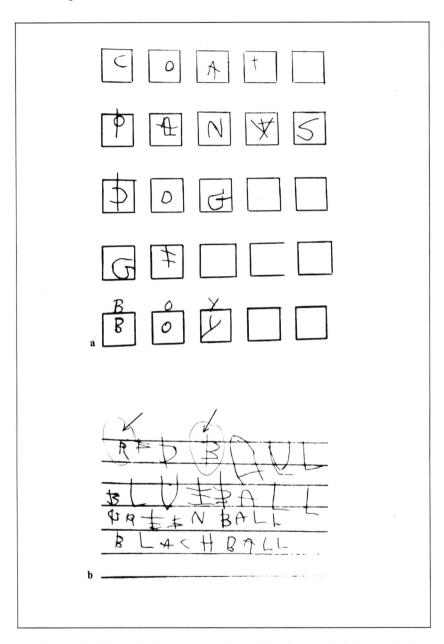

Fig. 8. Ronald. **a** Constructive apraxia-agraphia. Space orientation assisted by squares for individual letters (first stage of training). **b** Confusion of the letters R and B. Practice to write between lines as the second stage of training.

multi-digit numbers, although one-to-one correspondence and the concept of 'more' and 'less' may already be acquired.

By scrutinizing the mental operations required to read a multi-digit number we become aware of the technical differences from reading a word composed of several letters. *It is more complex to read a multi-digit number, than a word composed of an equal number of letters.*

When reading a word, in our culture, the scanning proceeds from left to right, in sounding out the word. One can read (sound out) the first half of a word on one page and the second half on the next page, without seeing the total gestalt at once like FA-THER. Furthermore, when seeing the total word as a gestalt, it makes sense even with minor 'spelling errors' (i.e., FA*HT*ER). It is 'readable' in spite of the transposition of the two middle letters.

Let us now consider a multi-digit number of only four digits: 3976. We must see and 'grasp' the whole picture of this gestalt before we can read it correctly as 'three thousand, nine hundred and seventy-six'. Why? Because unless we proceed first from right to left we cannot realize that in this constellation the six is six, but the seven which is at the left of the six, is actually (stands for) seventy, the nine is nine hundred and the three is really three thousand. This process is different from reading words where the letters do not have a relative 'position value' within the gestalt. This position value is implied in the relative distance of each digit toward the left from the last digit on the right (first, second, third place to the left of the last digit etc.).

The mental operation of reading multi-digit numbers requires more mental steps than reading a word. First step: scanning from right to left:

$$\overset{\leftarrow}{3} \quad \overset{\leftarrow}{9} \quad \overset{\leftarrow}{7} \quad \overset{\leftarrow}{6}$$

Second step: assigning position values to each digit:

3000	900	70	6
3	**9**	**7**	**6**

Third step: reading from left to right the whole number by keeping in mind the position value of each digit:

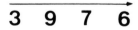

3   9   7   6

The readers can test themselves by attempting to read the following number: 4968000000000000000. You will indeed find yourself counting zeroes from right to left, before you even attempt to sound out the first four digits, although you recognize each digit separately.

In reading multi-digit numbers there is no way of having a data bank of gestalts (like a series of words) in memory, which can be recognized in spite of minor spelling errors. (FA*HT*ER can be correctly recognized as *the misspelled word FATHER*.)

Let us now consider these two numbers: 3976 (three thousand, nine hundred and seventy-six) and 3796; *3796 is not the same number as '3976' misspelled;* 3796 (three thousand, seven hundred and ninety-six) is a different number. The transposition of the two middle digits resulted in a 'new' number because of the new position value of each digit.

When operating with multi-digit numbers, each number must be decoded fully including both the right-left direction of decoding for position value and the left-right direction of reading it out.

Retardates with delayed right-left discrimination ability do not have the mental flexibility to perform these steps necessary for reading multi-digit numbers.

How do different cortical localizations produce the same end result of difficulties in recognizing numbers and of using them in various 'simple' operations?

Acalculia in parietal lobe deficit refers mostly to lack of number concept (e.g., five is more than four, and less than six) and the inability to perform operations with numbers (adding, subtracting, etc.).

In spacial agnosia the position value cannot be grasped. In the right-left discrimination disorder the above-described use of built-in directionality in the decoding is missing. In constructive apraxia the mental schema of sequencing the steps of writing multi-digit numbers is missing.

Each of these identifiable deficits may occur in retarded persons and they each require a different remedial technique. The more closely the cortical localization can be identified the more precise the remedial prescription can be.

Spacial Agnosia and Constructive Apraxia. For diagnosis, localization and testing, see tables IV and V and figure 5. *Spacial agnosia and constructive apraxia are probably the most frequently overlooked special developmental disabilities in mental retardation.* Usually, they are lumped together under the global labels of 'perceptual deficit' and 'eye-hand coordination disorder'.

Perceptual disturbance caused by spacial agnosia may be restricted to visual perception, or it may apply also to the disturbances of the tactile gestalt perception [*Jakab,* 1960] in cortical lesions of the angular gyrus and its surrounding region of the dominant hemisphere (fig. 5) or in subcortical lesions of the same areas in the nondominant hemisphere [*Hecaen and Angelergues,* 1963].

The intellectual qualitative growth from concrete thinking to abstract concept formation lies on the basis of organized space perception and constructive praxis. Retardates whose mental age remained permanently lower than 6 years never reach the developmental level of full orientation in the abstract visual space and they will miss the mental planning necessary for the sequences of complex manual tasks. In these cases the global retardation is responsible for the symptoms of space agnosia and constructive apraxia. In cases with the mental age over 7 years, the perceptual deficits and eye-hand coordination disorders should be further investigated for localization.

Differential diagnosis of space agnosia and constructive apraxia versus the perceptual disturbance and the eye-hand coordination disturbance caused by developmental delay. The developmentally delayed child has the ability to 'learn' to recognize a pattern by rote memory in a few trials and keep it in mind for immediate recall. In spacial agnosia, even though the details of a pattern are pointed out to the child, this knowledge is 'immediately lost' and not available for recall when the pattern is shown again. In constructive apraxia, similarly, this very 'learning' by simple repetition does not take place. The patient does not have the ability to acquire a mental schema required to complete the necessary steps of visual-manual tasks in order to arrive at the desired end product. Examples of such tasks are the items of the block design (WISC) where the subject is expected to copy a two-dimensional model with three-dimensional blocks.

The following steps are implied in solving the checkerboard design of red and white squares:

Step 1. Mentally analyzing the model into its elements:

Step 2. Identifying the surfaces of appropriate colors on the blocks (two red, and two white):

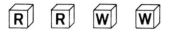

Step 3. Resynthesizing the gestalt with the blocks in the same pattern as the model so that the gestalt on the 'top' of the blocks would lie in the same orientation as the elements of the two-dimensional picture:

In step 3, the time sequence, in which the blocks are placed beside each other, is irrelevant. As long as the final pattern is correct, the subject can start with any of the four blocks and then place the others next to it.

In cases of global developmental delay with MA under 6 years the transfer of 'meaning' from the two-dimensional model to the three-dimensional blocks is not reached. Therefore, even if the examiner is drawing dividing lines into the two-dimensional model, the retarded child will not be able to proceed to step 2. In further assessing this case, the examiner should provide a three-dimensional model and thus, actually eliminate the need to mentally transfer the two-dimensional image into a three-dimensional concept. Now the child should be able to proceed to step 2 and step 3, unless he suffers from constructive apraxia.

On a lower level of developmental delay, even the three-dimensional model must be further 'analyzed' into its components by the examiner, i.e., distances between the pieces must indicate the boundaries of each element before they can be matched one-to-one with the blocks in step 2 and resynthesized by the child in step 3 (pushed together).

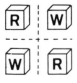

In this case the concrete level of thinking interferes with the performance without any specific cortical function deficit.

Remediation in these latter cases should follow maturational guidelines, instead of using techniques appropriate for perceptual disorders caused by localized cortical deficits.

In specific developmental disabilities (agnosia, constructive apraxia), any step of the required sequence for achieving the end product may be missing. The missing sequence can be identified and this will provide relevant information about the underlying cortical function deficit.

The three steps implied in solving a more advanced level of design are the following:

Step 1. The analysis of the gestalt is the ability to point out the different elements on the model picture. While in the checkerboard pattern the cross-dividing lines in the pattern were visually self-evident, this is not the case in the following pattern:

Here the subject must divide mentally this undivided picture.

Only after this mental analysis can the next step follow.

In space agnosia, step 1 is impaired. If the examiner draws the dividing lines, then the patient can complete the next step.

Step 2. Identifying the appropriate surfaces on the blocks to be used on a one-to-one correspondence with the elements of the model.

Step 3. Synthesis. Assembling the four blocks to form a pattern identical to the model picture:

This step requires again orientation in visual space perception and will be failed in space gnosia. A developmentally delayed child, Bobby (case 5), was unable to transfer the two-dimensional visual information onto the three-dimensional model. Even after being provided with four cubes in step 2, Bobby could not produce the correct pattern. He gave the following variations when tested:

  and

He was unable to 'see' the difference between his products and the model.

Remedial techniques consist in drawing dividing lines into composite pictures and teaching the patient to be alert to the need to mentally divide the gestalt, and to attempt to do so as a first step, instead of using only the trial and error method, while jumping step 1 and missing to provide a frame of reference in step 3.

By drawing an outline (like the board of a puzzle) which encloses the resynthesized pattern, step 3 can be achieved by patients with spacial agnosia. The examiner can teach them to work at first within the boundaries of a frame. This method helped Ronald (case 6) to learn how to write words, by providing him with individual squares for each letter before he reached the level of writing the letters between parallel lines (fig. 8).

In constructive apraxia the analysis of the gestalt (step 1) and the identification of similar three-dimensional elements is present (step 2) but the resynthesis (step 3) is missing. The individual pieces will be scattered in space at random in any direction, even with repeated attempts. For example, step 3 (resynthesis of the gestalt) of the above pattern as attempted by Ronald (case 6) resulted in these products:

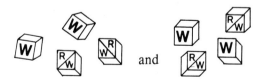 and

The proper remedial technique in constructive apraxia should emphasize the process of 'putting together'.

In cases of combined spacial agnosia and constructive apraxia, the remedial technique will have to be extended to all three steps of any construction.

In constructive apraxia, the final product will not resemble the model, it will be distorted in space even if the elements are present. Patients with constructive apraxia are unable to use a mental schema of sequences when solving a visual-manual task (puzzles, block design, three-dimensional building, folding paper and placing it in an envelope, copying geometrical shapes and figures, etc.) without having any actual deficits in recognizing the individual components on a model picture. This type of 'eye-hand coordination deficit', constructive apraxia, is caused by lesions of the parieto-occipito-temporal transitional areas (fig. 5). Copying is impaired in bilateral lesions. Apraxia and agraphia of the same hand may be selectively impaired in corpus callosum lesion [Gersh and Damasio, 1981].

The differential diagnostic considerations related to the localization of special developmental disabilities described above can help in designing treatment and educational methods.

Etiological Differential Diagnosis

The major etiological factors causing mental retardation are the following: (1) sociocultural deprivation (about 70% of all cases), which causes mostly mild to moderate retardation; (2) severe psychiatric disorders of childhood, may cause secondary mental retardation of different degree; (3) organic brain damage (about 20% of all cases), responsible for most cases of severe and profound levels of retardation.

The differential diagnostic discussion will be supported by case samples illustrating the strategies of treatment prescriptions, based on the etiological substratum of the retardation.

(1) Sociocultural Deprivation

Lack of appropriate environmental stimuli at an early age may hinder the development of the intelligence. Lack of parental interaction and verbal stimulation necessary for language development results in further intellectual handicap.

The etiology of Lila's (case 4, p. 95) severe mental retardation, withdrawal and language delay was related to the sociocultural deprivation during her formative years. Aphasia has been ruled out in the differential diagnostic procedure. Lila's rapid social improvement and verbal language acquisition during residential treatment have attested further to the correctness of the etiological diagnosis.

(2) Psychiatric Disorders

The etiological diagnosis of psychiatric disorders associated with retardation is covered in the section on psychiatric disorders (this book).

(3) Organic Brain Damage

An understanding of the neurodevelopmental phases and of the psychosocial and emotional maturational process is needed in the etiological differential diagnosis of mental retardation. For children special methods must be used to determine whether the low intelligence level is the result of arrest at a given level of maturation or the result of a constellation of multiple cortical-function deficits, while maturation in other areas is progressing. The prognosis of these cases is different, and they require different therapeutic interventions.

The etiological differential diagnosis helps in predicting the potential capacities of the developmentally delayed person. In the prognosis of mental retardation caused by brain damage it is important to differentiate progressive diseases from static consequences of early brain damage.

Genetic Metabolic Diseases

These diseases may be manifested already at birth, like Down's syndrome or phenylketonuria. Other central nervous system diseases may become evident clinically after a brief period of normal development in infancy, like the Tay-Sachs disease. In degenerative diseases the dementia is often revealed by a sequence of cortical deficits as each disease progresses. Aphasia is the most frequent early sign. The organic disorders may also be complicated by psychiatric symptoms during the clinical course, like in the case of acute optic hallucinosis described [*Villiez* et al., 1981] in a patient with Spielmeyer-Vogt disease. Psychosis in mongoloid patients is rare [*Cytrin and Lourie* 1967]. *Kety* [1978] discusses some single gene defects leading to retardation and psychosis.

Case sample: San Fillippo's disease with excessive aggression and self-abuse:

Case 7. Janet was referred for uncontrollable aggression and hyperactivity at the age of 7½ years to the John Merck Program. She was also self-abusing and became almost deaf in the last few months before admission. Neurological diagnosis of San Fillippo's disease has been established. The mother has reported that Janet was a well-behaved, pleasant child with slow motor developmental milestones. She spoke 3–4 words at the age of 3 years. Then at the age of 7 she became unmanageable at home and in school. By the age of 7½ in-patient admission was necessary to prevent self-injury and injury to others by Janet's indiscriminate aggression and abrupt episodes of self-abuse. During this acutely aggressive phase her symptoms were relieved by tranquilizers. The aggressive phase lasted for about 6 months only. Janet slowly became more passive and ultimately regressed to a level of total care. It was assumed that the progressive degenerative changes in the frontal lobes, the thalamic and hypothalamic areas contributed to the transitional behavioral symptoms during the progression of the dementing process.

Case sample: Trisomy 21 (Down's syndrome) with psychotic depression and basal ganglia calcification:

Case 8. Maria is a girl of Asian descent with Down's syndrome. At 19 years of age, she was referred to the John Merck Program because of psychotic depression with hallucinations of 1-year duration, extreme anxiety and regression to a symbiotic state with her mother. The differential diagnosis following a detailed developmental and family history revealed that the onset of depressive psychosis was related to the changes in the family constellation and caused by the departure from the family home of the patient's two sisters who started college overseas. The brainstem calcification (confirmed on CAT scan) and the Down's syndrome (trisomy 21) itself were considered as increasing the vulnerability of this youngster to psychological trauma. Intensive short-term psychiatric inpatient treatment aided by medication (Mellaril 50 mg, three times a day) and psychotherapy as well as family counseling produced lasting remission [*Jakab,* 1978]. At a 3-year follow-up she is still symptom free.

The reader should be alert to the danger of therapeutic nihilism due to insufficient differential diagnosis by disregarding the importance of environmental stress in similar cases of genetic disease with additional organic brain involvement.

Well-diagnosed reactive psychosis is treatable even in patients with unchangeable organic conditions.

Mental Retardation due to Prematurity, Perinatal Anoxia,
or Brain Injury

The most critical time for physical injury, or anoxia, is the perinatal period [*Jakab,* 1965]. Histologically proven, severe damages caused by anoxia due to status epilepticus in infancy are described by *Környey* [1955].

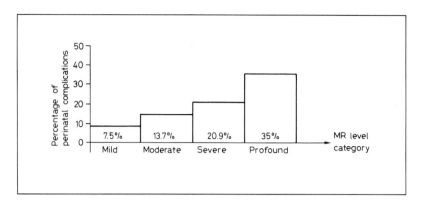

Fig. 9. Percentage of perinatal complications, total of 428 cases aged 2–14 years. Highest incidence (35 %) of perinatal complications were found in the category of profound retardates. From *Jakab* [1959].

He differentiates the acute symptoms of anoxia: unconsciousness, decorticated state, cortical excitatory signs, seizures, reflex and extrapyramidal disorders, from psychiatric disorders seen in the restitutional phase. An unusual case of lateralized EEG focal-motor abnormality in the acute comatous stage of carbon monoxide poisoning was reported by *Neufeld* et al. [1981]. *Schachter* [1950] in a comparative study of 199 anoxic infants and 100 normal deliveries found that anoxia was responsible for mental retardation. In a later study *Schachter* [1954] demonstrated that anoxia at delivery had more severe consequences than mechanical trauma by forceps. *Jakab* [1959] in a sample of 428 consecutive cases found a correlation between the severity of mental retardation and the perinatal complications including anoxia in children, without clinical neurological symptoms of brain damage (fig. 9). In another study [*Jakab,* 1965], the most frequent perinatal condition in the history of the mildly and moderately retarded children was prolonged delivery, over 24 h, with asphyxia (blue baby). High forceps, prematurity and neonatal apnea were found more frequently in the history of severely and profoundly retarded children. In cases of retardation without gross clinical neurological symptoms the history of perinatal complications would indicate the likelihood of early organic brain damage [*Brander,* 1955; *Enke,* 1955; *Tardieu,* 1954; *Tramer,* 1955]. Maternal eclampsia is considered to be a risk factor for the fetus by *Gavallér* et al. [1958].

Case sample: Retardation caused by anoxia complicated by symbiotic psychosis:

Case 9. Doris, a 5-year-old profoundly retarded white girl was evaluated at the John Merck Program in 1980. She was born with the umbilical cord around her neck, consequently, left hemiparesis developed. She was treated for 2½ years by 'patterning'. The mother felt very guilty 'for torturing her with the exercises' and cried with the baby while doing as many as 1,500 passive movements a day. The hemiplegia improved. By the age of 3 years, she was ambulatory and spoke in short sentences. Doris had an apneic seizure (went blue) at the age of 3½ years. At that time a corneal ulcer developed for which an eye patch was applied. Doris was carried around in her mother's arms for several months during all her waking hours 'to prevent pulling-off the patch'. From that time on Doris refused to walk or stand, withdrew, lost her speech and became 'zombie-like' not reacting to environmental stimuli. Presenting symptoms at admission: autistic-like withdrawal, negativism, stereotype hand play and self-abuse leading to ulceration of the left ankle from hitting it with her heel. Doris is a nonambulatory child with generalized hypotonia, positive Babinski on the left, and deep tendon reflexes 2+ on both lower extremities. EEG (11-20-80) was diffusely abnormal with multifocal paroxysmal outbursts. CAT scan was essentially normal, thus major structural abnormalities have not backed up her severely regressed state. She gave no eye contact and was negativistic (releasing objects placed into her hand, pushing away people and objects). She was able to stand for a few seconds, then went limp. The mother still carries this heavy child around in her arms. The etiology of the corneal ulcer is unknown. Herpes virus was suspected, thus, the possibility of undetected herpes meningoencephalitis should be considered. Severe anoxia during the apneic seizure of about 3-min duration may have increased the brain damage already sustained at delivery with the cord around her neck.

The differential diagnosis revealed: (1) mental retardation due to anoxia and possibly further aggravated by viral infection of the central nervous system; (2) symbiotic psychosis with autistic-like regressive features, secondary to the psychological experience of being carried around for 6 months by the mother at the age of 3½ years. Both the results of the organic brain damage and the psychosis had to be addressed by the treatment prescription. Brief therapeutic trial in a therapeutic education class and physical therapy have increased Doris's social awareness and signs of emerging independent unassisted sitting skills were observed. Her parents were included in the individually designed and performed therapeutic interventions.

Mental Retardation Caused by Encephalitis

Case sample: Herpes encephalitis complicated by anoxia due to cardiorespiratory arrest (caused by intravenous Valium injection to interrupt epileptic seizures). Mental retardation, unspecified psychosis and temporal lobe epilepsy were the long-term consequences of the illness:

Case 10. Chad, a retarded, 4-year-old Caucasian child was admitted to the John Merck Program in 1975 for uncontrollable aggression and panic attacks. Delivery was uneventful. (The film 'Chad, Who Has Far to Go', producer Gabor Nagy, 1979, presents Chad's illness and his rehabilitation and treatment.) Motor milestones and speech development were normal up to the age of 3½ years when he developed herpes encephalitis, which started by status epilepticus. The case was complicated by cardiorespiratory arrest caused by intravenous Valium administration, to control the seizures, which lead to a 21-day coma and was followed by a decorticated state (could not see, hear, speak or walk). Chad recuperated slowly, his verbal speech returned, he became ambulatory and toilet trained again. Shortly thereafter, he developed epileptic seizures again and became extremely aggressive to parents and siblings. He was destructive to objects and also hyperactive. These symptoms made inpatient admission necessary.

Differential diagnosis has established the following conditions. (1) By history: mental retardation due to herpes encephalitis aggravated by cerebral anoxia due to cardiovascular arrest. Technically, this was a case of dementia, since intellectual development was normal before the encephalitis. (2) EEG revealed temporal lobe epilepsy. (3) CAT scan showed massive encephalomalacia, especially in the left hemisphere, with large areas of tissue destruction in the parietal, temporal and occipital lobes and in the median aspects of the frontal lobes. Such devastating findings are not rare in herpes encephalitis [*DeLong* et al., 1981]. A different distribution of the severe lesions is also known [*Wildi,* 1961]. (4) Neuropsychological evaluation repeated at ages 5 and 6 years revealed amnestic aphasia (inability to learn new names); right-left disorientation; visual agnosia for pictures including human figures while his orientation in concrete space was good; he could name his body parts or the details of actual objects, but not the details on their picture. (5) Psychological testing at admission yielded an IQ of 32, short attention span, extremely low frustration tolerance, lack of time concept, lack of number concept and inability to recognize shapes on prereading level. (6) Psychiatric evaluation and observation revealed anxiety and rage attacks in addition to generally apprehensive mood (dysphoria) and negativism.

The above detailed differential diagnostic evaluation helped setting up the appropriate rehabilitation. It was established that the mental retardation was the result of diffuse, nonprogressive brain damage, with identifiable multiple focal cortical lesions leading to a mosaic of learning disabilities each requiring specific techniques of rehabilitation. General psychiatric treatment formed the matrix of the therapeutic interventions. These included milieu therapy, psychotherapy, special education, language therapy, physical therapy and drug treatment. Dilantin 100 mg twice a day kept his seizures under control. Stelazine (2 mg twice a day) was best tolerated and effectively decreased the child's pathological anxiety, without undue sedation.

After 3 years of intensive inpatient treatment and rehabilitation, Chad was discharged in a substantially improved state: no aggression, no temper tantrums, no epileptic seizures. Improved visual space perception and directionality concepts were also achieved. Chad's IQ increased by eleven points in the last year of treatment. With an IQ of 43, Chad reached the trainable range of retardation. This child's rehabilitation would not have been possible without accurate differential diagnosis of the conditions associated with, and etiologically contributing to, the mental retardation.

The etiological clarification is helpful in sexual and marital counseling of adult retardates. On one hand, there is no reason for a 'post-traumatic' retarded person to refrain from having offsprings, especially with a healthy spouse who can provide, or supplement the parenting skills during the early years of their child's development. On the other hand, retarded persons with a genetic, metabolic disease must be advised of the substantial risks of producing a defective offspring. 'Mental retardation in and of itself should not be a legal disqualification for marriage' (The President's Panel's Task Force on Law, 1963, p. 21) [*Tarjan,* 1973]. *Tarjan* reminds us that 'the onset of puberty, often even its anticipation, exacerbates parental conflicts particularly when the child is retarded'. The retarded child may still be completely unaware of the implications of sexual maturation, but the parents may already see signs of promiscuity or disbanded sexual aggressors around every corner. Parents may seek institutionalization as protection – sterilization. Medical advice and social support to the family of retarded youngsters is useful at this stage of growing up.

Completion of the Diagnostic Process

The diagnosis of mental retardation and associated conditions does not conclude the clinician's efforts. Discussing the etiology and the prognosis of the condition will alleviate some of the patient's and the family's distress, since 'the greatest source of emotional disturbance of parents is the uncertainty of just not knowing what has happened ... what can be done' [*Dybwad,* 1966].

The last phase of the diagnostic procedure includes the following details:

Imparting the diagnosis
Supporting the emotional reactions
Exploration of and referral to appropriate community resources
Advocacy and crisis prevention
Availability for guidance at times of inevitable crisis (divorce, death, in the family, etc.)
Assistance in important decision-making such as: the option of keeping the patient at home versus placement in a foster home, group care, institutionalization or deinstitutionalization.

Only after assuming these responsibilities can the clinician consider the diagnostic process to be completed.

Conclusions

Refined differential diagnosis is possible in most cases of mental retardation beyond establishing the presence of the three basic diagnostic criteria.

The labeling of mental retardation without further attempts at symptom-related and etiological differential diagnosis may lead to misguided therapeutic shortcuts through symptom suppression, rather than addressing the etiological components.

The *differential diagnosis* relies on the social and medical history with emphasis on the developmental history and on the sequence of the appearance of the symptoms. The detailed work-up may include specialized neurological and ancillary techniques such as EEG, CAT scan, metabolic screening, and neuropsychiatric, psychological and psychiatric evaluations.

The diagnostic procedure should not be considered completed without the physician's involvement in the management of the case at least by guiding the retarded person and his/her family, or the caregiving staff, to the appropriate resources.

The most brilliant differential diagnosis remains an exercise in the vacuum, not worth the patient's or the physician's time, unless it is followed by appropriate management and referrals for each aspect of the needed rehabilitation and treatment and/or genetic counseling and social environmental support.

Differential diagnosis in mental retardation is not only possible, but necessary for good medical practice.

References

Agranowitz, A.; McKeown, W. R.: Aphasia handbook, pp. 204–205 (Thomas, Springfield 1964).

Albert, M.S.; Butters, N.; Brandt, J.: Patterns of remote memory in amnesic and demented patients. Archs Neurol. *38:* 495–500 (1981).

Assal, G.; Perentes, E.; Deruaz, J.P.: Crossed aphasia in a right-handed patient. Postmortem findings. Archs Neurol. *38:* 455–458 (1981).

Balla, D.; Zigler, E.: Luria's verbal deficiency theory of mental retardation and performance on sameness, symmetry and opposition tasks: a critique. Am. J. ment. Defic. *75:* 400–413 (1971).

Bender, L.: The brain and child behavior. Archs gen. Psychiat. *4:* 531 (1961).

Blumberg, P.; Beran, R.; Hicks, P.: Myoclonus in Down's syndrome. Association with Alzheimer's disease. Archs Neurol. *38:* 453–454 (1981).

Brander, T.: Besteht ein Zusammenhang zwischen dem Geburtsgewicht und dem Intelligenzquotienten bei Frühgeborenen? Mschr. Kinderheilk. *63:* 341 (1955).

Brazelton, B.; Heidelise, A.: Early stages of mother-infant interaction, in Solnit. The psychoanalytic study of the child, pp. 349–369 (Yale University Press, New Haven 1979).

Breuning, S.E.: Analysis of single, double-blind procedures, maintenance of placebo effects, and drug induced dyskinesia with mentally retarded persons. A brief report. Proc. Psychopharmacol. Bull. *17:* 122–123 (1981).

'Chad, Who Has Far To Go'. Film (producer Gabor Nagy), text: Irene Jakab, 1979 (Source: Western Psychiatric Institute and Clinic, Pittsburgh.)

Corboz, R.: Die Psychiatrie der Hirntumoren bei Kindern und Jugendlichen (Springer, Wien 1958).

Crapper, D.R.; Dalton, A.J.; Skopitz, M.; Scott, J.W.; Hachinski, V.C.: Alzheimer degeneration in Down syndrome. Archs Neurol., Chicago *32:* 618–623 (1975).

Cytryn, L.; Lourie, R.: Mental retardation; in Freedman, Kaplan and Kaplan, Comprehensive textbook of psychiatry, pp. 817–856 (Williams & Wilkins, Baltimore 1967).

Dalton, A.J.; Crapper, D.R.; Schlotterer, G.R.: Alzheimer's disease in Down's syndrome: visual retention deficits. Cortex *10:* 336–377 (1974).

Das, J.P.: Patterns of cognitive ability in nonretarded and retarded children. Am. J. ment. Defic. *77:* 6–12 (1972).

DeLong, G.R.; Bean, C.; Brown, F.R.: Acquired reversible autistic syndrome in acute encephalopathic illness in children. Archs Neurol. *38:* 191–194 (1981).

Denes, G.; Caviezel, F.: Dichotic listening in crossed aphasia, 'paradoxical' ipsilateral suppression. Archs Neurol. *38:* 182–185 (1981).

Dennis, M.; Fitz, C.R.; Netley, C.T.; Sugar, J.; Nash-Harwood, D.C.F.; Hendrick, E.B.; Hoffman, H.J.; Humphreys, R.P.: The intelligence of hydrocephalic children. Archs Neurol. *38:* 607–615 (1981).

Detlerman, D.K.: Memory in the mentally retarded; in Ellis, Handbook of mental deficiency: Psychological theory and research; 2nd ed. (Lawrence Earlbaum Ass., Hillsdale 1979).

Deutsch, C.P.; Schumer, F.: Brain damaged children, p. 50 (Brunner/Mazel, New York 1970).

DSM III: Diagnostic and Statistical Manual of Mental Disorders; 3rd ed. (American Psychiatric Association/American Psychiatric Asociation, Washington 1980).

Duffy (quoted by Marx, L.): Evoked potential. Science *213:* 322 (1981).

Dutton, G.: Mental handicap (Butterworth, London 1975).

Dybwad, G.: The mentally hanicapped child under five. Oxford, England (Oxford and District Society for the Mentally Handicapped, 1966).

Eisenberg, L.: Psychiatric implications of brain damage in children. Psychiat. Q. *31:* 72–92 (1957).

Ellis, W.G.; McCullogh, J.R.; Corley, C.L.: Pre-senile dementia in Down's syndrome. Ultrastructural identity with Alzheimer's disease. Neurology *24:* 101–104 (1974).

Enke, W.: Mehrdimensionale Diagnostik bei erziehungsschwierigen Kindern. Z. Psychother. med. Psychol. *5:* 260 (1955).

Feldman, D. H.: Beyond universals in cognitive development, p. 60 (Alex Publishers, Norwood 1980).

Ford, F.R.: Diseases of the nervous system in infancy, childhood and adolescence (Thomas, Springfield 1946).

Freeman, B.J.; Ritvo, E.R.; Schroth, P.C.; Tonick, I.; Guthrie, D.; Wake, L.: Behavioral characteristics of high- and low-IQ autistic children. Am. J. Psychiat. *138:* 25–29 (1981).

Gallagher, J.J.: A comparison of brain injured and non-brain injured mentally retarded children on several psychological variables. Monogr. Soc. Res. Child Dev. *22,* Serial No. 65, no. 2, pp. 1–79 (1957).

Gavallér, J.; Orosz, E.; Séra, J.: Az eklampsia jelentösége a késöbb manifesztálodó magzatí idegrendszeri károsodások szempontjából. Orv. Hétil. *99:* 16 (1958).

Gersh, F.; Damasio, A.R.: Praxis and writing of the left hand may be served by different callosal pathways. Archs Neurol. *38:* 634–636 (1981).

Gevins, A.S.; Doyle, J. C.; Cutillo, B.A.; Schaffer, R.E.; Tannehill, R. S.; Ghannam, J. H.; Gilcrease, V. A.; Yeager, C. L.: Electrical potentials in human brain during cognition: new method reveals dynamic patterns of correlation. Science *213:* 918–922 (1981).

Goldstein, K.; Sheerer, M.: Abstract and concrete behavior. Psychol. Monogr. *53:* 1–151 (1941)

Greenspan, S.: Social intelligence in the retarded; in Ellias, Handbook of mental deficiency: psychological theory and research; 2nd ed. (Lawrence Earlbaum Ass., Hillsdale 1979).

Grossman, H.J.: Definition in manual on terminology and classification in mental retardation. Am. Ass. ment. Defici., pp. 11–14 (Pridemark Press, Garamond 1973).

Halstead, W.C.: Brain and intelligence (University of Chicago Press, Chicago 1949).

Hecaen, H.; Angelergues, R.: La cecite psychique (Masson, Paris 1963).

Heimburger, R.F.; Demyer, W.; Reitan, M.R.: Implications of Gerstmann's syndrome. J. Neurosurg. Psychiat. *27:* 52 (1964).

Heston, L.L.; Mastri, A.R.: The genetics of Alzheimer's disease: associations with hematologic malignancy and Down's syndrome. Archs gen. Psychiat. *34:* 976–981 (1977).

Humphreys, L.G.; Parsons, C.K.: Piagetian tasks measure intelligence and intelligence tests assess cognitive development: a reanalysis. Intelligence *3:* 369–382 (1979).

Jakab, I.: Rôle des tests psychologiques de l'intelligence en psychiatrie. Annls méd.-psychol. *108:* 585–606 (1950).

Jakab, I.: Les résultats des lobotomies. Congr. Rep. IInd World Congr. Psychiat., Zürich, vol: 2, pp. 459–465 (1957).

Jakab, I.: Complications obstétricales dans l'etiologie de l'oligophrénie. Annali Neuropsich. Psicoanal. *6:* 446–453 (1959).

Jakab, I.: Deux cas d'apraxie constructive avec agnosie spatiale. Rev. Neurosci *102:* 704–706 (1960).

Jakab, I.: The role of neonatal anoxia in mental retardation and its prevention. Acta paedopsychiat. *32:* 329–338 (1965).

Jakab, I.: The patient, the mother, the therapist: an interactional triangle in the treatment of the autistic child. J. Commun. Disord. *5:* 154–182 (1972).

Jakab, I.: Basal ganglia calcification and psychosis in mongolism. Eur. Neurol. *17:* 300–314 (1978).

Kamhi, A.G.: Developmental vs. difference theories of mental retardation: a new look. Am. J. ment. Defic. *86:* 1–7 (1981).

Kety, S.S.: Genetic and biochemical aspects of schizophrenia; in Nicholi, The Harvard guide to modern psychiatry, p. 94 (Belknap Press of Harvard University Press, Cambridge 1978).

Kolb, B.; Taylor, L.: Affective behavior in patients with localized cortical excisions: role of lesion site and side. Science *214:* 89–90 (1981).

Környey, S.: Histopathologie und klinische Symptomatologie der anoxisch-vasalen Hirnschädigung, p. 221 (Sec. edit. Akademiai Kiado, Budapest 1955).

Kurzberg, H.; Vaugham, D. (quoted by Marx, L.): Evoked potential. Science *213:* 322 (1981).

Lashley, K.S.: Studies of cerebral function in learning. XII. Loss of the maze habit after occipital lesions in blind rats. J. comp. Neurol. *79:* 431–462 (1943).

Laux, W.: Zur Genese der Angst nach Hirntraumen bei Kindern. Zchr. Psychother. med. Psychol. *15:* 12 (1965).

Luria, A.R.: Higher cortical functions in man (Basic Books, New York 1970).

Luria, A.R.: The working brain, p. 136 (translated by Haigh) (Basic Books, New York 1973).

Maggio, E.: Psychophysiology of learning and memory, p. 142 (Thomas, Springfield 1971).

Mahoney, G.; Glover, A.; Finger, I.: Relationship between language and sensorimotor development of Down syndrome and nonretarded children. Am. J. ment. Defic. *86:* 21–27 (1981).

Malamud, N.: Atlas of neuropathology, p. 294 (University of California Press, Berkely 1957).

Mapelli, G.; Pavoni, M.; Ramelli, E.: Emotional and psychotic reactions induced by aphasia. Psychiatria clin. *13:* 108–118 (1981).

Mercer, J.; Ysseldyke, J.: Designing diagnostic intervention programs, in Oakland, Psychological and educational assessment of minority children, p. 72 (Brunner/Mazel, New York 1977).

Milgram, N.A.: Cognition and language in mental retardation. A reply to Balla and Zigler. Am. J. ment. Defic. *76:* 33–41 (1971).

Neufeld, M.Y.; Swanson, J.W.; Klass, D.W.: Localized EEG abnormalities in acute carbon monoxide poisoning. Archs Neurol. *38:* 524–527 (1981).

Olson, J.I.; Shaw, C.M.: Presenile dementia and Alzheimer's disease in mongolism. Brain *92:* 147–156 (1969).

Ozer, M.N.: Solving learning and behavior problems of children, pp. 228–229 (Jarsey-Bass Publishers, San Francisco 1980).

Pearson, P.H.: The physician's role in diagnosis and management of the mentally retarded. Pediat. Clins N. Am. *15:* 835–859 (1968).

Pennsylvania Office of Mental Retardation: Some behavioral assessment tools, March 5, 1976, pp. 1–8 (Pennsylvania Office of Mental Retardation, Harrisburg 1976).

Piaget, J.: The origins of intelligence (International Universities Press, New York 1952).

Piotrowski, Z.: The Rorschach inkblot method in organic disturbances of the central nervous system. J. nerv. ment. Dis. *86:* 525–537 (1937).

Pirozzolo, F.J.; Hansch, E.C.: Oculomotor reaction time in dementia reflects degree of cerebral dysfunction. Science *214:* 349–351 (1981).

Pruyser, P. W.: The psychological examination, p. 84 (International University Press, New York 1979).

Ramsay-Graeme, R. M.: Language learning approach styles of adult multilinguals and successful language learners, pp. 73–96; in Teller, V.; White; J.: Studies in child language and multilingualism. Ann. N.Y. Acad. Scie. *345:* 74–92 (1980).

Ranschburg, P.: Zur Pathophysiologie der Sprech-, Lese-, Schreib- und Druckfehler. Psychiat. neurol. Wschr. *29:* Jan. 8, p. 15 (1927).

Reed, J.: Brain damage and learning disabilities; in Tarnopol, Learning disorders in children, pp. 320–321 (Little, Brown, Boston 1971).

Reiser, A.: Early detection of developing emotional and perceptual dysfunction. Psych. Ann. *11:* 39–43 (1981).

Reitan, R.M.: Psychological deficit. Am. Rev. Psychol. *13:* 415–444 (1962).

Richardson, S.O.; Normanly, J.: Incidence of pseudoretardation in a clinic population. Am. J. Dis. Child. *109:* 432–435 (1965).

Rorschach, H.: Psychodiagnostik (translated by Lemkov, Kronenberg) (Huber, Bern 1921).

Ross, A.O.: Conceptual issues in the evaluation of brain damage; in Khanna, Brain damage and mental retardation (Thomas, Springfield 1968).

Rossi, G.F.; Rossadina, G.: Experimental analysis of cerebral dominance in man; in Millikan, Darley, Brain mechanisms underlying speech and language (Grune & Stratton, New York 1967).

Sarason, S.B.: Psychological problems in mental deficiency (Harper & Brothers, New York 1959).

Sattler, J.M.: Assessment of children's intelligence (Saunders, Philadelphia 1974).

Schachter, M.: Observations on the prognosis of children born following trauma at birth. Am. J. ment. Defic. *54:* 456–463 (1950).

Schachter, M.: La querelle de la signification neuropsychique des asphyxies de la naissance. Annali Neuropsich. Psicoanal. *1:* 44 (1954).

Shapiro, I. L.: Visual perception and reading; in Faas: Learning disabilities p. 110 (Thomas, Springfield 1972).

Sipress-Goodwin, L.; Hellmann, J.; Vannucci, R.R.; Maisels, M.J.: Ventricular dimensions of the brain in premature and full-term infants. Archs Neurol., Chicago, *38:* 447–449 (1981).

Spitz, H.H.: Beyond field theory in the study of mental deficiency; in Elis, Handbook of mental deficiency, psychological theory and research; 2nd ed. (Lawrence Earlbaum Ass., Hillsdale 1979).

Tardieu, G.; Klein, M.R.; Held, J.P.; Trélat, J.: Les conséquences de l'anoxie néonatale. Ann. Neuropsychiat. Psicoanal. *1:* 44 (1954).

Tarjan, G.: Sex: a tri-polar conflict in mental retardation; in Zyman, Meyers, Tarjan, Sociobehavioral studies in mental retardation p. 175–183 (Monographs of the AAMD No. 1, 1973).

Tarnopol, L.: Introduction to neurogenic learning disorders; in Tarnopol, Learning disorders in children, pp. 320–321 (Little, Brown, Boston 1971).

Tonkonogy, J.; Goodglass, H.: Language function, foot of the third frontal gyrus, and rolandic operculum. Archs Neurol. *38:* 486–490 (1981).

Tramer, M.: Über aktuelle allgemeine Probleme der Kinderpsychiatrie. Schweiz. med. Wschr. *444:* (1955).

Turman, L.; Maud, M.: Stanford-Binet intelligence scale form L-M (Houghton Mifflin Company, Boston 1973).

Villiez, T.V.; Lagenstein, I.; Koepp, P.: Akute optische Halluzinose bei der juvenilen neuronalen Zeroidlipofuszinose (Spielmeyer-Vogt-syndrome). Acta paedopsychiat. *47:* 19–25 (1981).

Volpe, B. T.; Sidtis, J. J.; Gazzanigh, M. S.: Can left-handed writing posture predict cerebral language laterality? Archs Neurol. *38:* 637–638 (1981).

Walls, R. T.; Werner, T.; Bacon, A.; Zane, T.: Behavior checklists; in Cone, Hawkins, Behavioral assessment, pp. 77–146 (Brunner Mazel, New York 1977).

Watson, R.T.; Valenstein, E.; Heilman, K.M.: Thalamic neglect; possible role of the medial thalamus and nucleus reticularis in behavior. Archs Neurol. *38:* 501–506 (1981).

Wechsler, D.: A standardized memory scale for clinical use. J. Psychol. *19:* 87–95 (1945).

Wechsler, D.: The measurement and appraisal of adult intelligence. Baltimore: (Williams & Wilkins, Baltimore 1958).

Wechsler, D.: Wechsler intelligence scale for Children. (The Psychological Corporation, New York).

Wildi, E.: Herpes encephalitis in the newborn with unusual pathological findings, pp. 73–78 (Elsevier, Amsterdam 1961).

Winters, J.J.: Methodological issues in psychological research with retarded persons; in Bialer, Sternlicht, The psychology of mental retardation: issues and approaches (Psychological Dimensions, New York 1977).

Yannet, H.: Classification and etiological factors in mental retardation. J. Pediat. *50:* 266–230 (1957).

Zigler, E.: Developmental versus difference theories of mental retardation and the problem of motivation. Am. J. ment. Defic. 1969, *73:* 536–556 (1969).

5 Psychological Assessment of the Retarded

Craig Latham, Regina Yando

Pediatricians, psychiatrists, and family practitioners are among the physicians who come into frequent contact with retarded persons. Apart from diagnostic evaluations, physicians are often asked to provide counsel to individuals who face decisions about the education and care of a retarded member of their family. At such times, the physician will likely receive a psychological report or request a psychological evaluation. The value of that report to the physician, although largely determined by the competence of the psychologist, can be increased by the physician's knowledge of the assessment process.

The purpose of this chapter is to enhance the physician's ability to obtain and use psychological reports in diagnosing and recommending treatment for retarded individuals. To do so, we will focus on three major topics: (1) the referral process; (2) the measurement of intelligence and adaptation; and (3) the psychological report. First, however, we will briefly describe the nature of psychological assessment.

Psychological Assessment

Assessment is not the exclusive domain of the psychologist. Decisions such as whether to trust a friend with a secret, whether to believe a salesman's description of a used car, and whether to ask a person to do a job all involve assessing an individual's characteristics. Viewed simply as the process of trying to understand people, assessment is a process we all practice daily. In essence, psychological assessment is nothing more than a formalized attempt to understand people. Specialized knowledge, tools, and techniques are employed as aids in decision-making, and the basic method follows a pattern of scientific inquiry. That is, data concerning an individual's behavior are systematically gathered, organized, and interpreted. Standardized procedures are emphasized in data collection to maximize the reliability of the information, and psychological research and theory are used to guide the organization and interpretation of results.

There are numerous sources of assessment data. These include structured and unstructured interviews, rating scales, tests, personal documents, and the reports of family members, teachers and others who have had an opportunity to observe the individual. With specific data from these sources and general information from psychological theory and research, the psychologist formulates a set of hypotheses about the relative importance of cognitive, emotional, environmental, and, to the extent possible, biological factors in characterizing the individual's current functioning. She/he then considers the implications of these hypotheses, recommends procedures for intervention when appropriate, and, finally, makes the information available in a written report.

Referral Process

The extent to which a psychological report contains information that is useful to the physician is strongly influenced by the adequacy of the communication between the physician and psychologist at the time of referral. A referral may be requested verbally or through a referral form. In either case, the physician is expected to state why the individual is being referred, and the psychologist is expected to provide a report. It is important for the physician to note that a request for a psychological evaluation is very different from requests for laboratory test information. When ordering a laboratory test, such as a white cell count, the physician does not specify why (i.e., the hypotheses related to a disease state) she/he wants a particular test, nor do these reasons influence the test procedure or the way in which results are reported. The reasons for the referral, as well as the questions asked, however, serve to focus a psychological evaluation. To a great extent they determine the choice of assessment methods as well as the information contained in the final report. It is, therefore, important that the physician clearly formulate the questions she/he wants answered and define the kinds of information she/he desires.

Psychologists are asked to evaluate retarded individuals for any number of reasons. The information requested and the format of the response will obviously vary according to the needs of physicians in different settings, such as private practice, clinics, hospitals, or institutions. The questions most commonly asked of psychologists can be grouped as follows:

(1) Diagnosis: Is the individual retarded in either cognitive or adaptive capabilities? Is there psychological evidence of some type of organic disorder? Are there concommitant psychiatric symptoms? (2) Placement: Where can the individual's needs best be met – in the home, in special classes, in sheltered workshops, in an institution, or in some combination of placements? (3) Treatment: Are there emotional disturbances that indicate a need for psychotherapy? Are there behavioral problems that require specific management techniques? (4) Education: Are there specific perceptual, motor, or cognitive deficits that require special attention in school or in training? (5) Legal decisions: Is the individual competent to stand trial, make decisions about hospitalization, or manage his or her own affairs?

Two general categories of questions emerge: questions regarding the individual's functioning and questions related to decisions about the individual. Psychologists are best equipped to answer the first category of questions. That is, the psychologist has at his/her disposal a wide variety of tests and techniques to obtain information on most aspects of individual functioning. It is particularly helpful to the psychologist, though, if the physician delineates why she/he desires information about a particular function. For example, a physician may want to know if there is psychological test information that suggests a person has central nervous system damage. Even if the assessment indicated such a possibility, it would not necessarily follow that the findings were related to the problem the person presents (e.g., hyperactivity). The point is that the psychologist will be able to provide more specific and useful information if she/he is aware of the problem the physician is trying to solve as well as the physician's reasoning about the problem.

Questions about an individual's innate capacity or potential, in contrast to an individual's current functioning, cannot be answered through a psychological assessment. For this reason the second category of questions, those related to decisions about individuals, are much more difficult to answer. This is not to say that a psychologist cannot make predictions about an individual's future behavior. Many people expect, however, that a psychological evaluation can provide *accurate* predictions of future behavior. This, in general, is not true. Predictions are always probabilistic statements, the accuracy of which is highly dependent upon knowledge of both the individual and his/her environment. Stated somewhat differently, most psychologists believe that behavior is a function of person and environment. To best predict future behavior, then, a psychologist must have information about the individual and the individual's current and future environments. Unfortunately, this usually does not happen.

While it is impossible to fully describe an individual's environment, it is possible to specify decisions that have to be made about an individual's situation (e.g., whether or not to provide special education). Since the changes that might be considered are limited by economics, by what is available, and by what the individual or his/her guardian will tolerate, it is often possible to specify all of the environments into which the individual could be placed (e.g., special class, day school, or residential care facility). Given such information the psychologist can better assess the individual's needs and predict his/her behavior in the proposed environments. Since we know that person characteristics are not overtly manifest in all situations and, conversely, that behavior is never totally situation-specific, the predictions are usually stated in a conditional form: If a person with X characteristics enters a situation that has Y characteristics, then such-and-such behaviors will probably occur. If, on the other hand, the same person enters a situation that has Z characteristics, other behaviors are more likely to occur. With this type of information, the physician should be better able to help those individuals who have sought his/her help in the decision-making process.

Retardation - Criteria

Although a psychological evaluation is rarely conducted solely to classify an individual as either retarded or not, frequently it is just such a classification that determines whether services to that individual are offered or withheld. The *definition* of retardation, then, becomes quite important for a largely economic reason. The third edition [1978] of the *Diagnostic and Statistical Manual of Mental Disorders* (DSM III) lists the essential features of mental retardation (based upon the American Association on Mental Deficiency [AAMD] 1973 definition) as follows: (1) significantly subaverage general intellectual functioning (as defined by an IQ score obtained from an individually administered intelligence test); (2) concurrent deficits in adaptive behavior (as defined by the individual's ability to function independently and to assume the social responsibilities appropriate to his or her age and culture); and (3) onset before the age of 18 (APA, 1978; parenthetical insertions ours). Likewise, the diagnosis of mental retardation is very important, again not because the label will affect the type of treatment and placement that may be recommended, but because it can determine the treatment and placement that will be funded.

Since the diagnosis of mental retardation must involve the use of at least one standardized test – the intelligence test – and it typically involves several more, it is essential that physicians with the responsibility of making such a diagnosis understand the use and limitations of psychological tests. Rating scales have become nearly as important in this context because they are the primary means to evaluate adaptive behavior and environments. Accordingly, the following sections on measurement will focus on the standardized tests and rating scales commonly used in diagnostic and management decisions with retarded individuals, rather than on clinical material that may be more relevant to the individual's therapist.

The Measurement of Intelligence and Adaptation

The scientific study of individual differences began in the 19th century, due in large part to the stimulation provided by Darwin's theory of evolution. Most notable among the early investigators in the field was Darwin's half-cousin, Sir *Francis Galton,* whose interest in demonstrating the inheritance of mental capacity led him to invent a large number of physical and 'mental tests' as a method to assess intellectual functioning. Galton applied the mathematical procedures of *Adolph Quetelet* to the data obtained from tests. He then proposed that the relative position of a person's test score in a statistical frequency distribution of other scores was measure of that individual's intelligence. Although Galton devised an ingenious battery of tests to measure a wide variety of abilites, such as visual and auditory discrimination, muscle strength, and breathing power, few of these tests are recognized today as measures of 'intelligence'. Nonetheless, Galton initiated the method of testing and, more importantly, laid the foundation for the use of statistical procedures as a means of defining individual differences.

The first successful intelligence test was constructed by *Alfred Binet* and *Theodore Simon,* 1905. Prior to that time, Binet and his colleagues, although impressed with Galton's work, proposed that to measure intelligence one had to look at complex behavior such as reasoning, memory, and judgement. They further suggested that intelligence was an age-related phenomenon. In 1904, the Minister of Public Instruction in Paris commissioned Binet to devise a method to evaluate children who could not profit from ordinary public school education. The Minister wanted to place these 'mentally retarded' children in special classes on the basis of both medical and psychological evaluations. Binet's response to this request was cautious and thorough. The 1905 scale, which emphasized both scientific rigor and humane concern, was based upon a decade of research with normal and retarded children. Binet's investigations were geared not only toward discovering 'intellectual tests' that measured differences among children, they also considered how age, school attainment, and teacher's evaluation of children related to test performance.

The success of the Binet scales (which he revised in 1908 and 1911), and for that matter most other intelligence and ability tests that rapidly followed, lay not in their contribution to our understanding of intelligence, but rather in their usefulness in meeting social needs. Compulsory education and the need to provide children with special education, for example, demanded an objective and relatively convenient method to detect children who had difficulty in learning. Tests provided a means to accomplish such goals. Whether tests, however, actually measure 'intelligence' is a matter of controversy and is a topic well beyond the scope of the present chapter [for reviews, see *Cronbach,* 1975; Harvard Educational Review, 1969; *Tuddenham,* 1966]. Suffice it to say that although tests indeed have been misused, as yet no viable alternative to identify children with special needs has been constructed.

Despite the overwhelming success of IQ tests, most professionals working with retarded individuals never accepted the IQ score as the sole basis for diagnoses and decision-making. Widespread acceptance of the social competence or adaptation factor existed prior to and certainly after the advent of testing. As early as 1913, a Mental Deficiency Act was established in England which ruled that a person could be considered 'feebleminded' only if she/he lacked the ability to manage his/her own affairs as well as an 'ordinary' person. Interestingly, the author of the major textbook on retardation in the 1950s, *A.F. Tredgold,* considered social incompetence a necessary and sufficient condition to make a diagnosis of retardation. He, in fact, rejected standardized IQ test performance. The exclusive reliance on behavioral maladaptation as the criterion of mental retardation, however, is frought with problems. Social criteria are relative, changeable, and value-laden. Moreover, few standardized instruments have been developed to measure adaptation.

The first widely accepted instrument, designed by Doll in 1953, was the Vineland Social Maturity Scale. Doll's scale is similar in format to the Binet, but consists of items related to social adjustment rather than intellectual performance (e.g., 9 to 10 year level: 'cares for self at table'). More recently, however, attention has been given to the development of standardized measures and a number of new scales have emerged. Nonetheless, the evaluation of adaptation is still dependent more on the clinical sensitivity and skills of the examiner than on well-established population data.

Proper use of measurement techniques should increase objectivity. If theories are to be tested and techniques and treatments evaluated, it is necessary to specify concepts in a measurable form. A statement by *Thorndike* [1918, p. 194] speaks directly to these concerns: 'Whatever exists at all exists in some amount. To know it thoroughly involves knowing its quantity as well as its quality.' Simply knowing a 'quantity' (e.g., IQ score) without understanding the derivation and application of measurement, however, can result in an overreliance on and misuse of quantitative information. For this reason, we now turn to a discussion of measurement concepts.

Basic Concepts of Measurements

Test

A psychological test is a tool that elicits a specific type of behavior under carefully controlled conditions. In addition to the test material itself, some information must be provided that establishes the relationship of the test behavior, either directly or indirectly, to other behaviors of interest such as school performance or the ability to function in a community. Some means must also be provided to allow comparisons between individuals and appropriate reference groups.

Tests can be conceptually divided in two ways. The first division can be made according to the type of behavior elicited, or the content of the test. Although tests have been constructed to measure nearly every imaginable characteristic of human behavior (*Buros* Mental Measurements Yearbook [1978] lists over 1,200 tests currently in use), they can nevertheless be divided into three general categories. These are: (1) tests of general intellectual development; (2) tests of specific aptitudes or abilities, such as reading, music, or mechanical engineering; and (3) tests of personality, including attitudes, interests, values, and problem-solving styles.

Tests can also be divided according to the nature of the stimulus, or the way in which the behavior is elicited. Objective tests are those in which the intended meaning of the stimulus can be specified exactly, and in which responses can be directly compared to some standard, either absolute or normative. Examples of objective stimuli include instructions to copy designs, solve math problems, hop on one foot, read a paragraph, or assemble a puzzle. In each of these examples, as with all objective tests, individuals are assumed to have enough common experience so that variations in responses from person to person are attributed to factors other than the individual's interpretation of the stimulus.

Associative or projective tests, in contrast, are those in which the meaning of the stimulus is deliberately made ambiguous. The response is then obviously determined to a large extent by the particular interpretation made by the individual. If the performance aspect of the response can be made sufficiently simple, such as reporting what a picture looks like rather than composing a song about the feeling it evokes, one can discount the performance component as a source of variation and assume the behavior elicited by the test is that of organizing and interpreting ambiguous stimuli. One of the oldest and most widely-known examples of a projective stimulus is the instruction to report what the Rorschach inkblots bring to mind. Various aspects of the pattern, content, and form of the response to this and other projective stimuli are interpreted as characteristic of the way in which an individual organizes his perceptions, approaches ambiguous situations, and deals with impulses. Further evaluation may be based on the number of various response types in comparison with a reference group. In either case, variations in responses from different individuals are assumed to be due to differences in past experiences that have led to a characteristic way of viewing and organizing perceptions.

Test Scores

Virtually all test performances – both objective and projective – are evaluated at least in part by comparing an individual score with scores obtained by an appropriate reference group. Raw scores, such as the length of time spent on a test, the number of items completed, or the average number of errors per trial, are not very useful in and of themselves because they do not incorporate any information about the individual's relative standing. Furthermore, it is not possible to compare performances among tests with only raw scores because the units represented by the scores are different for each test. It is, therefore, necessary to convert raw scores into a format that does contain information about relative standing and that is based on a standard scale.

Table I. Hypothetical grade-equivalent conversion table for raw test scores

Raw score	Grade equivalent	Raw score	Grade equivalent	Raw score	Grade equivalent
1	K.1	16	2.5	31	4.8
2	K.2	17	2.6	32	5.0
3	K.4	18	2.8	33	5.1
4	K.7	19	3.1	34	5.2
5	K.9	20	3.2	35	5.3
6	1.1	21	3.3	36	5.5
7	1.2	22	3.4	37	5.7
8	1.3	23	3.5	38	5.9
9	1.4	24	3.6	39	6.1
10	1.6	25	3.8	40	6.2
11	1.7	26	4.0	41	6.3
12	1.8	27	4.1	42	6.5
13	2.1	28	4.2	43	6.7
14	2.2	29	4.4	44	6.8
15	2.4	30	4.6	45	6.9

There are two general formats for this conversion, age- or grade-equivalent scores and percentile ranks. Age-equivalent scores indicate the age of the individuals for whom a given score was the average score. The test authors determine the average score for every age group with which the test may be used, usually in increments of fractions of years, by administering the test to a large sample population. An individual score can then be compared to these age means to determine the age at which that score was the average in the reference group. Table I is an example of a grade-equivalent table constructed on these principles. According to this table, the grade equivalent of a raw score of 32 would be fifth grade, independent of the actual grade or age of the individual. The interpretation, however, would focus on any discrepancies between actual grade or age and the test equivalent, rather than on the scores themselves. Age- and grade-equivalent scores may be compared to other such scores, providing the reference groups from which the norms were taken were similar.

Percentile ranks indicate the percentage of individuals in the comparison group whose performance fell below a given score. If, for example, a 10-year-old child took 47 s to assemble a puzzle, and 70% of the comparison group of 10 year olds took 48 s or more (longer times represent less adequate performances in this context), the raw score of 47 s corresponds to the 70th percentile. In general, percentiles and several other scores based on frequency distributions (discussed below) represent the percentage of individuals in a *same-age* reference group whose performance was *different* – in this case, lower – than the individual score, whereas age- or grade-equivalent scores are based on comparisons of an individual score to reference groups of *many ages* to determine the age *most representative* of that particular score.

Percentile scores are thus derived from the range or frequency distribution of the test scores within a same-age reference group. Almost all tests have frequency distributions with essentially the same shape, which is important in this context because in makes comparisons easier and because some of the difficult calculations involved in deriving percentile scores do not have to be repeated by authors of new tests. The *particular* shape that all of these distributions take – the familiar bell-shaped or normal distribution – is only important because it is so common in the study of complex random variables and because the calculations that do have to be done by test authors are relatively straightforward with the normal distribution.

Two parameters are necessary to describe a distribution: a measure of central tendency and a measure of spread. The most common measure of central tendency in symmetric distributions such as the normal distribution is simply the arithmetic mean or average, $\overline{X}$.[1] It is computed by summing all the individual scores ($X_1 + X_2 + X_3 \cdots + X_N = \Sigma (X)$) and dividing by the total number of scores, $\overline{X} = \Sigma (X)/N$.

The spread is a measure of the variability in scores. One could simply use the range of scores, from the highest to the lowest, but a more precise statistical measure of variability in distributions is the standard deviation, S. This measure is calculated by obtaining the difference or deviation of each score from the mean ($D = X - \overline{X}$), squaring each deviation (D^2), summing the squared deviations ($D_1^2 + D_2^2 + D_3^2 \cdots + D_N^2 = \Sigma (D^2)$), dividing by the number of cases[2], and taking the square root of the quotient: $S = \sqrt{\Sigma (D^2)/N}$. The standard deviation may be conceptualized as the average difference from the mean.[3] It is a useful measure because with normal distributions, a known *percentage* of the scores fall within each standard deviation from the mean, regardless of the particular raw score scale or the values of the mean and standard deviation. This can be seen in figure 1, along with the relationship of percentile ranks to the normal distribution.

[1] Readers with knowledge of statistics may be aware that two other measures of central tendency – the mode and median – equal the mean in the normal distribution.

[2] If the number of cases is small, approximately 40 or less, dividing by N–1 rather than by N is a common, theoretically motivated adjustment.

[3] This is not technically correct. While the average difference from the mean is a conceptually appealing measure, it is mathematically difficult to work with; one problem is differentiating the absolute value function. The standard deviation has been created as a more manageable substitute.

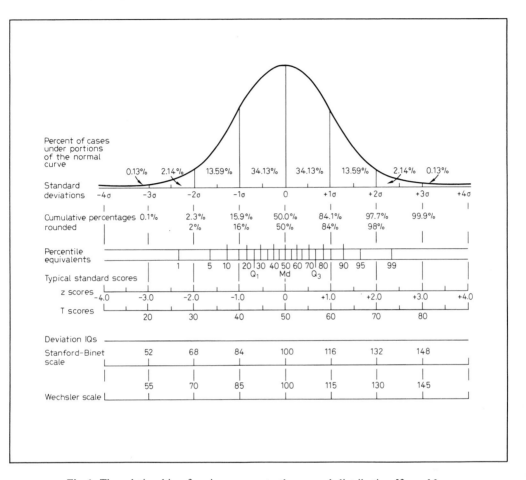

Fig. 1. The relationship of various scores to the normal distribution [from *Munn*, 1961].

Standard deviations (or fractions thereof) are also used as measurement units that are independent of the raw score scale to describe the distance between individual scores and the mean. This distance is usually expressed as the ratio of the unscaled difference to the standard deviation, $(X–\overline{X})/S$ or D/S, and is called a z score. There is an adaptation of the z score that is designed to eliminate negative numbers and decimal points, the T score. T scores are calculated by multiplying z scores by an arbitrary constant, usually 10, and then adding some other constant, usually 50: $T = 10z + 50$. Thus, a raw score of 25 on a test with a mean of 30 and a standard deviation of 10 yields $z = (25–30)/10 = -0.5$ (0.5 standard deviations below the mean) and $T = (10 \times -0.5) + 50 = 45$. The relationship of z and T scores to the normal distribution is also shown in figure 1.

There is one additional test score that, at least historically, was a combination of age-equivalent and percentile type scores, and that is the IQ. Before 1944, raw IQ scores were transformed to age-equivalent scores that were interpreted as measures of absolute mental capacity or mental age (see, for example, the test manual for the Wechsler Adult Intelligence Scale). To make performances of different-age individuals more directly comparable and to include information about the rate of mental growth, the quotient of mental age divided by chronological age, or intelligence quotient, was computed. Like the T score, these ratios were multiplied by an arbitrary constant – in this case, 100 – to eliminate fractional IQ scores. For example, a child with a chronological age (CA) of 5 and a mental age (MA) of 6, an acceleration of 1 year above the average in 5 years of mental growth, has an IQ of $(6/5) \times 100 = 120$. A child with a CA of 10 and an MA of 11, also an acceleration of 1 year but this time over a 10-year period, has an IQ of $(10/11) \times 100 = 110$.

Serious theoretical objections developed to this use of the mental age concept in deriving IQs (Wechsler's discussion of these issues can be found in the Wechsler test manuals). MA-based IQ scores fluctuated from year to year, and large differences in the standard deviations in the various age groups made comparisons across age groups statistically invalid. More recent versions of the Wechsler scales, the Stanford-Binet, and several newer tests use a scoring system based on Wechsler's 1944 revision. This revision compares raw scores to same-age reference group scores and converts them directly to IQs as though they were percentile scores. This eliminates the need for the mental age in deriving IQ scores.

The mental age as a simple age-equivalent score has, however, become enormously popular because of the ease with which it can be explained to parents and teachers. It has also been a very effective tool to use in describing what to expect from an individual. On a more theoretical level, the functioning of nonorganically impaired retarded persons can often be meningfully compared to that of an average younger child [*Ziegler,* 1967]. In these cases, the constellation of abilities may be similar, but the retarded individual's rate of mental growth is slower. Since mental age is still widely used as an age-equivalent score, it is often reported along with the new form of IQ score.

Notice that there is no explicit information about relative standing in an IQ score. Many psychologists have, however, developed a sense of the practical implications of various IQ scores in the same way most of us have with the Fahrenheit temperature scale (when the temperature is below 65, we need a sweater; an IQ below 85 implies special needs). The fact that the new scores are not in the actual percentile form is strictly a matter of convention. Intelligence tests are arguably the oldest psychological instruments in current use, and IQ scores were established long before the need to use a standard format for test scores became apparent. As is shown in figure 1, these scores can easily be converted to percentile, z, or T scores when necessary. The Wechsler scales now have a mean of 100 and a standard deviation of 15, and the Stanford-Binet has a mean of 100 and a standard deviation of 16. (Since these are both arbitrary scales, it is unfortunate they were not arbitrarily made the same.) To distinguish these from the scores that were derived from mental age, the new scores are termed 'deviation' IQs.

Rating Scales

We have described tests as tools that sample specific types of behavior under carefully controlled conditions. Test behaviors are selected to be representative of some larger set of behaviors, and they serve as the basis for inferences about that larger set. There are some aspects of functioning, though, that can be evaluated directly – without samples, inferences, or generalizations. This is more often the case in medicine than in psychology. In an evaluation of hearing or visual acuity, for example, the behavior of interest is tested directly and virtually in its entirety, and the results can be stated in a relatively brief and unambiguous manner.

Adaptive behaviors are important examples of psychological functioning that can be directly evaluated. Such behaviors may be described with a clinical narrative, or they may be enumerated with rating scales such as the Vineland Social Maturity Scale or the AAMD Adaptive Behavior Scale. These are lists of self-help skills, social skills, and personal skills that can be observed and, perhaps with some elaboration, rated as either present or not. The ratings are often converted to age-equivalent or percentile scores as were the test scores described previously. Another important use of the ratings is in evaluating the suitability of particular environments for an individual. The question in this case is not 'How does this individual compare numerically with other individuals', but 'In my judgement, does this individual have the skills to get along in this environment', regardless of the functioning of others in the environment. This latter approach is called criterion-referenced evaluation.

Reliability and Validity

Assessment information from tests and rating scales is judged by two criteria: reliability and validity. Reliability simply means the extent to which the information would be the same if it could be obtained again under identical conditions. There are basically two techniques to determine reliability. The first, test-retest reliability, involves administering a test (or filling out a rating scale), waiting some period of time, and then repeating the same procedure with the same group of people. If one assumes the behaviors were stable over time, the results should be more or less the same. Test-retest reliability is appropriate only when the behavior in question is not expected to change due to maturation or some intervention, and when the experience of having taken the test once will not affect the outcome of a second administration of the same test (practice effect). If both of these conditions are not met, reliability can be determined in a manner similar to that used to evaluate clinical laboratories that perform blood tests: take a single sample, divide it into two presumably identical halves, and compare the results when each half is evaluated separately. If the halves were, in fact, identical, and if the procedures were reliable, the results should be nearly identical. This is called split-half reliabilty.

Validity is the extent to which a test or rating scale accomplishes its stated goals. The American Psychological Association [1966] has defined three types of validity in its *Standards for Educational and Psychological Tests and Manuals:* content validity, criterion-related validity, and construct validity. These are enormously complicated issues, and most of the controversy surrounding specific tests and testing in general can be traced to questions of validity. While a thorough discussion is beyond the scope of this chapter, we will nevertheless define the three types of validity if only to point out some of the ways in which tests may fall short of the ideal. For a more complete discussion, the reader is referred to *Cronbach* [1970] or *Anastasis* [1976].

Content validity is the extent to which a test obtains a representative sample of the behaviors in question. Math achievement tests, for example, would not be representative of general math skills if the questions only concerned calculus. Although this is largely a subjective judgement, empirical techniques can be used to support it. Matched forms of the test can be administered before and after some event generally thought to affect the behavior, such as a course of algebra instruction. If the test content is valid, the results should be different (better, in this case) after the intervention.

Criterion-related validity refers to the match between the test results and whatever independent means exist to evaluate the same behavior. Tests that are used to select candidates for medical school, such as the Medical College Admission Test (MCAT), could be compared to the successful applicants' later medical school performance. Or, results from medical specialty board exams could be compared to senior physicians' ratings of the same individuals' performances. These two examples, which differ only in the timing of the comparisons, illustrate predictive and concurrent forms, respectively, of criterion-related validity. Since there may be explanations other than that the test was invalid if the results of the test and the independent evaluation do not agree, this type of validity is also in part a subjective judgement.

Construct validity, which is probably the most difficult of these types to evaluate, refers to the success of a test in measuring what it was intended to measure. More specifically, it is an evaluation of the chain of inferences connecting the observed behavior to the abstract concept or construct it supposedly taps. Some tests, such as achievement tests, require very little inference in moving from the test behavior to interpretation. Projective and intelligence tests, however, involve considerable inferential leaps between the behaviors that are actually seen and the functions ascribed to them. A further complication lies in the fact that these tests are intended to reflect functions that few psychologists can agree on how to define, let alone how to measure. Fortunately, it is not necessary to abandon tests because their construct validity is open to some question. When they do have a well-established utility in predicting some important behaviors, such as school performance in the case of intelligence tests, that utility can be appreciated in the absence of an explanation of the mechanism.

The measurement concepts described above should enable the reader to understand better the tests and scales used in the assessment of retarded individuals. A brief description of several of the instruments most commonly used to assess intelligence and adaptation are given below. Space limitations preclude a discussion of tests used to assess personality and specific problem areas (e.g., neurological functioning), even though such tests are often used in the assessment of retarded individuals. The reader is referred to *Anastasi* [1976] for a description of these tests.

Assessment Instruments

Stanford-Binet Intelligence Scale
The Binet Scale was translated into English in 1916 by *L.M. Terman* at Stanford University. Now known as the Stanford-Binet, the test is among the most successful instruments of its type. The most recent version was designed in 1960 to incorporate the best features of two earlier versions, forms L and M. The new form, designated L-M, is for individuals who range in age from 2

years through adulthood. Updated norms were last obtained in 1972 from a comparison group that was carefully selected to be representative of the ethnic, economic, and geographic distributions in this country.

The tasks are grouped in levels of difficulty that correspond to half-year intervals between the ages of 2 and 5, yearly intervals between the ages of 5 and 14, and four adult levels (average adult and superior adult I, II, and III). There are six tasks for each age level with the exception of average adult, which has eight. Tasks at the younger age levels involve manipulation and identification of objects and various forms of eye-hand coordination. The upper age level tasks are primarily verbal items that include vocabulary, sentence completion, and analogies.

The Stanford-Binet, which yields both an MA and an IQ score, is generally considered one of the most reliable standardized intelligence tests. It is more reliable for older (over 6 years) than younger children, and also for lower than for higher IQs. Numerous tests of concurrent and predictive validity also rank the Stanford-Binet as one of the best tests of general intelligence.

Wechsler Scales

There are three Wechsler scales in current use: the Wechsler Adult Intelligence Scale (WAIS), the Wechsler Intelligence Scale for Children – revised form (WISC-R), and the Wechsler Preschool and Primary Scale of Intelligence (WPPSI). They are, respectively, for individuals from 16 years to adult, from 5 to 15 years, and from about 4 years to about 7 years.

Although they were designed to serve many of the same functions as the Stanford-Binet, these scales differ in several ways. The tasks on the Wechsler scales are grouped by content into subtests of similar items, with each subtest arranged in order of increasing difficulty. The Stanford-Binet has varied items arranged in discrete age-level tests. The Wechsler scales, in addition to a mental age, yield verbal, performance, and full-scale IQs. The subtest scores are also tabulated separately to suggest specific areas of strength or weakness.

The WAIS has eleven subtests; six verbal and five performance. The verbal subtests are information, comprehension, arithmetic, similarities, digit span, and vocabulary. The performance subtests are digit symbol, picture completion, block design, picture arrangement, and object assembly. Each subtest yields a scaled score with a mean of ten and a standard deviation of three. Verbal, performance, and full-scale IQs are computed by summing the appropriate subtest scores. The WAIS and Stanford-Binet are essentially equal in reliability and validity, although older and less able individuals tend to score higher on the WAIS than on the Stanford-Binet. Norms for the WAIS were obtained in 1955 from a reference group that was selected on the basis of 1950 census data. Although they were representative when they were published, these norms should be updated to reflect population changes in ethnic balance, education, and geographic distribution.

The organization and form of the WISC-R and the WPPSI are virtually identical to the WAIS. Each scale has the same verbal and performance subtest areas, with only age-appropriate adjustments of the tasks. Scoring, reliability, and validity are also similar among the scales. The Stanford-Binet again yields higher scores for younger and brighter individuals, while retarded individuals score slightly higher on the WISC-R. Norms for both the WISC-R (1974) and the WPPSI (1967) are fairly recent. They have been very carefully prepared and are among the best available with any standardized test.

Nonverbal Intelligence Tests

Although the Binet and Wechsler scales are most often used to measure intellectual functioning, several other individually administered IQ tests should be mentioned. These are the Peabody Picture Vocabulary Test (PPVT), The Columbia Mental Maturity Scale (CMMS), and the Leiter International Performance Scale. These are tests of nonverbal intelligence and, as such, are often used with retarded individuals who have language, sensory, and/or motor problems. The best standardized and, for the most part, most reliable and valid test is the third edition of the CMMS. This test is designed to evaluate children between the ages of 3 years 6 months and 9 years 11 months. The child's task is to select one drawing on each card (92 in all) that is different from the other drawings on the card. The task requires perceptual discriminations that involve color, shape, size, missing parts, function, number, and symbolic material.

The least satisfactory among the three tests, although it is often used, is the Leiter. The test has unsatisfactory reliability and validity, and the standardization sample is poorly defined. A somewhat better designed test than the Leiter is the PPVT, which is perhaps the most widely used of the three instruments. It should be noted that retarded children receive slightly higher IQ's on the PPVT than on the Stanford-Binet and Wechsler scales.

Vineland Social Maturity Scale

The first measure of adaptive behavior to gain wide popularity was the Vineland Social Maturity Scale, which was designed by Doll in 1953. As we described previously, the form of the scale is similar to the Stanford-Binet intelligence test. Items are grouped in levels of difficulty that correspond to discrete age levels, with only a few items per level. The content, of course, is related to specific areas of social adjustment rather than intellectual performance. The Vineland Scale, like most instruments of this type, can be used to obtain age-equivalent scores. These scores have also been used to derive the adaptive equivalent of an IQ: the social quotient (SQ). This measure is subject, though, to the same criticisms that applied to the old MA-based IQ scores (see page 132). Unfortunately, the Vineland Scale norms were obtained from a geographically isolated and therefore nonrepresentative reference group.

Adaptive Behavior Scale (ABS)

The ABS is gaining popularity as the 'official' scale of the AAMD. It consists of a two-part checklist with 28 general areas of functioning. The first part deals with ten areas considered important in independent daily living, each with several specific behaviors to rate. The ten areas include self-help skills, such as toileting and eating; physical and social development; language; and socialization. Part two is concerned with the frequency of various inappropriate behaviors exhibited by an individual, such as violent or destructive acts, withdrawal, stereotyped behavior, or self-abusive behavior.

The scores from the various ratings can be used as an adaptive profile to compare the individual with an appropriate reference group. Percentile conversions are available for eleven groups ranging from three years of age through late adulthood. Although the ABS is widely used in community settings, it was originally standardized on an institutionalized population. *Baumeister and Muma* [1975, p. 298] point out that, in this regard, the authors of the ABS assume 'that the determinants of adaptive capacity are exclusively within the province of the individual's faculties ... This position simply attributes retardation to a person without due regard to the functional context in which he lives ...'. Recent norms for children, at least, are based on a more representative sample of normal individuals: boys and girls of various ethnic groups from regular and special school programs in different geographic areas. Since adaptive behavior can only be defined in terms of a particular environment, the most useful application of the ABS may be in a criterion-referenced evaluation of specific treatment or management decisions.

The Psychological Report

The psychological report is not a simple compendium of test findings, despite our emphasis on tests and measurement. Rather, a report represents an interpretative statement of psychological data obtained from observation, interviews, and tests. As stated previously, the quality of the interpretation depends upon the psychologist's knowledge of human behavior and his/her skill as a clinician. However desirable it might be to eliminate subjective judgement, it remains an essential ingredient at all levels of assessment. The psychologist interprets (1) the referral request in order to choose appropriate assessment techniques and to formulate meaningful hypotheses; (2) the data obtained; (3) how the data interrelate and correspond to data from other sources; and (4) the meaning of treatment in order to define the possible effects of alternative solutions to the problem in question. The final assessment report, then, represents the psychologist's professional judgement. Nonetheless, the physician's knowledge of the assessment process can aid him/her in judging the quality of the psychological report.

In general, a psychological report is organized within a rather standard format. It begins with a concise statement of the reasons for the referral, followed by a list of tests employed and a brief description of the conditions of the testing sessions (general observations). The physician should first review the referral statement to determine if his/her questions and concerns were accurately interpreted. Secondly, the physician can review the tests administered not only for test scores, but also to obtain an understanding of the types of reference groups the psychologist used as a basis for interpreting the data. (The physician interested in understanding more about a particular test will find the Buros Mental Measurement Yearbooks an invaluable source of information.)

The testing conditions section is used to briefly describe the person's behavior throughout the assessment. Such factors as whether or not the person was involved in the tasks, understood instructions, accepted being in the situation, and his/her interaction with the examiner are reported. Other factors that may have biased the assessment (e.g., recent death in the family, removal from school) are also taken into account. In general, the purpose of the section is to indicate whether or not the assessment could be considered a reliable and valid sample of the individual's behavior. A person may, for example, have been acutely anxious during the assessment, thereby reducing the likelihood that the test performance was representative of behavior under stress-free conditions. Such factors obviously will have a bearing on the interpretation of test results and on the final recommendations.

The major body of the report is devoted to a description of the person's current functioning and developmental level. The data from all assessment methods are integrated and the 'facts' are presented. No one piece of datum can stand alone; the total body of data must be correlated and interpreted before it can be related to the questions of interest. It should be noted that a good psychological report is jargon-free and written about the person assessed rather than the tests administered. That is, the report should focus on the individual and not on raw data from test findings. In general, then, the person's cognitive, emotional, and interpersonal functioning is discussed in the body of the report. This includes not only the obvious types of test information, such as reasoning skills and general factual knowledge, but also cognitive style (e.g., how a person attends to and organizes information), strategies used to cope with impulses and environmental stress, and the person's perception of self. In brief, a 'picture' of the person's total functioning, including both his/her strengths and weaknesses, should emerge within this section.

The final section of the report is perhaps most important to the referring physician. It is here that diagnostic impressions are specified and the information obtained about the individual's functioning is related to environmental (or treatment) considerations. That is, the reasons for referral are addressed. The psychologist's primary responsibility in writing an assessment report is to provide the information requested and to respond to the questions posed in the referral. If a question could not be answered, the reasons why it could not should be specified. If the referral requested information about a change in a person's environment, the question of whether or not the change is related to the problem should be delineated. For example, if the decision to move a child from a regular class to a special day school program had to be made, the relationship between the child's problem (e.g., acting-out behavior) and his inability to understand the school work, as compared to any number of other factors such as family discord, should be specified. Finally, a projection of how the child might function in the proposed and/or alternative environment(s) should be given. That is, the conditional propositions (see page 124) are outlined.

As stated previously, the final interpretation of the assessment data must be made relevant to the questions to be answered and the decisions to be made. Because of this, it is evident that the psychologist and physician must work closely together. We hope this chapter will better enable the physician to communicate his/her needs to a psychologist and to evaluate critically and use the information obtained in a psychological report.

References

Anastasi, A.: Psychological testing; 4th ed. (Macmillan, New York 1976).

American Psychiatric Association: Diagnostic and statistical manual of mental disorders; 3rd ed. (Washington 1978).

American Psychological Association. Standards for educational and psychological tests and manuals (Washington 1966).

Baumeister, A.S.; Muma, J.R.: On defining mental retardation. J. spec. Educ. 9: 293–306 (1975).

Buros, O.K.: Mental measurements yearbooks (Gryphon Press, Highland Park, 1938–1978).

Cronbach, L.J.: Essentials of psychological testing; 3rd ed. (Harper & Row, New York 1970).

Cronbach, L.J.: Five decades of public controversy over method testing. Am. Psychol. 30: 1–14 (1975).

Environment, Heredity, and Intelligence: Harvard Educational Review, Reprint Series No. 2 (Cambridge, 1969).

Munn, N.L.: Psychology, p. 747 (Houghton Mifflin Company, Pittsburgh, 1961).

Thorndike, E.L.: The nature, purposes and general methods of measurements of educational products; in 17th ybk. Nat. Soc. Study of Education. II. Measurement of Educational Products (Public School Publishing Company, Bloomington 1918).

Tuddenham, R.D.: The nature and measurement of intelligence; in Postman, Psychology in the making. (Knopf, New York 1966).

Yando, R.: Psychological assessment; in Talbot, Kagan, Eisenberg, Behavioral science in pediatric medicine (Saunders, Philadelphia 1971).

Zigler, E.: Mental retardation. Current issues and approaches; in Hoffman, Hoffman, Review of child development research, (Russell Sage Foundation, New York 1967).

6 A Behavioral Approach to the Treatment of the Mentally Retarded
Regina Yando

Behavioral treatment in clinics, schools and institutions is commonplace today. Controversy surrounding such treatment prevailed a decade ago. Professionals within these settings who have no training in the behavioral sciences, however, may still become perplexed with their 'behavioral' colleagues. This is not surprising, since they are faced with an often bewildering array of persons, techniques, and approaches that are subsumed under the term behavioral.[1]

It is the purpose of this chapter to provide the nonbehaviorally trained professional with a general outline to guide his/her understanding of the field. Although the chapter will focus on one major behavioral approach used in the treatment of the mentally retarded, it seems prudent to begin with a brief history[2] of the major developments in the area. This historical orientation hopefully will help the reader discriminate among the various approaches and techniques currently in use.

A Brief History

Psychology is a young science. Established by *Wilhelm Wundt* in 1860, 'experimental physiological psychology' was the result of a union between philosophical psychology and physiology. Influenced by British associationism and Kantian subjectivism, *Wundt* defined the subject matter of psychology to be immediate experience and its method to be introspection. The goal of psychology was the analysis of consciousness. Among the psy-

---

[1] For convenience and clarity throughout this chapter, the term 'behavioral psychology' will be used generically to include all approaches that have historical ties to objectivism.

[2] For a more complete history of psychology and the development of behavioral approaches see *Boring* [1950] and *Kazdin* [1978]. The author is indebted to them for their excellent historical research.

chological problems studied in Wundt's laboratory were vision, audition, sensation, perception, and reaction time, problems which had earlier been concerns of physiology, physics and astronomy.

Less than 50 years after Wundt had established psychology as an independent 'scientific discipline', a movement within the field served greatly to alter the course of its development. 'Behaviorism' began as a reaction to both the method and the data of Wundt's psychology. Introspection and consciousness were to be replaced with conditioning and behavior. The 'new' psychology was to be objective.

'Objectivism' developed within the tradition of French philosophical psychology. Two schools of thought, positivism and Cartesian materialism provided behaviorism with its philosophical underpinnings: the rejection of subjective experience as admissible data, and the view of man as a 'machine'. Of even greater importance to the development of the movement, however, were advances that had taken place in science. The growth of experimental physiology in Russia and widespread acceptance of evolutionary theory permitted the behavioral movement effectively to challenge the 'experimental psychology' of Wundt.

Reflexology – The Russian School

Prior to the mid-nineteenth century, theoretical analyses dominated Russian physiology. The emphasis on experimental physiology in the latter part of that century was due primarily to the work of three well-known physiologists: *Ivan Sechenov, Ivan Pavlov,* and *Vladimir Bekhterev.* Their contribution to behavioral psychology resulted from their empirical investigations of the nervous system and their strong advocacy of objectivism.

Sechenov (1829–1905) introduced the field of reflexology by proposing that psychological problems could be studied through the application of experimental methods developed in the area of neurophysiology. His proposal evolved from his interest in psychology, his dissatisfaction with the introspective method, and his experimental work on reflexes.

Sechenov's research on the inhibitory action of the cerebral cortex on spinal reflexes led him to believe that all behavior, voluntary and involuntary, was reflexive. In *Reflexes of the Brain*, published in 1863, *Sechenov* [1965] argued that thinking and problem-solving, even though emanating from the brain rather than the spinal cord, were in origin dependent on environmental stimulation and, therefore, were reflexes. Complex human behavior, he hypothesized, was basically reflexive and acquired through learning.

Somewhat later *Sechenov* proposed a methodological approach to the study of psychical phenomenon in a paper entitled, 'Who Must Investigate the Problems of Psychology and How?' In that work, he declared that since behavior (cognition) could be explained as reflexive, it could therefore be examined scientifically. Not surprisingly, he concluded that experimental physiologists were best trained to 'investigate the problems of psychology'. Even though he did not attempt to demonstrate his assumptions, his arguments were persuasive and greatly influenced *Pavlov* who successfully established an 'objective' method for the study of learned behavior.

Although *Pavlov* (1849–1936) received the Nobel prize for his research on the physiology of digestion, he is best known as the 'father of classical conditioning'. *Pavlov's* [1957] famous series of conditioning experiments began as an attempt to control for the appearance of confounding variables in animal studies on the relationship of digestive processes to physical stimulation. In that research, he used surgical techniques to route salivary and stomach secretions away from the digestive tract and to the surface of the body. In doing so he could observe and measure how the flow of digestive juices related to substances placed into the mouth or other parts of the digestive tract. During the course of his studies, he observed that secretions could be evoked without physically stimulating the system. That is, secretions began when the animal simply looked at food or at the experimenter. *Pavlov* initially labelled this phenomenon 'psychical secretion', and attempted to understand it by imagining the subjective state of the animal. The futility of the subjective method led him to observe systematically the phenomenon, and subsequently to redefine it as a 'conditioned reflex'.

The subjects for *Pavlov's* research on conditioning were dogs; the response selected for study was the salivary reflex. The basic research procedure to establish the conditioned reflex was as follows. The stimulus (e.g., food) that elicited the salivary reflex and a neutral nonreflex-evoking stimulus (e.g., a bell) were simultaneously and repeatedly presented to the animal. When the reflex was elicited solely by the presentation of the neutral stimulus, that reflex was considered to be 'conditioned'. The components of this procedure, now known as the classical or respondent conditioning paradigm, were defined as: (1) an automatic reflex response called the unconditioned response (UCR); 2) a stimulus, referred to as the unconditioned stimulus (UCS), that can elicit the UCR; and (3) a neutral stimulus which under ordinary circumstances does not elicit the UCR. Once the neutral stimulus (e.g., a bell) has gained the power to elicit the automatic reflex (e.g., salivation), the neutral stimulus is regarded as a conditioned stimulus (CS). Similarly, the automatic reflex (e.g., salivation) which was the UCR to the UCS (e.g., food) becomes the conditioned response (CR) to the CS (e.g., bell).

The importance of *Pavlov's* research was not in discovering the conditioned reflex, however, but rather in carrying out a systematic program that defined the characteristics of learned responses. In studying the relationships between stimuli and responses under varying conditions, *Pavlov* was the first to describe a number of principles governing these relationships. For example, he defined the CS and UCS pairing process as reinforcement, and the principle for establishing a conditioned or learned reflex, as repeated reinforcement. He also identified the principle of extinction; that is, a CS will lose the ability to elicit a CR if the CS (e.g., the bell) is repeatedly presented in the absence of the UCS (e.g., food). Among the other principles he described were spontaneous recovery, generalization, and discrimination. In fact, the systematic nature of his research yielded a description of most of the stimulus and response relationships that were to be more fully explored by later researchers.

The influence of *Pavlov's* research on the development of behavioral psychology was substantial. Even today, an emphasis on overt behavior and a concern for experimental methodology, as well as Pavlovian terminology, characterize the field of behavioral psychology. His contribution was, however, primarily methodological. Although he conceptualized the application of conditioning to human pathology, he did not attempt to define or engage in the treatment of human problems.

The use of conditioning as an approach to the treatment of psychiatric disorders was of central interest to *Bekhterev* (1857–1927) who, in addition to being a physiologist, was a psychiatrist of considerable stature. In 1907, *Bekhterev* opened a psychoneurological institute and established within it a program of experimental and applied research.

Bekhterev's research program at the Institute was related to his earlier work on reflexive motor behavior. In that work, he observed, as had *Pavlov* in his work with the digestive system, that motor reflexes could be evoked by a variety of 'neutral' stimuli. *Bekhterev,* too, began detailed studies of the phenomenon, which he called 'associative reflexes'. In his research, the associative reflex was established by pairing shock, which evoked muscle flexion, with a neutral stimulus which did not. *Bekhterev* demonstrated, first with animals and then humans, that a wide variety of auditory, visual, and tactile stimuli could acquire the power to evoke the reflex. Perhaps not surprisingly, he soon hypothesized that complex human behavior comprised a series of learned motor reflexes.

Bekhterev's [1933] combined clinical and research work led him naturally to propose that the study of personality would be conducted through the objective analysis of the relationship between a person's behavior and environment. Such an approach, which he called 'reflexology', would represent a 'new science', a science that he believed should and would replace the discipline of psychology.

Bekhterev's influence on the course and substance of behavioral psychology was not as great as that of *Pavlov*. His concern, and indeed his attempts to apply conditioning to the treatment of psychiatric disorders, however, did forecast the future of the field.

Animal Psychology – Learning Theory

In 1859, 4 years before *Sechenov* published *Reflexes of the Brain*, *Darwin* published *The Origin of Species*. The impact of evolutionary theory on psychology was multifaceted and far-reaching. It initiated not only the study of individual differences and mental testing, but also comparative and animal psychology as well. These latter areas flourished as the result of *Darwin's* proposition that continuity of both mental and physical functioning existed between human and animal species. Animal research could now be brought to bear on the understanding of human functioning.

Initially, the central focus of animal research, particularly in England, was to understand the animal 'mind'. Nonexperimental approaches characterized this work. In contrast, American researchers, no less interested in the 'mind', began to employ experimental methods and to focus on behavior. Animal 'learning' became an active area of investigation in American laboratories.

Historically, one major difference developed between the proponents of learning theory and the Russian school of conditioning. Central to the research of *Pavlov* and *Bekhterev* was the question of how various stimuli acquired the power to elicit reflexive behavior. Learning theorists, on the other hand, were concerned with the question of how specific stimuli acquired varying responses. The importance of this distinction by researchers in both traditions, however, was not discerned for several decades. In general, the differences between as well as among the theorists within the two schools were minimized in light of their similar emphasis on obtaining objective evidence through experimentation and the rejection of introspection.

The most prominent theory of learning[3] in the history of American psychology was that proposed by *Edward L. Thorndike* (1874–1949) in *Animal Intelligence* [1911]. Working primarily with cats, he identified a type of learning which he initially called 'trial-and-error'. He hypothesized that the basis of such learning was the association or 'connection' between sense impressions (stimuli) and impulses to action (responses). In a typical experiment, *Thorndike* placed a hungry cat into a locked 'puzzle box' that had a concealed mechanism operated by a latch. Food was placed outside the box. When the animal correctly manipulated the latch, the door would open and the cat would gain access to the food. Repeated placements of the cat into the box revealed that the random behavior and errors that characterized the first trial (length of time to solution) gradually decreased over trials until the animal was able to solve the problem without errors.

The 'connections' between a stimulus in the animal's environment (e.g., floor of box) and the animals response (e.g., clawing), *Thorndike* reasoned, was not established unless the response (e.g., pushing) produced an effect (e.g., gaining access to food). These latter responses, which he called 'instrumental behaviors', were learned because they were instrumental in leading the animal to its goal. *Thorndike* defined three 'laws' that governed such learning: the laws of Readiness, Exercise, and Effect. Central to his theory was the Law of Effect which, simply stated, referred to the strengthening or weakening of connections (stimulus-response or S-R learning) as a result of its consequences. That is, if a connection is accompanied or followed by a satisfying state of affairs (reward) the connection is strengthened (i.e., will recur); if the connection has been made and is followed by discomfort (punishment) the connection will be weakened. *Thorndike* later rejected the Law of Exercise and revised the Law of Effect by renouncing the proposition that punishment has weakening effects.

He came to believe that the laws governing animal learning were also fundamental to human learning. He also considered it important to explain complex human learning in terms of the simple learning manifested by animals, and he devoted considerable effort defining the application of his theory to problems of educational and social importance.

---

[3] Space does not permit an extended discussion of the many important figures in the field of learning theory. Among the major learning theorists whose contributions also added substantially to the development of behavioral psychology were: *Edward Tolman, Edwin Guthrie* and *Clark Hull.*

Thorndike is perhaps best known for his achievements in educational psychology. Although he was a rigorous experimenter and his research was objective, he, unlike the reflexologists, introduced concepts into his work that alluded to 'subjective states'. Consequently, he is often not recognized as a behaviorist. His emphasis on motivation and his use of such terms as 'satisfaction' and 'discomfort' led *Watson,* for example, to ignore the behavioral implications of *Thorndike's* work. Nonetheless, *Thorndike's* proposition that the consequences of a response will serve to alter that response was a substantial contribution to behavioral psychology.

Behaviorism

The 'behaviorist manifesto' was published in 1913 by *John B. Watson* (1878–1958). In it, he delivered a frontal attack on introspection, and argued that psychology should be an 'objective experimental science' whose goal was the 'prediction and control' of behavior. Despite the increasing acceptance of objectivism by psychologists both in the United States and abroad, *Watson's* declaration marked the beginning of behaviorism.

Watson's work, although highly influenced by both *Bekhterev* and *Pavlov,* developed independent of reflexology. He accepted the method of conditioning, but rejected the narrowly focused content area of reflexology. In the belief that psychologists should investigate more than discrete physiological responses, he turned his attention to verbal and emotional behavior. He considered these complex behaviors to be made up of integrated combinations of simple reflexes and proposed that the complex behavior as well as simple reflexes could be experimentally investigated.

The classic study of 'Little Albert' is *Watson's* final (he left the field for a career in advertising) and perhaps best known research. *Watson* hypothesized that three emotional responses (rage, fear and love) were unlearned and therefore basic to all complex emotional behavior. For example, the unlearned response of fear would naturally be evoked by such stimuli as loud sounds; more complex phobic fears, however, could be understood as conditioned responses originating from the unlearned response. To demonstrate this, *Watson and Rayner* [1920], selected a 9-month-old child (Albert) as the subject for their experiment. Three questions were posed: (1) could Albert be conditioned to fear an animal; (2) could the fear be generalized; and (3) how long would the fear persist? Initially, Albert was tested to determine that he was unafraid of a variety of animals (e.g., dog, rabbit, rat) and objects (e.g., blocks). Further, they demonstrated that the clang of a steel bar behind Albert's back would evoke a startle (fear) response from the child. 2 months later, they attempted to condition Albert to fear a white rat. To do so, the steel bar was hit each time Albert attempted to touch the rat. After a week of sound/rat pairings, Albert withdrew in fright when the rat was presented without the sound. Generalization of this response to other furry objects, including the white rabbit and the dog, was next demonstrated. Further, the conditioned fear reaction was specific to items similar to the rat (e.g., furry) and not to objects distinctly dissimilar (e.g., blocks). Testing a month later showed some persistence of the 'conditioned fears'.

Despite the methodological problems, the 'Albert' experiment proved to be a dramatic example of *Watson's* position. *Watson* had not only firmly established behaviorism in American psychology, but also furthered the movement toward the application of conditioning to human problems.

Operant Conditioning

Few movements, political or scientific, are born full term. Watsonian behaviorism was no exception. It was marked by a shortage of facts as well as premature and exaggerated claims about its future. The growth and development of the field resulted from the simplification of its objectives, the clarification of existing contradictory data, and the meticulous collection of systematic data. Major credit for these accomplishments belongs to *Burrhus F. Skinner,* a man whose name has become synonymous with behaviorism.

By the late 1930's the differences between the learning paradigms of Pavlov and Thorndike had been recognized and explained by a number of theorists [e.g., *Hull,* 1937]. Skinner's articulation of the differences between the paradigms and the ambiguities they presented, however, substantially changed the course and substance of behaviorism. *Skinner* [1935] asserted that two response classes could be distinguished in the paradigms; classes which he termed respondent and operant. The characteristics of these classes are as follows. Respondent behaviors are: (1) elicited by stimuli; (2) related to new and varied stimuli; (3) conditioned through reinforcement correlated with the stimulus; and (4) measured by the strength of their association to the new stimuli. Operant behaviors, on the other hand, are: (1) spontaneously performed or 'emitted'; (2) related to a given stimulus; (3) conditioned through reinforcement correlated with the response; and (4) measured by their frequency of occurrence.

Based upon the function of reinforcement in the learning paradigm, *Skinner* defined the conditioning of respondent behaviors as type S conditioning (reinforcement correlated with *stimulus*), and the conditioning of operant behaviors as type R (reinforcement correlated with *response*) conditioning. Type S or respondent conditioning is synonymous with Pavlovian or classical conditioning. Type R or operant conditioning refers to the paradigm defined by *Thorndike* in the Law of Effect. *Skinner* further noted that although an operant response could become stimulus-related, the stimulus does not elicit the response as a stimulus can elicit a reflex, but rather serves as a cue for reinforcement. For example, when the animal learns that pressing a lever will be followed by food, the lever (stimulus) will become the cue that food (reinforcement) will be dispensed if the lever is pressed (response).

Althouth *Skinner* clearly articulated the distinction between the two types of conditioning, he also elucidated the difficulties that existed in separating both the models and the responses in actual research. For example, a respondent behavior, such as a child's crying in fright, may be maintained by the consequences to that behavior. That is, if a parent gave considerable attention to the child's crying, the response (crying) could become an operant (crying to gain attention) as well as a respondent (crying elicited by a loud noise) behavior. Despite the ambiguities present in the models, however, the distinction that *Skinner* outlined had significant effects. Prior to *Skinner's* work, behavioral researchers had emphasized respondent conditioning as the explanatory basis of behavior. *Skinner* succeeded in shifting this emphasis to a focus on operant behavior. Further, his own detailed and programmatic investigations of operant conditioning provided the experimental foundations for contemporary behaviorism.

Operant conditioning is today the major behavioral approach used in the treatment of mental retardation. A more detailed discussion of operant conditioning, therefore, will be presented later in this chapter. It is important to note, however, that the principles and techniques employed in treatment are derived from experimental laboratory research, most of which was originally defined by *Skinner*. Unlike previous workers in the field, he was adamantly opposed to theory. His research program focused upon describing the lawful relationships between environmental events and behavior.

Applied Behavioral Psychology

The application of laboratory-derived behavioral principles and techniques to the *treatment* of clinical problems in humans, although initiated by *Bekhterev,* was greatly influenced by *Pavlov's* research on experimental neuroses in animals. *Pavlov* and his colleagues demonstrated that neurotic-like reactions in animals could be induced through experimental manipulations. These findings not only defined the role of learning in the development of emotional responses, but also suggested that maladaptive emotional behavior could be unlearned.

The demonstration of conditioned emotional responses in a human infant was reported in 1920 by *Watson and Rayner* (see p. 148). They also outlined, but did not evaluate, a number of therapeutic techniques that could be used to eliminate fear reactions. The investigation of these techniques was undertaken by *Mary Cover Jones* [1924], a student of *Watson.* Working with institutionalized children who had demonstrated fear reactions, *Jones* found that two techniques, direct conditioning and social imitation, could be used to eliminate a child's fear.

The use of conditioning to treat a wide variety of disorders, including addiction, alcoholism, and hysteria, became fairly common both in Europe and the United States during the 1920s and 1930s. Nevertheless, the systematic development of treatment techniques and etiological formulations based on learning theory were rarely reported. A notable exception was the work of *Mowrer and Mowrer* [1938] on enuresis. Working from a Pavlovian model, they derived a treatment technique and evaluated its effects on a large group of enuretic children. They also conceptualized the problem (i.e., inadequate habit training) and treatment of enuresis within a model of learning and contrasted that interpretation with a psychoanalytical formulation.

Throughout the 1940s, an increasing number of writers began to advocate learning approaches as conceptual and treatment alternatives to the dominant psychoanalytic position. During the 1950s concern over the split between clinical and experimental psychology led a number of theorists to attempt to integrate learning and psychoanalytic theory. *Dollard and Miller* [1950], for example, proposed a comprehensive theory. Although a classic in exposition, the work failed to generate research and did little to curtail the growing antagonism between 'applied behavioral' and clinical psychology.

The applied behavioral psychology movement was fully realized in the work of *Joseph Wolpe.* A South African psychiatrist, *Wolpe* became dissatisfied with the use of psychoanalytic techniques in the treatment of emotional disorders. Influenced by the work of *Pavlov* and *Hull, Wolpe* began to conduct research on experimental neuroses in cats. As a result of that work, *Wolpe* [1958] formulated the principle of reciprocal inhibition: i.e., the occurrence (induction) of a response antagonistic to anxiety in the presence of an anxiety-producing stimulus will serve to weaken the bond between the anxiety response and the stimulus. He used this principle as the basis for developing techniques (specifically, systematic desensitization) to treat neurotic reactions in humans.

Outstanding in many respects, his work was marked by clearly defined and testable hypotheses regarding therapy. It not only provided clinicians with behavioral techniques for the treatment of neuroses, but also stimulated an enormous amount of research as well.

The application of the principles and techniques of operant conditioning to clinical populations also began in the 1950s. Methodological rather than treatment goals, however, characterized applied operant work during that decade. Nevertheless, behavioral changes in the populations studied (mainly institutionalized psychotic and retarded individuals) led investigators to become increasingly interested in treatment. By the mid-1960s, operant procedures were widely used in the treatment of retarded and psychotic individuals.

Contemporary Applied Behavioral Psychology

Terminology

Today, behavioral psychology offers a number of treatment approaches that vary widely in conceptualization and methodology. Three somewhat broadly defined groups can be delineated: behavior therapy, operant conditioning, and cognitive behavior therapy. A number of other commonly used identifiers can be related to these groupings. For example, although the term *behavior modification* is often used interchangeably with behavior therapy, it is most commonly associated with the operant conditioning approach. *Cognitive behavior modification,* however, is more similar in conceptualization to cognitive behavior therapy than it is to operant conditioning. *Applied behavioral analysis* was introduced as a term to distinguish applied from basic operant research. Although the term can be considered synonymous with operant conditioning, not all behavioral psychologists who employ operant treatment techniques adhere to the philosophical or specific methodological requirements of applied behavioral analysis. Therefore, the term 'operant conditioning' seems more appropriate for classifying purposes.

Finally, *biofeedback* and *behavioral medicine* are best considered as distinct from the three above-identified groups. Biofeedback is primarily defined by the use of a specific apparatus as part of the treatment procedures. In general, data regarding a person's ongoing internal physiological functioning (e.g., heart rate) is 'fed-back' to the person by means of an apparatus (e.g., polygraph) in order to aid the person in changing the physiological response. Although initial work in the area relied upon extrapolations from the classical conditioning model (characteristic of the behavior therapy approach), operant methods are now commonly used. Most recently, the role of cognitive processes in biofeedback has received considerable attention [e.g., *Meichenbaum*, 1976; *Hoon* et al., 1977].

Behavioral medicine can perhaps best be described as an emerging field of study. In 1978, *Schwartz and Weiss* defined it as 'the interdisciplinary field concerned with the development and integration of behavioral and biomedical science knowledge and techniques relevant to the understanding of health and illness and the application of these techniques to prevention, diagnosis, treatment, and rehabilitation'. To some extent, behavioral medicine can be seen as evolving from the successful use of biofeedback in the treatment of medical problems. As the use of behavioral techniques unassociated with biofeedback apparatus (e.g., the use of operant techniques to 'treat' the problem of noncompliance with medication regimes) has become more common, other 'working' definitions of the field have been offered [see *Pomerleau*, 1979, for a review].

Commonalities and Differences among Approaches

Contemporary applied behavioral psychology is richly variegated. Nevertheless, all approaches within the field share at least one common feature. That is, the treatment of clinical problems is undertaken within an analytical and empirical framework. In general, treatment procedures are generated from psychological research and/or theory, and rely upon experimental findings. Outcome evaluation is considered a necessary component of treatment, and is conducted, at least in part, through the use of direct behavioral measures. Finally, behavioral psychologists assume that the acquisition, maintainance and modification of behavior is governed by principles of learning that are similar for both adaptive and maladaptive behavior.

Behavioral approaches differ along several dimensions. Among the most salient are: theoretical orientation, behavioral emphasis, treatment techniques, and methods of evaluation. Examples of the treatment techniques and procedures included within the three approaches are presented in table I. (Operant techniques are emphasized because of their use with retarded individuals.) The other distinctions are described below.

Table I. Examples of techniques within different behavior approaches

General behavioral approach	Technique	Procedure	Use
Behavior therapy	aversion	pair unwanted stimulus (e.g., cigarettes) with aversive stimulus (e.g., shock)	alter valence of a stimulus (e.g., cigarettes) to decrease behavior (e.g., smoking)
	covert sensitization [Cautela, 1967]	imagine engaging in unwanted behavior with negative consequence; followed by imagining alternative adaptive behaviors with positive consequences	decrease maladaptive avoidance and approach (e.g., drugs) behaviors, as well as substitute adaptive behaviors
	flooding [Marks, 1972]	repeated exposure to intense anxiety-provoking stimuli (real or imaginary)	decrease avoidance and anxiety-based maladaptive behaviors
	implosion [Stampfl and Levis, 1967]	same as flooding except psychodynamically relevant material, presented by the therapist, is used as the imaginary stimuli	decrease avoidance and anxiety-based maladaptive behaviors
	systematic desensitization [Wolpe, 1958]	pair relaxation with progressive series of anxiety-provoking images	decrease avoidance and anxiety-based maladaptive behaviors
Cognitive behavior therapy	anxiety-management training [Suinn and Richardson, 1971]	use systematic desensitization to teach a person to use relaxation as a self-control skill	develop coping skills
	disputing irrational beliefs [Ellis, 1971]	person instructed to self-ask and answer (on tape or written) 6 questions on irrational beliefs (e.g., can I rationally support this belief?	decrease irrational thinking
	modeling [Bandura, 1969]	therapist demonstrates ways to effectively manage a problem situation	develop adaptive behavior
	self-instruction [Meichenbaum, 1975]	therapist 'thinks aloud' with verbal statements designed to control behavior; person is taught to develop self-instructional verbalizations (first aloud, then covertly)	decrease maladaptive behaviors; learn new behaviors
	testing cognitions [Beck et al., 1976]	teach person to discriminate between thought and reality, and to treat thoughts as hypotheses rather than fact	decrease maladaptive thought processes

Operant conditioning	backward chaining	teach last element in determined complex behavioral sequence first–proceed backwards until complex behavior is learned (e.g., making a bed)	develop behavioral chain
	differential reinforcement of other behaviors (DRO)	reinforce any response individual makes except for one specific response; that is, person receives scheduled reinforcement except when engaged in the particular specified behavior	decrease maladaptive behavior
	errorless discrimination	arrange sequence of stimuli in such a manner as to insure correct response	develop behavior
	extinction	reinforcement of a previously reinforced behavior is discontinued	decrease maladaptive behavior
	imitation	match behavior of a model	develop new behaviors
	negative reinforcement	removal of unpleasant stimulus	increase/maintain adaptive behavior
	over-correction and restitution	perform response (hang clothes) to correct the consequences (e.g., clothes all over the floor) of an inappropriate behavior; repeated rehearsal of appropriate behavior	decrease maladaptive behavior
	punishment	contingent presentation of aversive stimulus	decrease maladaptive behavior
	reinforcement	contingent presentation of a positive stimulus	increase adaptive behavior
	reinforcement schedules	reinforce some responses, but *not* all, of a specific behavior – use of a 'schedule' (e.g. fixed ratio, variable ratio) to determine which response	maintain adaptive behavior
	reinforcer sampling	permit person to experience positive aspects of a stimulus	develop new reinforcers
	reinforcing incompatible behaviors	reinforce behavior that cannot co-exist with a 'maladaptive' behavior	decrease maladaptive behavior, increase adaptive behavior
	response cost	contingent withdrawal of specified available reinforcers	decrease maladaptive behavior
	shaping	systematic reinforcement of 'successive approximations' of the desired behavior	develop/extend new behavior
	stimulus change	the use of a stimuli that elicits or inhibits specific behaviors	decrease or increase behavior
	time out	removal of person from the opportunity to obtain access to reinforcement for a specified time	decrease maladaptive behavior

Behavior Therapy. Arnold Lazarus [1958], a student of *Wolpe,* introduced[4] the term 'behavior therapy' to describe the use of 'objective, laboratory-derived tools' in addition to traditional techniques in the treatment of neurotic patterns of behavior. In general, the term now refers to those behavioral approaches that employ techniques based upon the experimental and theoretical work of *Pavlov, Guthrie, Hull, Mowrer* and *Wolpe.* Mediational constructs, which explain the relationship between stimuli and responses (e.g. anxiety), are central to theory and treatment. The application of the principles of classical conditioning and counterconditioning are emphasized. Although covert behavior is often used in treatment procedures, such behavior is defined within a strict stimulus-response model. That is, unobservable constructs, such as imagined anxiety-provoking events, have been operationally defined and tied to stimulus-response reference points. Psychophysiological studies, for example, have shown that imagining a fear stimulus produces an autonomic arousal similar to that elicited by the actual stimulus. Behavior therapists tend to treat adults with neurotic disorders or addiction problems. Between-group research designs and statistical analyses are employed to evaluate treatment outcome.

Operant Conditioning. Applied operant techniques are derived primarily from the empirically established principles of operant conditioning elaborated by *Skinner.* Among the psychologists who employ these techniques, only applied behavioral analysts strictly adhere to *Skinner's* [1974] doctrine of radical behaviorism. In brief, *Skinner* rejects theory and considers covert behavior and cognitive processes as inappropiate data for study. Overt behavior alone is acceptable for scientific investigation, and the environmental influences on behavior are emphasized. A distinctive method of treatment evaluation is employed; single-subject designs[5] in which an individual's behavior is repeatedly measured over a period of time. For example, two or more behaviors of a given individual will be observed and measured prior to treatment. Once the usual patterns of behavioral activity are determined, intervention is implemented successively for each behavior. Treatment is considered effective if each behavior changes only when

---

[4] To be precise, the term 'behavior therapy' was first used by *Skinner* in 1953 to describe the studies he and his colleagues were conducting on the applicability of operant conditioning with psychotic patients. *Lazarus'* definition, which referred to techniques derived from *Wolpe's* work, was initially more widely accepted.

[5] A detailed discussion of the experimental designs employed in applied behavior analysis can be found in *Hersen and Barlow* [1976].

intervention is specifically implemented for that behavior. Operant conditioning has been used primarily in the treatment of children, institutionalized psychiatric patients, offenders, and retarded persons. A more extended discussion of this approach will be presented in the next section.

Cognitive Behavior Therapy. The role of cognition in learning was not ignored, and in fact was emphasized by many early learning theorists (e.g., *Tolman).* Nevertheless, the development of behavior change techniques that focus on the 'manipulation' of private, covert events is recent. The applied cognitive approach has been strongly influenced by the growth of the 'cognitive movement' in experimental psychology [*Neisser,* 1967]. Cognitive therapies are research-oriented and stress the role of cognitive processes (e.g., perception and thought) in the development of maladaptive behavior. A large number of investigators and techniques are included within this group, and three subdivisions have been identified by *Mahoney and Arnkoff* [1978]. These are: (1) rational psychotherapies, as represented by *Albert Ellis* [1962] and *Aaron Beck* [1976]; (2) coping-skills therapies, such as *Meichenbaum's* [1973] stress inoculation; and (3) the problem-solving therapies of, for example, *Spivack* et al. [1976]. Cognitive therapy has been used with a wide variety of problem behaviors. Statistical analyses and between-group research designs are used to evaluate treatment.

It should be noted that today, applied behavioral psychologists do not necessarily use techniques from one of the above-described approaches. Likewise, no *one* approach is solely used with the retarded population. Modeling and relaxation techniques, for example, can be used with retarded as well as with nonretarded individuals. Nonetheless, operant conditioning is by far the most widely used approach in the field. Therefore, a somewhat more detailed discussion of that approach is presented below.

Treatment of the Mentally Retarded

The successful use of operant conditioning techniques with retarded individuals has been well-documented [for reviews see, *Birnbrauer,* 1976; *Forehand and Baumeister,* 1976]. 'Treatment' goals with the retarded have focused primarily on the development of behavioral skills in the self-care, language, academic, social, and work areas. A wide variety of maladaptive behaviors have also been successfully treated with operant techniques. Among these are self-injurious behavior [e.g., *Peterson and Peterson,* 1968], aggressive behavior [e.g., *White* et al., 1972], and rumination [e.g., *Kohlenberg*, 1970].

Operant techniques and systems (e.g., token economies and contingency contracting) are derived from the basic experimentally-defined principles of operant conditioning [*Skinner*, 1953]. Reinforcement, punishment, extinction or the combination of these principles are the basis for most applied techniques (see table I).

In general, a principle describes the relationship between a behavior and its environment and is stated in terms of the effect of an environmental event (action/object) on the behavior. If an event has the effect of *increasing or strengthening* the behavior immediately preceding it, the effect is called the principle of *reinforcement*. There are two types of reinforcement. Positive reinforcement refers to the increase of a response that is followed by a 'positive' event (e.g., a child makes his bed and is *presented* with an allowance). Negative reinforcement refers to the increase of a response that is followed by the *removal* of a 'negative' event (e.g., a child who is being teased by another child, tells the teacher who removes the teasing child from the classroom). In both instances, the behavior (bed-making; telling teacher) will be strengthened. If a behavior is followed by the *presentation* or *removal* of an event that *decreases* the probability of the recurrence of that behavior, the environmental effect on that behavior is called the principle of *punishment*. Spanking a child (presentation – 'aversive' event) or taking away television privileges (removal of 'positive' event) are examples. (It should be noted that if an event does *not* have the desired effect, the event is *not* considered to be a 'reinforcer' or 'punishment'. Although a spanking may be a punishment for one child, it may not be for another.) Finally, the absence of a relationship between a behavior and an environmental event (i.e., no consequence follows the behavior) will also result in *decreasing* the strength of that behavior. In other words, if a previously reinforced behavior is no longer reinforced, the behavior will weaken (e.g., the child who makes faces at the teacher, a behavior that had previously received attention, is ignored). This effect is referred to as the principle of *extinction*. Reference to the procedure section of table I should help clarify these principles.

As can be seen in table I, a wide variety of operant techniques have been developed. The following abbreviated example is given to illustrate how a technique is chosen and used in the treatment of a retarded person. Typically, the initiation of programs to alter behavior proceeds through the following stages.

(1) *Description of the problem:* In the case of a simple or a complex problem, the first task for the behavioral specialist and the client (and/or their guardian) is to decide what needs to be changed. To do so, the problem is analyzed and defined in terms of observable and measurable *behaviors.* For example, a child's problem of 'hyperactivity' may include behaviors such as: not staying in seat during school, not completing school assignments, not following directions, biting nails, running around the room, and hitting other children.

Once the behaviors have been described, the relationship of the behaviors to each other as well as their effect on the overall adaptive functioning of the child are considered. For example, since remaining seated and following directions are necessary to completing an assignment, these behaviors should be altered before trying to change the assignment behavior. Further, staying seated will reduce running around the room behavior, and possibly hitting other children. Finally, the importance of changing these behaviors is determined by the effect they have on the child's school progress.

(2) *Observation and measurement:* Once the behavior(s) *(target behavior)* has been chosen and the general goal (e.g., remain seated) set, the behavior is observed and charted in order to measure its current status *(baseline).* The observations can be recorded in a number of ways. For example, one could count the number of times *(frequency)* a child left his/her seat during the entire school day *(total observation)* or during selected class times *(interval observation).* Likewise, one may measure the length of time *(duration)* a child stays in his seat. No intervention is introduced during the collection of baseline data (usually 1 or 2 weeks). The data is then used to specify the change desired and eventually to analyze whether the change has occurred as the result of the intervention. For example, a child may leave his seat on the average of 15 times a half an hour during a week of observation. Once intervention has begun, progress can be determined if the frequency of the behavior decreases from 15.

In addition to charting the behavior, attention is given to the environmental events that precede and follow a behavior since such information is useful in defining the intervention. The teacher's attention to this behavior, for example, may be reinforcing to this particular child. Altering the teacher's behavior would then be necessary.

(3) *Selection of goals and procedures:* The baseline data is used to specify the criteria to determine change. Terminal goals (remain in seat during class hours) are broken down into easily manageable small steps on the

basis of that data. If, for example, the child was in his/her seat only on the average of 4 min at one time, the first step criterion might be set for 5 min. Behavior change is not immediate, and the successful completion of short-term goals is reinforcing.

The target behavior and the type of change desired (e.g., increase or decrease), as well as the nature of the environment, suggest the type of procedure (see table I) chosen for intervention. For example, the child who does not remain in his seat is in fact seated at some time. Choosing a procedure to increase 'sitting' behavior (e.g., *reinforcement*) may produce the desired results. If one wanted to change the child's behavior of 'hitting other children', two procedures in combination could be tried, *reinforcing incompatible behaviors* (e.g., playing with others) and *time out*.

(4) *Selection of reinforcers and definition of contingencies:* Even if one is using a procedure that is not based on reinforcement (e.g., extinction), one rarely, if ever, designs an intervention that does not include reinforcement. Reinforcers are selected as appropriate to the individual being treated. Often the best way to do so is simply to ask the person who will receive it. Reinforcers vary with individuals and can range from a cookie to playing baseball.

The relationship between the targeted behavior and its environmental consequences as specified by the procedure (contingency) are next defined. That is, when the child sits in his seat for 5 min (targeted criterion behavior) he will be given a star on his chart. The reinforcer, then, is contingent upon performance of the response. It is given *immediately and consistently* after the response is performed.

(5) *Monitoring and modifying the program:* Once the intervention begins, the baseline data previously collected serves as the measure by which behavior change can be determined. During intervention the behavior is continually charted to determine the effectiveness of the program. Interventions are most often not immediately effective. In fact, the frequency of undesirable behaviors usually increases in the initial phase. Therefore, a reasonable period must elapse before a program is judged ineffective. If the person's behavior fails to change, a number of program features, such as weakness of reinforcer, lack of consistency, or inappropriate goals, may be at fault. If the program is successful, a change in reinforcement schedules (from continuous to intermittent) will serve to maintain the behavior.

The brief overview of operant conditioning given above is by no means intended to serve as a guide to action. Many aspects of the process have been de-emphasized (e.g., data recording and analyses) and many nuances of operant technology have simply been omitted. The outline has been presented in an effort to aid the reader to better understand the behavioral programs with which she or he might come into contact.

Postscript

Understanding is basic to communication. Retarded individuals, perhaps more than other persons in need of service, come into contact with a large number of service professionals from a variety of disciplines. The quality of service received by these clients is enhanced by our ability to effectively communicate with each other. To further that end, it is hoped that this chapter has provided the reader with a context for understanding.

References

Bandura, A.: Principles of behavior modification (Holt, Rinehart & Winston, New York 1969).

Beck, A.T.: Cognitive therapy and the emotional disorders (International Universities Press, New York 1976).

Beck, A.T.; Rush, A.J.; Kovacs, M.: Individual treatment manual for cognitive/behavioral psychotherapy of depression (University of Pennsylvania, Philadelphia 1976).

Bekhterev, V.M.: General principles of human reflexology. An introduction to the objective study of personality (Translation). (Jarrolds, London 1933).

Birnbrauer, J.S.: Mental retardation; in Leitenberg, Handbook of behavior modification and behavior therapy (Prentice-Hall, Englewood Cliffs 1976).

Boring, E.G.: A history of experimental psychology; 2nd. ed. (Appleton-Century-Crofts, New York 1950).

Cautela, J.R.: Covert sensitization. Psychol. Rep. *20:* 459–468 (1967).

Dollard, J.; Miller, N.E.: Personality and psychotherapy. An analysis in terms of learning, thinking, and culture (McGraw-Hill, New York 1950).

Ellis, A.: Rational-emotive therapy; in Jurjevich, Directive psychotherapy (University of Miami Press, Miami 1971).

Ellis, A.: Reason and emotion in psychotherapy (Lyle Stuart, New York 1962).

Forehand, R.; Baumeister, A.: Deceleration of aberrant behavior among retarded individuals; in Hersen, Eisler, Miller, Progress in behavior modification, vol. 2 (Academic Press, New York 1976).

Hersen, M.; Barlow, D.H.: Single case experimental designs. Strategies for studying behavior change (Pergamon Press, New York 1976).

Hoon, P.W.; Wincze, J.P.; Hoon, E.F.: The effects of biofeedback and cognitive mediation upon vaginal blood volume. Behav. Ther. *8:* 694–702 (1977).

Hull, C.L.: Mind, mechanism, and adaptive behavior. Psychol. Rev. *44:* 1–32 (1937).

Jones, M.C.: The elimination of children's fears. J. exp. Psychol. *7:* 382–390 (1924).

Kazdin, A.E.: History of behavior modification (University Park Press, Baltimore 1978).

Kohlenberg, R.J.: The punishment of persistent vomiting. A case study. J. appl. behav. Analysis *3:* 241–245 (1970).

Lazarus, A.A.: New methods in psychotherapy. A case study. S. Afr. med. J. *32:* 660–664 (1958).

Mahoney, M.J.; Arnkoff, D.: Cognitive and self-control therapies; in Garfield, Bergin Handbook of psychotherapy and behavior change; 2nd ed. (Wiley, New York 1978).

Marks, I.M.: Flooding (implosion) and allied treatments; in Agras, Behavior modification. Principles and clinical applications (Little, Brown, Boston 1972).

Meichenbaum, D.H.: Cognitive factors in behavior modification. Modifying what clients say to themselves; in Franks, Wilson, Annual review of behavior therapy. Theory and practice vol. I, pp. 416–431 (Brunner/Mazel, New York 1973)

Meichenbaum, D.H.: Cognitive factors in biofeedback therapy. Biofeedback Self-Regul. *1:* 201–215 (1976).

Meichenbaum, D.H.: Self-instructional methods; in Kanfer, Godstein, Helping people change. A textbook of methods (Pergamon Press, New York 1975).

Mowrer, O.H.; Mowrer, W.M.: Enuresis. A method for its study and treatment. Am. J. Orthopsychiat. *8:* 436–459 (1938).

Neisser, U.: Cognitive psychology (Appleton-Century-Crofts, New York 1967).

Pavlov, I.V.: Experimental psychology and other essays (Translation). (Philosophical Library, New York 1957).

Peterson, R.F.; Peterson, L.R.: The use of positive reinforcement in the control of self-destructive behavior in a retarded boy. J. exp. Child Psychol. *6:* 351–360 (1968).

Pomerleau, O.F.: Behavioral medicine. The contribution of the experimental analysis of behavior to medical care. Am. Psychol. *34:* 654–663 (1979).

Schwartz, G.E.; Weiss, S.M.: Behavioral medicine revisited. An amended definition. J. behav. Med. *1:* 249–251 (1978).

Sechenov, I.M.: Reflexes of the brain. An attempt to establish the physiological basis of psychological processes (Translation). (MIT Press, Cambridge 1965).

Skinner, B.F.: Science and human behavior (Macmillan, New York 1953).

Skinner, B.F.: About behaviorism (Knopf, New York 1974).

Skinner, B.F.: Two types of conditioned reflex and a pseudo type. J. gen. Psychol. *12:* 66–77 (1935).

Spivack, G.; Platt, J.J.; Shure, M.D.: The problem-solving approach to adjustment (Jossey-Bass, San Francisco 1976).

Stampfl, T.G.; Levis, D.J.: Essentials of implosive therapy. A learning-theory-based psychodynamic behavioral therapy. J. abnorm. Psychol. *72:* 496–503 (1967).

Suinn, R.M.; Richardson, F.: Anxiety management training. A nonspecific behavior therapy program for anxiety control. Behav. Ther. *2:* 498–510 (1971).

Thorndike, E.L.: Animal intelligence. Experimental studies (Macmillan, New York 1911).

Watson, J.B.: Psychology as the behaviorist views it. Psychol. Rev. *20:* 158–177 (1913).

Watson, J.; Rayner, R.: Conditioned emotional reactions. J. Psychol. *3:* 1–14 (1920).

White, G.D.; Nielsen, G.; Johnson, S.M.: Timeout duration and the suppression of deviant behavior in children. J. appl. Behav. Analysis *5:* 111–120 (1972).

Wolpe, J.: Psychotherapy by reciprocal inhibition (Stanford University Press, Stanford 1958).

Suggested Reading

The reader who wishes to gain a more sophisticated knowledge of behavioral psychology will find the following journals and books helpful.

Journals
Applied Behavior Analysis, Journal of
Behavior Research and Therapy
Behavior Therapy
Behavior Therapy and Experimental Psychiatry, Journal of
Behavioral Medicine, Journal of
Biofeedback and Self-Regulation, Journal of
Cognitive Therapy and Research
Experimental Analysis of Behavior, Journal of

Books
Bandura, A.: Principles of behavior modification (Holt, Rinehart & Winston, New York 1969).
Beck, A.T.: Cognitive therapy and the emotional disorders (International Universities Press, New York 1976).
Franks, C.M.: Behavior therapy. Appraisal and status (McGraw-Hill, New York 1969).
Lazarus, A.A.: Behavior therapy and beyond (McGraw-Hill, New York 1971).
Meichenbaum, D.H.: Cognitive behavior modification (Plenum Press, New York 1977).
Pomerleau, O.F.; Brady, J.: Behavioral medicine. Theory and practice (Williams & Wilkins, Baltimore 1979).
Skinner, B.F.: About behaviorism (Knopf, New York 1974).
Skinner, B.F.: Science and human behavior (Macmillan, New York 1953).
Yates, A.: Theory and practice in behavior therapy (Wiley, New York 1975).

For behavioral materials such as films, training manuals, and books for parents, the reader is referred to the Research Press catalog, Box 317730, Champaign, IL 61820 (USA).

7 Applications of Psychological Evaluation Methods

Vivian T. Harway, Edward Shapiro [1]

I. Psychological Methods in the Diagnosis of Mental Retardation

The current definition of mental retardation in the DSM III (1981) and the definition of the AAMD [*Grossman,* 1973] present mental retardation as a complex condition involving both intellectual subnormality and impairment in adaptive behavior and having its onset in the developmental years (i.e., before age 18). 'Mental retardation refers to significantly subaverage general intellectual functioning existing concurrently with deficits in adaptive behavior, and manifested during the developmental period.' This definition differs from traditional approaches in that it does not require that mental retardation be considered as essentially incurable and there is not an absolute insistence on regarding mental retardation as related to organic factors. 'Adaptive behavior' refers to functioning in the following areas:

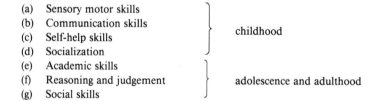

(a) Sensory motor skills
(b) Communication skills
(c) Self-help skills   childhood
(d) Socialization
(e) Academic skills
(f) Reasoning and judgement   adolescence and adulthood
(g) Social skills

This paper will consider briefly the role of the psychologist in the diagnostic process, to assist the physicians, in working effectively with the psychologist.

---

[1] Part I of this contribution was prepared by *Vivian T. Harway* and part II by *Edward Shapiro.*

It is necessary for impaired adaptive functioning to be associated with subnormal intelligence in order for an individual to be considered mentally retarded.

The psychologist thus is called upon to make this 'differential diagnosis' through the assessment of the adaptive level and the assessment of the intellectual level. A variety of methods and techniques are available to assist in evaluation and in planning for the treatment and habilitation of individuals considered to be mentally retarded. A list of tests commonly used in asessment is to be found in table I compiled by E. Shapiro.

Traditionally, Mental Retardation has been Considered Primarily as a Disorder Involving Subnormal Intellectual Functioning

From the pioneer work of Binet and Simon evolved the widely used Stanford-Binet intelligence scales, and the concept of the IQ as an expression of the ratio of an individual's observed level of functioning to the expected functional levels for his age-group. This also had the effect of defining intelligence for future researchers as a fundamental, innate and relatively unchangeable trait of human behavior. Extreme trust was placed in the IQ and as is usually the case when more is demanded of something than it can produce, it let people down. The IQ is a simple objective statement of a numerical relationship. It is as good as the normative sample from which it is derived. Its reliability is subject to vagaries of mood, climate and physical condition and to changes in environmental factors. It is subject to a statistical range of error (standard error of measurement). Different patterns of skills may contribute to a given IQ score, and this will have an important bearing on the assessment of the child's adaptive capabilities.

The IQ has fallen into disrepute in some areas and this is undeserved, too – it is a useful tool but not the only tool. Very good interpretive considerations for the Stanford-Binet L-M and the WISC tests are to be found in *Sattler's* book [1974, pp. 175–190].

For the complete psychological evaluation the intelligence tests are complemented by projective and other personality tests.

This traditional testing approach results in a report being written in a certain way – this is what this individual is like. This is his intellectual level. These are his needs, this is how he structures his world, how he responds to pressure, how he handles conflict, this is what makes him anxious, what motivates him.

Table I. Tests commonly used in assessment (compiled by *Edward Shapiro*)

Name of test	Age range	Type of test
Arthur point scale of performance tests	5–15 years	nonlanguage performance test of general ability (I)
Bayley infant scales of development	2–30 months	infants' general ability (I)
Blacky pictures	5 years and over	projective technique (I)
Bender visual-motor gestalt test	children and adults	diagnostic: intellectual impairment associated with organicity (I)
Cattell infant intelligence scale	3–30 months	infants' general ability (I)
Children's apperception test	3–10 years	projective technique (a downward extension of the TAT; I)
Culture fair intelligence test (Cattell)	4 years to adult	nonculture test of general ability; not dependent on language ability (G)
Durrell analysis of reading difficulty	grades 1–6	achievement test: comprehension of oral and silent reading, rate, word recognition and analysis (I)
Gates-McKillop reading diagnostic tests	grades 3–10	diagnostic: reading disabilities (I)
Gesell developmental schedules	4 weeks to 6 years	infant behavior development (I)
Goldstein-Scheerer tests of abstract and concrete thinking	children and adults	diagnostic: intellectual impairment (I)
Goodenough-Harris drawing test	5–15 years	nonverbal general mental ability (G)
Illinois test of psycholinguistic abilities	4–10 years	abilities and disabilities associated with communication (I)
Interim Hayes-Binet test for the blind	2 years to adolescent	special test for the blind: general mental ability (I)
Kuder preference record – vocational	grades 9–16, adult	vocational interests (G)
Leiter international performance scale	2–18 years	nonculture test for foreign-born and deaf children (I)
Lincoln-Oseretsky motor development scale	6–14 years	motor development: coordination and motor speed (I)

Test	Age range	Description
Machover draw-a-person test	children and adults	projective technique (I)
Make-a-picture-story test (MAPS)	6 years and older	projective technique (I)
Merrill-Palmer scale of mental tests	18 months to 6 years	nonverbal mental ability (I)
Minnesota multiphasic personality inventory (MMPI)	older adolescents and adult	self-report personality inventory (G)
Portous maze test	3 years to adult	nonlanguage test of mental ability
Progressive matrices (Raven's)	8 years to adult	nonverbal general ability (I, G)
Rorschach	children and adults	projective technique (I)
Rosenzweig picture frustration test	4 years to adult	projective technique (I)
Rotter incomplete sentences blank	adolescents and adults	projective technique (I)
Stanford-Binet scale (revised) 1973 – Terman and Merrill forms L and M 1960 – form L-M	2 years to adult (not standardized for older adults)	general ability (intelligence) (I)
Thematic apperception test (TAT)	children and adults	projective technique (I)
Vineland social maturity scale	birth to maturity, especially children	social maturity (I)
Wechsler adult intelligence scale (WAIS)	16 years to adult	general ability (intelligence) verbal and performance scales (I)
Wechsler-Bellevue intelligence scale, forms I and II	10 years to adult	general ability (intelligence) verbal and performance scales (I)
Wechsler intelligence scale for children (WISC)	5–15 years	general ability (intelligence) verbal and performance scales (I)
Wechsler preschool and primary scale of intelligence	4 ½ years; bright 3, dull 7 and over	general ability (intelligence) verbal and performance scales (I)
Wide-range achievement test	kindergarten to college	achievement in reading, spelling and arithmetic (I, G)

I = Individually administered; G = group administered.

The psychological report can 'zero in' on specific problem areas if these have been raised in the referral questions (and vagueness should be avoided in referrals) and can also recommend plans for remediation or resolution of problems.

Behavior Modification and the Mentally Retarded
This approach results from regarding the retarded individual from a viewpoint which emphasizes social adaptation skills rather than subnormal intellectual functioning.
Principles of learning from which behavior modification is derived:
(1) Behavior is controlled by its consequences. (2) Behaviors which are reinforced (rewarded) tend to be strengthened (repeated). (3) In the absence of reinforcement, behaviors will weaken and eventually fail to be emitted.
The principles and the application of behavior modification are presented in details elsewhere in this volume *(Yando; Latham and Yando)*.

Behavior approaches versus the more dynamic/analytic approaches:
Emphasis is on present level of the individual and future potential, rather than on past history. Emphasis is on what adaptational demands this individual's environment is placing on him and how the behavior may be 'shaped' to meet these demands, rather than on individual skills in coping with environment.

In the case of undesirable, unadaptive behavior, a study is made of what factors in the individual's environment are providing reinforcement (perhaps subtly and indirectly) for this behavior. Observation, record-keeping and manipulation of environmental reinforcement are key techniques. In the case of the child, often the parent may be used as an important observer, recorder, and also reinforcing agent. Standardized psychological tests are not often utilized.

Behavior modification techniques are not new. *Itard's* reports on the 'Wild Boy of Averyron' are classics of behavioral analysis. *Lightner Witmer's* case of 'Donnie' (1919) sounds almost 'modern' in his descriptions of trying to find out what would and would not motivate this small psychotic 5-year-old boy to turn his attention toward the outer world. What is 'new' is the systematization in the field of behavior modification, which has occurred only in the past 10–15 years.
The integration of behavioral and dynamic approaches in clinical practice is possible and often desirable.

The following three case vignettes illustrate the importance of supplementing traditional psychological assessment with a consideration of behavioral factors, and the opportunity for and nature of behavioral reinforcers in the background and present life situation of the child. Placement recommendations may then be made which truly reflect the childs' needs. All of these children were given a full battery of psychological tests.

Case 1. Amy, seen at 7 years, 2 months – eldest of 2 children in a close-knit three-generational rural family. Considered solely from the viewpoint of subnormal intellectual functioning, Amy was appropriately placed in a special class for the educable retarded. Her IQ on the Stanford-Binet was in the 50–75 range, although an accurate measure was never obtained because of wide variablitiy in interest and cooperation. In behavioral terms, Amy was noted to be quite articulate on the subject of animals, but to avoid responses to direct questions in almost all other areas. However, when direct questions were rephrased into shorter, highly structured integrating phrases, she was able to frame a brief, appropriate response before becoming rambling and tangential. Her play was highly idiosyncratic, and she resisted interpersonal interactions. Behaviorally, her performance more closely resembled a severely disturbed child who was having difficulty responding to usual social reinforcements, but who could be helped to learn to value a wider range of reinforcing experiences in her day-to-day life. A total, therapeutic behaviorally, oriented learning environment was recommended as more appropriate for Amy. Her response was positive. After 3 years she returned in a substantially improved state to a special class for emotionally disturbed children in her home school district.

Case 2. Marshall, seen at age 4 years, 11 months, with a history of severe environmental deprivation and neglect during the first 3 years of his life. Marshall was in institutional care in a children's shelter when he was seen. Expressive language was limited to single words, pointing and vivid gestures. He had severe articulation problems. Although his IQ was in the retarded range (Stanford-Binet IQ = 63), Marshall's behaviors in the testing situation suggested that he had been able to make good use of the limited range of positive reinforcements available to him in his early life to achieve close to age-level performances on tasks involving eye-hand coordination and visual discrimination. His learning patterns seemed to rely upon visual-motor experience rather than auditory-verbal experience. However, he did respond alertly and positively to praise for listening with persistent attempts to follow and reproduce auditory-verbal inputs. Placement in specialized foster care, plus enrollment in a language-enriched preschool were recommended. He remains in foster care and is adjusting well in a special class for learning disabled children.

Case 3. Lisa, seen at age 6 years, 11 months – youngest of 5 children, siblings aged 10–23 years – from an upper middle class family with highly stimulating home environment. Lisa was sociable and ingratiating in the testing situation. Her best performance was on vocabulary and language comprehension. She also was able to make simple visual discriminations, and could recognize and name letters of the alphabet. On cognitive, problem-solving tasks, Lisa was quite concrete in her conceptualizations on both verbal and nonverbal tasks. Her skills seemed to reflect a positive response to consistent environmental enrichment and positive social reinforcements, but the overall impression of problems in cognitive adaptation was supported by the wide range of tests administered. Lisa has adjusted well to placement in a special class for educable retarded children.

II. Steps toward Formulating a Behavior Management Program and Illustrative Case Samples

The following is an outline of the steps toward formulating an individualized behavior management program.

(1) Identify

(a) Target Behavior. Clearly define the behavior you wish to change. The behavior should be specified so that independent observers, not familiar with the child, can accurately observe the same behavior. For example, 'poor eating habits' is not a good behavioral definition. An acceptable alternative would be 'when eating with a fork, child drops 8 of 10 forkfulls on the floor, table, or clothing.'

(b) Reinforcers. The type of reinforcer that is useful in behavior management programs varies with each child. All individuals have specific likes and dislikes. Anything a child enjoys can be used as a reinforcer. This means games, academic tasks, gross motor activities, etc., as well as candy and other treats. Be aware through observation of what is reinforcing to each child.

(c) Goal of the Program. Decide before you start a program the criterion by which you determine success or failure. This will allow you to accurately assess your program in an objective manner.

(2) Baseline

(a) Behavior before the Program. It is important to know how bad is the situation you are trying to change before you start changing it. Therefore, it is necessary to establish a baseline rate of behavior. This tells you how often the behavior occurs in the natural environment before any manipulation is made to change it. In addition, a baseline may indicate that the behavior is not occurring as often as you thought and may not involve an elaborate program.

(b) Observe Antecedants and Consequences before the Program Starts. Many times we are not aware of *Why* a child does things. Instead, we concentrate on what *Maintains* the behavior. It is important to notice whether a child displays the target behavior only in certain places, in front of certain people, or after certain events. In short, what happened before and after the behavior occurred.

(3) Procedure

(a) Decide What the Procedure Will Be. Decide how the reinforcers will be applied. You need to state after what behaviors the reinforcer will be used as well as procedures to deal with periods of inappropriate behavior. Spell out *Exactly* how the procedures are to be followed.

(4) Data Recording

(a) Use a Method of Recording That Is Suitable to the Target Behavior. There are a multitude of ways to record data. The procedure used in each program should be the most efficient to allow one to observe the target behavior. For example, a simple frequency count (number of times the behavior occurs) would be good for a behavior that does not happen often during the day. However, a frequently occurring behavior may best be counted by only observing for short periods of time but repeating those observations several times per day. Be sure the method of recording used is feasible for the environment in which the data is being recorded.

(5) Re-Evaluation

(a) Decide before Starting How Long You Will Wait before Re-Evaluating. Before beginning a program, decide how long you will wait before changing anything. A good suggestion is to wait 3–4 weeks. At that time, observe the trend established by the data see whether the program is working. If it is not, re-think the program by changing one element at a time. For instance, if after 3 weeks a program has not decreased the target behavior, one would first change reinforcers, then look at antecedants, and finally change the contingencies. Each step is done alone and then evaluated before the next step is tried. If one change in the program proves successful, then the program is implemented fully.

   The following clinical cases illustrate the practical application of behavioral programs at the John Merck Program (at the Department of Psychiatry, University of Pittsburgh), an inpatient setting for emotionally disturbed mentally retarded children.

   The following case study *(E. Shapiro)* represents the first report of successful long-term elimination of aggressive-disruptive behavior treated with overcorrection, and is similar to findings of studies where self-stimulatory behaviors were reduced in children [*Freeman* et al., 1977; *Luiselli* et al., 1977]. In contrast to the adult studies of *Matson* et al. [1979] and *Rollings* et al. [1977], the target behavior in this study remained at a zero rate for 18 months without specific programming for maintenance.

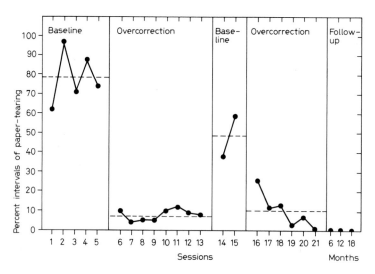

Fig. 1. Percentage of intervals in which paper-tearing was observed. From *Shapiro* [1978].

Case 1

Jane, a 5½-year-old, moderately mentally retarded, nonverbal girl, spent much of her free time shredding paper. In addition, she was frequently aggressive, often hitting and kicking. During the 4 weeks prior to implementing this procedure, she had destroyed many books on the unit. Previous unsuccessful attempts to alter the paper tearing behavior included making her stand in a corner immediately after ripping books and getting her interested in an alternate activity.

The procedure which was implemented in a reversal design to assess the effects of the treatment, consisted of restitutional overcorrection and positive practice. Immediately after Jane was observed tearing paper, she was instructed to pick up all paper she had torn and then clean the area for 2 min by placing all toys in the toy box and putting clothes in their proper place (restitution). This was followed by 5 min where Jane and the child care worker practiced looking through books without tearing them (positive practice).

Figure 1 displays the successful outcome of this procedure which was maintained over 18 months post-treatment.

Case 2 [from Shapiro and Klein, 1980]

Four children, aged 6–9 years (mean 8), functioning in the moderate to mild range of mental retardation, were selected for inclusion in a study to teach self-management of classroom behavior. All children were assigned three academic tasks to complete within a 30-min session. Tasks consisted of various developmentally appropriate activities such as sorting, matching, and identifying colors. Children were initially rewarded with tokens on a variable-interval schedule contingent upon being on-task as each interval ended. Tokens were exchanged for a variety of back-up reinforcers following each day's session.

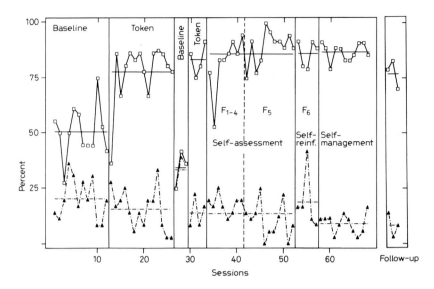

Fig. 2. Group mean scores for on-task (□) and disruptive (▲) behavior across phases. From *Shapiro* [1979].

Once the children had responded effectively to the teacher-based reward system, the children were trained in self-assessment and self-reinforcement through a series of verbal instruction phases. For the final phase, the teacher prompting and verbal instruction were faded and the children managed their token economy by themselves.

Results of the study displayed in figure 2 show that the mentally retarded, behaviorally disturbed children were capable of maintaining high levels of on-task behavior after being trained in self-management strategies.

Case 3 [from Barret and Shapiro, 1980]
Annie was a 7½-year-old, severely mentally retarded nonverbal girl, who has been observed to pull individual hairs from her head and ingest them. Attempts to eliminate the behavior through the use of verbal reprimands and redirection to activities that required the use of both hands proved ineffective.

After initial assessment found the behavior to occur mostly in the classroom, a treatment program was proposed. The procedure involved a verbal warning followed by positive practice overcorrection. Each time Annie pulls her hair, she is taken into an adjoining bathroom and required to brush her hair for 2 min. Prior to beginning the program, however, during a home visit the weekend before the program was to begin, Annie's parents shaved her head (a 'treatment' designated as response prevention) reportedly out of frustration. After a 3-month period, as Annie's hair grew back, she resumed pulling her hair and the program was implemented.

Results of the program were successful elimination of hair pulling. In addition, it was anecdotally reported that reductions in hair pulling had generalized to the unit and home.

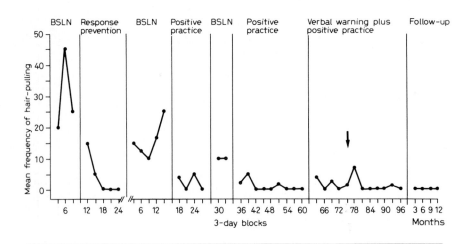

Fig. 3. Mean frequency of stereotyped hair-pulling per school day (9:00 a.m. to 12:00 p.m.) in 3-day blocks across all phases. Since the subject's head had been shaved, data collected within the response prevention phase of 'treatment' represents the mean frequency of attempts to pull hair. Interruption in the data collection following the 24th school day represents an actual time period of 3 months, during which the subject's hair was quite short and in the process of regrowth. The arrow at school day 75 indicates when the positive practice overcorrection procedure was implemented unit-wide and by parents on weekend home visits. From *Barret and Shapiro* [1980].

Follow-up data collected up to 12 months post-treatment found a continued elimination of the response (fig. 3).

Case 4 [from Barrett *et al., 1981]*

Two moderately retarded, behaviorally disturbed children, both nonverbal, were treated for stereotyped behavior. Julie (age 5), was frequently observed to suck her right index finger, resulting in chronic suppuration and infection of her fingernail. Jack (age 9), frequently exhibited tongue protrusion which contributed to a bizarre unsocialized appearance and a severe dermatologic condition (topical fissures) during the winter months.

Fig. 4. Tabulation of the results of behavioral program versus no treatment for stereotyped finger sucking. From *Barrett* et al. [1981].

Fig. 5. Tabulation of the results of behavioral program versus no treatment for stereotyped tongue protrusion. From *Barrett* et al. [1981].

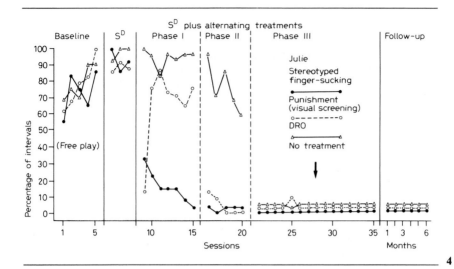

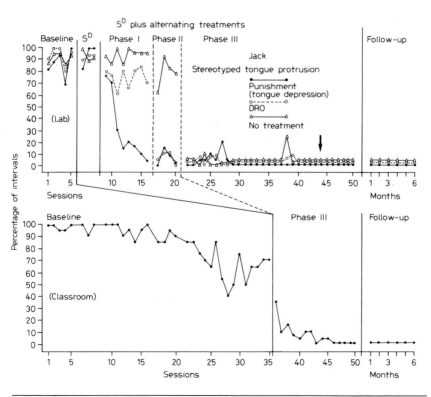

Unsuccessful attempts by the unit staff to reduce the behavior consisted of scoldings, Jack's parents used spankings, also, and praise for not engaging in the behavior.

Two treatments were designed to reduce the behavior. In each case, one treatment consisted of differential reinforcement of other behavior (DRO) in which a primary reinforcer (sugared cereal) was given contingently upon 10 s of nonoccurrence of the target behavior. The other procedure consisted of a type of punishment. For Julie, a contingent visual screening procedure was used. Each time she placed her finger in her mouth, the therapist placed his hands over her eyes for 10 consecutive seconds. For Jack, each time tongue protrusion was observed, the therapist placed a sterile tongue depressor lightly against Jack's tongue until Jack retracted his tongue into his mouth.

An alternating treatment design was used to evaluate the relative effectiveness of the two procedures in contrast to a no-treatment condition.

Results of the study can be seen in figures 4 and 5. For both Jack and Julie, both procedures were more effective than no treatment. More importantly, the punishment in both cases was much more successful in reducing the behavior than DRO alone. Follow-up data collected up to 6 months post-treatment found maintenance of the elimination of the behavior. In addition, in Jack's case, the tongue depression procedure when implemented in the classroom resulted in immediate suppression of tongue protrusion.

In summary, the use of psychological testing and behavioral modification methods are useful both in the differential diagnosis of mental retardation and in the treatment of retarded persons.

References and Recommended Reading

Anastasio, H.: Developing appropriate classroom behaviors in a severely disturbed group of institutionalized kindergarten-primary children utilizing a behavior modification model. Am. J. Orthopsychiat. *37:* 313–314 (1967).

Ayllon, T.; Azrin, N.: The token economy: a motivational system for therapy and rehabilitation (Appleton-Century-Crofts, New York 1968).

Azrin, N.H.; Foxx, R.M.: Toilet training in less than a day (Simon & Schuster, New York 1974).

Azrin, N.; Lindsley, O.R.: Reinforcement of cooperation between children. J. abnorm. soc. Psychol. *52:* 100–102 (1956).

Balthazar, E.E.: Balthazar scales of adaptive behavior for the profoundly and severely mentally retarded (Research Press, Champaign 1971).

Bandura, A.: Principles of behavior modification (Holt, Rinehart & Winston, New York 1969).

Barrett, R.P.; Shapiro, E.S.: Treatment of stereotyped hair pulling with overcorrection: a case study with long-term follow-up. J. Behav. Ther. exp. Psychiat. *11:* 317–320 (1980).

Barrett, R.P.; Matson, J.L.; Shapiro, E.S.; Ollendick, T.H.: A comparison of punishment and DRO procedures for treating stereotypic behavior of mentally retarded children. App. Res. ment. Retard. (in press 1981).

Becker, W.C.: Parents are teachers: a child management program (Research Press, Champaign 1971).

Bradfield, R.H. (ed.): Behavior modification of learning disabilities (Academic Therapy Publications, San Rafael 1971).

Browning, P.L.: Mental retardation rehabilitation and counseling (Thomas, Springfield 1974).

Carlin, A.S.; Armstrong, H.E.: Rewarding social responsibility in disturbed children: a group play technique. Psychotherapy: theory, Res. Pract. 5: 169–175 (1968).

Clark, F.W.; Evans, D.R.; Hamerlynck, R.A.: Implementing behavioral programs for schools and clinics: third Banff int. Conf. Behavior Modification (Research Press, Champaign 1972).

Ferster, C.B.; Perrot, M.C.: Behavior principles (Appleton, New York 1968).

Fischer, C.: On the way to psychological assessment as human science, (Xerox Publishers, Pittsburgh, 1974).

Gardner, J.E.; Pearson, D.T.; Bercovici, A.N.; Bricker, D.E.: Measurement, evaluation, and modification of selected social interactions between a schizophrenic child, his parents, and his therapist. J. consult. clin. Psychol. 32: 543–549 (1968).

Gardner, W.I.: Behavior modification in mental retardation (Aldine Atherton, Chicago 1971).

Gelfand, D.M.; Hartmann, D.P.: Behavior therapy with children: a review and evaluation of research methodology. Psychol. Bull. 69: 204–215 (1968).

Grossman, H.J.: Manual on terminology and classification in mental retardation (American Association on Mental Deficiency 1973).

Guerney, B.F.; Jr. (ed.): Psychotherapeutic agents: new roles for nonprofessionals, parents and teachers (Holt, Rinehart & Winston, New York 1969).

Haring, N.G.; Phillips, E.L.: Analysis and modification of classroom behavior (Prentice Hall, Englewood Cliffs 1972).

Harway, V.T.: Psychological assessment of the learning disabled child: a guide for parents, (Association for Children with Learning Disabilities 1971).

Hawkins, R.P.; Peterson, R.F.; Schweid, E.; Bijou, S.W.: Behavior therapy in the home: amelioration of problem parent-child relations with the parent in a therapeutic role. J. exp. Child Psychol. 4: 99–107 (1966).

Hewett, F.M.: The emotionally disturbed child in the classroom: a developmental strategy for educating children with maladaptive behavior. (Allyn & Bacon, Boston 1968).

Homme, L.E.; et al.: How to use contingency contracting in the classroom. (Research Press, Champaign 1969).

Johnson, S.M.; Brown, R.A.: Producing behavior change in parents of disturbed children. J. Child Psychol. Psychiat. 10: 107–121 (1969).

Knowles, P.L.; Prutsman, T.D.; Raduege, V.: Behavior modification of simple hyperkinetic behavior and letter discrimination in a hyperactive child. J. School Psychol. 6: 157–160 (1968).

Kozloff, M.A.: Educating children with learning and behavior problems. (Wiley, New York 1974).

Kuypers, D.S.; Becker, W.C.; O'Leary, K.D.: How to make a token system fail. Exceptional Children. 35: 101–109 (1968).

Lazarus, A.: Behavior therapy and beyond (McGraw-Hill, New York 1971).

Leff, R.: Behavior modification and the psychoses of childhood: a review, Psychol. Bull. *69:* 396–409 (1968).

Mager, R.: Preparing instructional objectives (Fearon Publishers, Palo Alto 1962).

Mitroff, I.: The subjective side of science, part 3 (American Elsevier, New York 1974).

Ney, P.: Symposium: therapy in child psychiatry; combined psychotherapy and deconditioning of a child's phobia. Can. psychiat. Ass. J. *13:* 293–294 (1968).

O'Leary, K.D.; O'Leary, S.: Classroom management (Pergamon Press, New York 1972).

Patterson, G.R.: Behavioral intervention procedures in the classroom and in the home; in Bergin, Garfield, Handbook of psychotherapy and behavior change (Wiley, New York 1971).

Phil, R.O.: Conditioning procedures with hyperactive children. Neurology *17:* 421–423 (1967).

Popovich, D.: Effective educational and behavioral programming for severely and profoundly handicapped students. A manual for teachers and aides (Paul Brooks, Baltimore 1981).

Poser, C.M. (ed.): Mental retardation; diagnosis and treatment (Holber, New York 1969).

Risley, T.; Wolf, M.: Establishing functional speech in echolalic children. Behavi. Res. Ther. *5:* 75–88 (1967).

Sarason, S.B.; Doris, J.: Psychological problems in mental deficiency; 4th ed. (Harper & Row, New York 1969).

Sattler, J.: Assessment of children's intelligence (Saunders, Philadelphia 1974).

Shapiro, E.S.: Self-management in educating mentally retarded, emotionally disturbed children (Unpublished doctoral diss., University of Pittsburgh, 1978).

Shapiro, E.S.: Restitution and positive practice overcorrection in reducing aggressive-disruptive behavior: a long-term follow-up. J. Behav. Ther. exp. Psychiat. *10:* 131–134 (1979).

Shapiro, E.S.; Klein, R.D.: Self-management of classroom behavior with retarded/distrubed children. Behav. Modification *4:* 83–97 (1980).

Skinner, B.F.: About behaviorism (Knopf, New York 1974).

Staats, A.W.; Minke, K.A.; Butts, P.: A token-reinforcement remedial reading program administered by black therapy-technicians to problem black children. Behav. Ther. *1:* 331–353 (1970).

Sulzer-Azaroff, B.; Roy, G.: Applying behavior analysis procedures with children and youth (Holt, Rinehart & Winston, New York 1977).

Tharp, R.G.; Wetzel, R.J.: Behavior modification in the natural environment (Academic Press, New York 1969).

Thompson, T.: Behavior modification of the mentally retarded (Oxford University Press, New York 1972).

Wetzel, R.: Use of behavioral techniques in a case of compulsive stealing. J. consult. Psychol. *30:* 367–374 (1966).

Williams, C.D.: The elimination of tantrum behavior by extinction procedures. J. abnorm. Soc. Psychol. *59:* 269 (1959).

Zifferblatt, S.M.: You can help your child improve study and homework behaviors (Research Press, Champaign 1970).

Yule, W.; Carr, J. (eds): Behavior modification for the mentally handicapped (University Park Press, Maryland 1980).

Films on Behavior Modification

All of the films below are 16 mm and sound.

Achievement Place. 30 min, b/w. Rental $5. The University of Kansas, Bureau of Visual Instruction, 6 Bailey Hall, Lawrence, KS 66044. Teaching family approach; small group home for delinquent children operated on very precise behavioral regime.

Behavior Modification: Teaching Language to Psychotic Children. 60 min, color. Rental $30. Appleton-Century-Crofts, 440 Park Avenue South, New York, NY, 10016. Can be borrowed from Behavioral Education Projects, Inc. An in-depth look at Lovaas' language training program; expands upon the segment in 'Reinforcement Therapy'. Not too good for beginners or parents; good for staff, with back-up discussion; raises issues of punishment.

Behavior Therapy with an Autistic Child. PHS No. MIS 895. About 20 min, b/w. Audio Visual Facility, Communicable Disease Center, Atlanta, GA 30333. An early film, demonstrating speech conditioning with one child; generally poor compared with Lovaas' films; adds nothing for experienced staff.

Chad, Who Has Far to Go ... 27½ min, color. Rental – inquire Dr. Irene Jakab, Western Psychiatric Institute and Clinic, 3811 O'Hara St., Pittsburgh, PA 15261. Through Chad's case, information is provided on the feasibility and the methods of psychiatric treatment and special education of double handicapped mentally retarded-emotionally disturbed children.

Changes Behavior Modification for the Mentally Retarded. 15 min, b/w. Rental $25. Sensory Systems, 4314 Abbott Ave., Minneapolis, MN 54410. Behavior modification in an institutional setting, primarily for attendant staff; similar to 'Teaching the Mentally Retarded' though not as good.

David. 28 min, color. Sale $400.00, rental $40.00. Distribution: Film-makers Library Inc., 133 East 58th St., Suite 703A, New York, NY 10022. David is spirited, verbal 17-year-old with Down's Syndrome, whose parents refuse to have him institutionalized. With support from his family and school, plus his own perseverance, he leads a rich life. He enjoys sports, makes friends easily and goes about independently. He shows success in his starring role in a TV drama about Mongolism.

Help for Mark. 20 min, color. Appleton-Century-Crofts, 440 Park Ave., South. New York, NY 10016. Demonstrating for parents a feeding and dressing program for their child; well done, with good introduction to step-wise teaching. Good introduction for parents.

Reinforcement Therapy. About 45 min, b/w. Rental, free, though long wait. Smith, Klein and French (Film Center), 1500 Spring Garden Street, Philadelphia, PA 19101. Three early behavior modification programs for autistic children, retarded children, and psychotic adults. First two, illustrating language training program (Lovaas) and programmed classroom (Birnbrauer) are excellent.

Rewards and Reinforcements in Learning. 25 min, b/w. Rental $15. Association for Precision Teaching, c/o Joyce Fridell, 316 Hamilton, Evanston, IL 60202. Behavioral techniques in remedial classroom for 'disadvantaged' and skill-learning for retarded. Despite some good demonstrations, not too useful; adds nothing new, and appeared to us as somewhat racialistic.

Step Behind Series. Three films: color. Rental $20/day. 'Genesis', 25 min. 'As Just for Little Things', 20 min. 'I'll Promise you Tomorrow', 20 min. Max Brachen, Hallmark Films, 1511 E. North Ave., Baltimore, MD 21213. The most complete step-by-step analysis of skill teaching we have seen; a bit tedious to the experienced, but very good for training. Films cover self-help, communication, and social skills.

Teaching the Mentally Retarded. 25 min, b/w. Southern Regional Education Board (Bensberg). Owned by the Federal State School (Mr. Mike McCoy, Director of Media Services). Made for training attendant staff; focuses on feeding, dressing and toileting severely retarded children. Good for basics.

The Broken Bridge. 60 min, color. Rental $44. Time-Life Films, New York. (Will soon be available from Behavioral Education Projects, Inc.) Language training of severely speech-deficient children; focuses on involving parents. Studies 3 children and centers around the approach of Dr. Irene Kassorla; novices in behavior modification will need a supplementary discussion to partial out what is behavior modification and what is Irene's striking, forceful style. A good film to stop mid-way, discuss, and then finish reviewing.

Sex Education Series. Educational Division, Hallmark Films and Recordings, Inc., 1511 East North Ave., Baltimore, MD 21213.

I. The ABC of Sex Education for Trainables (20 min/color/16 mm; rental $25, purchase $250). Brand new, enthusiastically received-sensitive and direct treatment of the how's and why's of training in this frequently neglected area – low on moralizing; high on credibility and information.

II. The How and What of Sex Education for Educables (20 min/color/16 mm; rental $25, purchase $250). Somewhat more sophisticated treatment including what to do on a date, at a dance, in a bed – and how to say no! – honest, clear presentation, will generate useful discussion.

III. Fertility Regulation for Persons with Learning Disabilities (18 min/color/16 mm rental $20, purchase $200). Most informative of the three methods of contraception, but mainly a lecture which might as well be presented in written form. Some implicit advocacy of sterilization. Provocative.

8 The Pediatric Neurologist's Approach to the Child with Mental Retardation

Raymond S. Kandt, Bernard J. D'Souza

Definition of Mental Retardation

'Mental retardation refers to significantly subaverage general intellectual functioning existing concurrently with deficits in adaptive behavior, and manifested during the developmental period' [29]. This definition specifically does not include comment about etiology or prognosis but instead refers to the current behavior. To be significantly subaverage, the intelligence quotient (IQ) must be less than 70 on the Wechsler Intelligence Scale for Children (Revised) and the child must be unable to meet the standards of personal independence and social responsibility expected of his age and cultural group. In the older child, examples of adaptive behavior include concepts of time and money, self-directed behaviors, social responsiveness and interactive skills [29].

Although there is agreement on the IQ score used to define mental retardation (IQ less than 70), there is disagreement as to the subtype classifications (table I).

Table I. Subtype classifications of mental retardation (MR)

Subtypes of MR	IQ Level	
	American Psychiatric Association [4]	American Association on Mental Deficiency [29]
Mild	50–70	55–69
Moderate	35–49	40–54
Severe	20–34	25–49
Profound	19 and below	24 and below

Identification

In early childhood, developmental milestones are well standardized, and failure to achieve these milestones reflects either a static or progressive deficit. Important milestones reflecting intellectual ability are the language milestones. Although motor milestones such as sitting and walking are easily remembered by parents and frequently asked about by physicians, they are much less helpful in the identification of mental handicap than are the language milestones. Most children with mild or moderate mental retardation have normal motor milestones unless there is concomitant cerebral palsy or a degenerative process involving the motor system. Hence, identification of the mentally impaired younger child is achieved by asking the parents about the language milestones (table II) [1].

In the older child, rather than reviewing each milestone, it may be more valuable to ask the parent general questions such as whether or not the child was slow in smiling or speaking. This is because the further one gets from the age at which the milestone was achieved, the more faulty is the mother's memory [33]. Parents are generally concerned when a milestone is delayed [33], even if they do not recall the exact age of its achievement. Since speaking in sentences is generally remembered as occurring earlier than it actually does [33], a history that the child was late in speaking in sentences may be especially significant. It is also very helpful to ask of a child's caretaker a question such as, 'How old a child does John act (or think) like?' It is remarkable how accurate the parent's estimate of mental age can be.

Table II. Language milestones

Language milestones	Attainment
Social smiling	6 weeks
Cooing	3 weeks
Babbling	6 months
'Mama' or 'dada' (used indiscriminately)	8 months
'Mama' or 'dada' (used appropriately)	10 months
First word (other than the name of a person)	11 months
Two-word sentences	2 years
Three-word sentences and also the use of pronouns, plurals and prepositions	3 years
Counts to 3 and knows two to three colors	4 years
Follows three-step commands	5 years

In the school-age child, poor school achievement is an obvious way to identify the impaired child. One may ask the child to read simple selections or to perform simple math problems. However, at this age (school age), mental processes have reached such complexity that psychological testing should be performed if one is suspicious about the child's intellectual function. Frequently, psychometric testing has already been performed in the school.

Many children are referred to the psychiatrist because of behavioral problems and/or inadequate school achievement. Although these may be independent, the behavioral problem is frequently due to the child's frustration and may be alleviated by proper educational placement. Specific learning disabilities frequently present in this way as may degenerative processes of the central nervous system. Children with hepatolenticular degeneration (Wilson's disease) may manifest many types of psychiatric disturbance (e.g. adolescent-adjustment reaction, bizarre behavior, anxiety-neurosis, mania, depression, psychosis, hysteria, schizo-affective disorder, or even schizophrenia) and are often seen primarily by a psychiatrist [9, 17, 55, 76]. Neuronal ceroid lipofuscinosis (Batten's disease), subacute sclerosing panencephalitis, and congenital syphilis may present primarily as psychiatric disturbances and/or school failure.

Evaluation

History

Having identified a mental impairment, it is essential to determine the onset and progression. Drawing a graph with the parents while taking the history is quite helpful (fig. 1). In this way, it is easy to define either a static process with onset prenatally, postnatally, or at birth and associated with absent or slow development versus a degenerative process. It is somewhat more difficult to determine the static versus progressive nature of a process if the child was initially normal and then stopped progressing. Although the child has not yet begun to regress (i.e. lose milestones), lack of progress, when considering the dynamic nature of development, may represent the onset of a slowly degenerative disease. Repeated examinations are frequently required to make this distinction.

While taking the history, one can categorize the disorder chronologically with regard to onset. Useful chronological divisions include prenatal, perinatal, postnatal and undecided age of onset [70]. For example, a

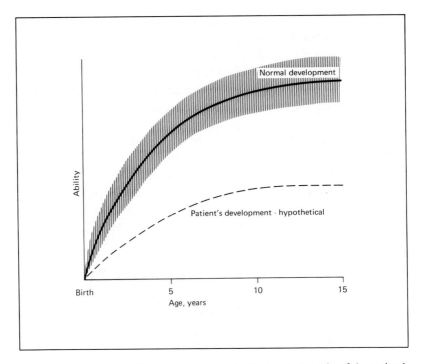

Fig. 1. A graph such as this may be used to clarify the relationship of the patient's development to normal development. It may also be helpful when explaining the situation to the parents [from 22].

Table III. Classification of mental impairment by *apparent* age at onset [67]

I.   Prenatal problem in morphogenesis (53% of cases)
     A. Single defect in development of brain (33% of category I)
        1. Microcephaly, primary
        2. Hydrocephaly
        3. Hydranencephaly
        4. Defect of neural tube closure
        5. Other types of cerebral dysgenesis
     B. Multiple major and minor non-CNS malformations (66% of category I)
        1. Chromosomal abnormalities (27% of category I)
           a. Trisomy 21 (most common)
           b. Fragile-X syndrome (added to the table by the current authors)
           c. Others
        2. Known nonchromosomal syndromes (12% of category I)
        3. Unknown patterns of malformation (27% of category I)

Table III (cont.)

C. Enzymatic defects of metabolism (the rare disorders of Leroy I-cell disease and generalized gangliosidosis present in the perinatal period, however, almost all other metabolic disorders have the onset of dysfunction in the postnatal phase)
D. Prenatal infectious diseases
E. Hypothyroidism

II. Perinatal insult to brain (3% of cases; neonatal maladaptation may be secondary to a prenatal defect)
   A. Hypoxemia
   B. Kernicterus
   C. Neonatal hypoglycemia
   D. Intracerebral hemorrhage
   E. Meningitis
   F. Sepsis
   G. Prematurity
   H. Prenatal infectious diseases
   I. Hypothyroidism

III. Postnatal brain dysfunction (4% of cases)
   A. Environmental insults
      1. Trauma
      2. Meningitis
      3. Encephalitis
      4. Hypernatremia
      5. Water intoxication
      6. Severe hypoxemia
      7 Lead intoxication
   B. CNS degenerative disorders
   C. Enzymatic defects of metabolism
      1. Amino acids (including phenylketonuria)
      2. Carbohydrates
      3. Uric acid
      4. Mucopolysaccharides
      5. Brain lipids
   D. Prenatal infectious diseases
   E. Hypothyroidism

IV. Undecided age at onset (40% of cases)
   A. Hypothyroidism
   B. Prenatal infectious diseases
   C. Sex chromosome abnormalities (e.g., Klinefelter's syndrome, XXX, etc.)
   D. Phenylketonuria
   E. Unknown cause (majority of cases in group IV are in this category)

retarded child whose history reveals decreased fetal movements during pregnancy, delayed milestones from the onset, and whose examination shows multiple non-central nervous system (CNS) malformations can easily be placed in the category of prenatal onset. In contrast, a child whose milestones were normal until the age of 3 years when he suffered meningitis with resultant halting of intellectual progress clearly fits in the category of postnatal onset. Various disorders occur relative to these chronological divisions (table III). Most mentally retarded children will be classified in the prenatal (44–53%) or undecided (40–41%) age of onset categories [39, 70]. It should be noted that prenatal infectious diseases and hypothyroidism may present clinically in any of these chronological categories of onset [70]. Although a perinatal event may appear to be causative, a primary defect in brain morphogenesis or an intrauterine insult (e.g. infection) often predisposes to neonatal adaptive problems such as apnea, hypoglycemia, hypoxia, hyperbilirubinemia, etc. Clues to a primary prenatal defect include a history of depressed fetal activity, the presence of non-CNS malformations, and intrauterine growth retardation.

Important historical features include: (1) the course and duration of the pregnancy with reference to toxins (such as maternal use of alcohol or other drugs, radiation exposure), maternal infections, trauma, onset and quality of fetal activity, and polyhydramnios; (2) labor and delivery; (3) immediate neonatal course (Apgar score, weight, head circumference, cyanosis, jaundice, seizures, vomiting, congenital malformations, duration of postnatal hospital stay – a child who has gone home at age 2–3 days rarely has had significant neonatal problems); (4) developmental milestones; (5) CNS infections such as meningitis, encephalitis or brain abscess; (6) head trauma; (7) medical conditions that may have caused CNS damage, such as hypoxemia secondary to cardiopulmonary disease or electrolyte imbalance secondary to various infections; (8) abnormal behavior such as teeth grinding (bruxism), aggression, self-injury, head-banging or other stereotyped movements, excessive masturbation, etc.; (9) associated conditions such as epilepsy, cerebral palsy, deafness, or blindness; (10) family history; (11) psychosocial history; (12) toxin exposure (e.g. lead).

Since most inherited degenerative diseases of the central nervous system exhibit recessive inheritance or represent sporadic mutations, family history is likely to be negative. However, parental consanguinity, a maternal or family history of stillbirths, or institutionalized siblings increases the risk of an inherited condition. Huntington's chorea, a dominantly inherited condition, may occur in children, and the family history will usually be positive.

In most cases, mild mental retardation is due to psychosocial factors, low socioeconomic level with its associated poor learning environment and poor medical care, or polygenic inheritance [26]. Chronic lead intoxication, however, can be manifest as mild retardation or behavioral problems similar to those of the attentional deficit disorder [53]. When confronted with a family in which there are multiple mildly retarded children, the mother should be tested for phenylketonuria [10, 25, 41, 45]. In contrast to mildly retarded children who often come from deprived environments, severely, and profoundly retarded children come from all socioeconomic classes [26].

Physical Examination

Complete physical examination is necessary. Measurement of head circumference should never be omitted. When plotted on a growth chart, the head circumference curve should follow the same trend as the weight curve [36]. Since children who suffer central nervous system disease after 1 year of age generally have normal head circumference, microcephaly suggests the onset of the disease process prior to 1 year of age [36].

When evaluating a child, it is good to formulate an overall gestalt. That is, does the child appear sick or healthy, good-looking or funny-looking (dysmorphic), or does the child have an abnormal affect? If a child with mental retardation has three or more major plus minor anomalies, there is a high likelihood that the retardation had a prenatal onset. 71 % of the minor anomalies can be discovered by examining the hands, eyes, face, mouth, and ears [69]. Examples of such minor anomalies include epicanthal eyefolds, slanted palpebral fissures, protruding and slanting ears, low-set ears, narrow maxilla (high-arched palate), moderate micrognathia, simian crease of the palm (fig. 2), clinodactyly of the fifth finger.

Some specific disorders and syndromes associated with mental retardation can be identified or suspected by physical examination. Hypothyroidism is the most common endocrine cause of mental retardation and is characterized by short stature with increased upper-to-lower ratio, dry brittle hair and dry skin, depressed nasal bridge, coarse face, thick tongue and thick eyelids, and sometimes a goiter. Congenital hypothyroidism occurs in 1 out of 3,500–4,000 births [24] and in the neonatal period the child may not have the typical features listed above. Neonatal screening for hypothyroidism is performed in many areas of the United States at the time of phenylketonuria screening. Neurofibromas and café au lait spots are typical of neurofibromatosis which may also be associated with mental retardation and/or seizures. Features of tuberous sclerosis include the classical triad of seizures, mental retardation, and skin lesions (angiofibromas – incorrectly called adenoma sebaceum, depigmented nevi, shagreen patches, and subungual fibromas). However, it has now

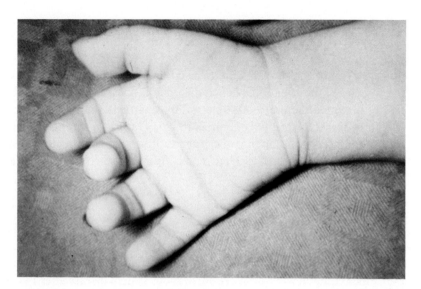

Fig. 2. Single midpalmar crease (simian crease).

become apparent that many children with tuberous sclerosis are not mentally retarded [28]. Coarse facial features, vertebral and other skeletal anomalies, corneal opacities, cherry-red spots of the retinal maculae, or visceromegaly should suggest a hereditary storage disorder. An abnormal skin or urinary odor suggests an aminoaciduria or an organic aciduria. Wiry or brittle hair occurs in kinky hair disease (Menke's disease) and argininosuccinic aciduria.

The only relatively common metabolic disorder associated with mental retardation is phenylketonuria, which may have the features of eczema, hyperactivity, seizures, hypotonia, and autistic-like behavior. With widespread neonatal screening and early treatment, phenylketonuria has markedly decreased as a cause of mental retardation.

Both autosomal and sex chromosome abnormalities are associated with mental retardation. The most common recognizable syndrome associated with mental retardation is trisomy 21 (synonyms include Down's syndrome and mongolism). This autosomal chromosome syndrome is usually associated with severe mental retardation, but uncommonly, the retardation may be mild [14, 26]. Characteristic features of trisomy 21 include hypotonia, flat face, upward slanting palpebral fissures (mongoloid slant), Brushfield spots of the iris (fig. 3), prominent tongue and small ears. A simian crease of the palms occurs in 45% and incurving of the fifth digit (clinodactyly) in 50%. The nose is generally small with a depressed nasal bridge and the eyes have a tendency toward inner epicanthal folds [67]. Trisomy 13 and trisomy 18 will not be reviewed here because the mental retardation is profound and most of these infants die by 2 years of age. The chromosome deletion syndromes are extremely rare but should be identified because many of them result from a parent with a balanced translocation. In this situation, genetic counseling is very important. The mental retardation ranges from severe to mild. Although variable, frequent physical findings in the chromosomal deletion syndromes include microcephaly, hypoto-

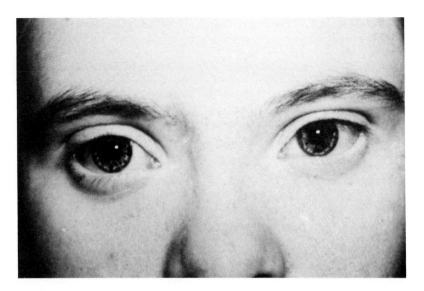

Fig. 3. Brushfield's spots of the iris.

nia, hypertelorism, epicanthal folds, slanting of the palpebral fissures, ear abnormalities, imperforate anus, congenital heart disease and short stature.

A relatively recently recognized sex chromosome condition is that of X-linked mental retardation caused by the fragile-X syndrome. It has been estimated that this is the second most common cause of mental retardation that can be specifically diagnosed [27], the most common cause being trisomy 21. Features suggestive of the fragile-X syndrome include enlargement of the testes in a postpubertal boy and a family history of retarded boys. 75% of the boys with the fragile-X syndrome are mildly retarded (IQ 50–70) while 25% have an IQ less than 50 [30]. Approximately 20–30% of females heterozygous for the fragile-X chromosome will be mentally retarded [73]. Antenatal diagnosis of this condition is not currently availabe. After the fragile-X syndrome, Klinefelter's syndrome (XXY genotype) is the most common of the male phenotype sex chromosome abnormalities associated with mental retardation. It has the features of hypogenitalism, gynecomastia, long legs, and behavioral problems.

The most common sex chromosomal abnormality in the phenotypic female is XXX. Minor physical anomalies such as epicanthal folds, clinodactyly, and wide-set eyes may be noted. The association of XXX with mental retardation has been biased by screening for chromosomal abnormalities in institutions for the mentally retarded. The proportion of normal females with the XXX genotype is unknown. The very rare female genotypes of XXXX and XXXXX are all associated with mental retardation and have similar minor anomalies as those listed for the XXX genotype. Radioulnar synostosis and congenital heart disease may be additional findings in the multi-X genotypes. Turner's syndrome (XO genotype) is much less commonly associated with mental retardation and has the characteristic features of female phenotype, ovarian dysgenesis with absent secondary sexual

Table IV. Dysmorphic conditions (nonchromosomal) associated with mental retardation [5, 13, 15, 34, 38, 67]

Condition	Etiology	Common physical findings
Cerebral gigantism	unknown	macrocephaly, prenatal onset of excessive size, downslanting palpebral fissures, coarse face, large hands and feet
Seckel's bird-headed dwarfism	AR	severe short stature, facial hypoplasia and prominent nose, microcephaly
Rubinstein-Taybi syndrome	unknown	broad thumbs and toes, strabismus, downslanting palpebral fissures, narrow palate, beaked nose, very short stature
Prader-Willi syndrome	unknown	'H$_3$O': hypotonia, hypogonadism, hypomentia and obesity
Lawrence-Moon-Biedl syndrome	AR	obesity, retinitis pigmentosa, polydactyly and/or syndactyly, hypogenitalism
De Sanctis-Cacchione syndrome	AR	Xeroderma pigmentosa, microcephaly, hypogonadism, mental deterioration
Smith-Lemli-Opitz syndrome	AR	microcephaly, toe syndactyly (less commonly polydactyly), hypospadias, anteverted nostrils
Cornelia de Lange syndrome	unknown	synophrys (fusion of the eyebrows), increased body hair, thin upper lip, short or small limbs, short stature
Oral-facial-digital syndrome	dominant (autosomal or X-linked)	clefts of lip, tongue, or palate; pseudohypertelorism, shortening and incurving of digits; variable intelligence with average IQ of 70; lethal in the male, hence, all cases are female
Oculocerebrorenal syndrome of Lowe	X-linked	cataract, hypotonia, renal dysfunction, and osteoporosis
Pseudohypoparathyroidism	probably X-linked dominant	short fourth and fifth metacarpals, short stature, poor tooth enamel, obesity, subcutaneous calcification, variable hypocalcemia with seizures, variable intelligence with average IQ of 60
Acrocephalosyndactyly syndromes (Apert's and Carpenter's syndromes)	AR and AD	craniostenosis, syndactyly, irregular mental retardation
William's syndrome	unknown	prominent lips, hoarse voice, variable cardiac anomalies, outgoing and loquacious personality, average IQ 56, 1/6 with severe behavior problems, outturning of great toe

Table IV (cont.)

Condition	Etiology	Common physical findings
Noonan syndrome	unknown	males only, webbing of the neck, pectus excavatum, cryptorchidism, pulmonary stenosis, short stature
Multiple lentigines syndrome (LEOPARD)	AD	*l*entigines (freckles), *E*KG abnormalities, *o*cular hypertelorism, *p*ulmonic stenosis, *a*bnormal genitalia, *r*etardation of growth, *d*eafness, irregular mental retardation
Cockayne's syndrome	AR	senile-like appearance, retinal degeneration, moderate deafness, skin photosensitivity, weakness with peripheral neuropathy, microcephaly
Fetal alcohol syndrome	maternal alcoholism	growth deficiency, mild to moderate mental retardation, irritable infant and hyperactive child, short palpebral fissures, hypoplastic philtrum (the infranasal depression); thinned upper vermilion, short nose
Fetal hydantoin syndrome	maternal phenytoin (Dilantin) use during pregnancy	growth deficiency, hypoplastic nails, microcephaly, mental deficiency, broad or depressed nasal bridge (syndrome occurs in 11% of infants exposed to phenytoin in utero)
Fetal trimethadione syndrome	maternal trimethadione use during pregnancy	variable malformations with cardiac defects; mild midface hypoplasia; unusual upslanting eyebrows, growth deficiency
Fetal warfarin syndrome	maternal warfarin use during pregnancy	hypoplastic nasal cartilage, stippled epiphyses, variable hypotonia and seizures
Congenital rubella syndrome	maternal rubella infection during pregnancy	microcephaly, deafness, cataract, patent ductus arteriosus

AR = Autosomal recessive inheritance; AD = autosomal dominant inheritance.

characteristics, short stature, 'shield' chest with widely spaced nipples, webbed neck, and short fifth metacarpals.

There are many other dysmorphic syndromes associated with mental retardation. The number of recognized dysmorphic and metabolic conditions has so increased in the past few decades that it is nearly impossible for any physician to memorize them all [26]. A catalogue such as *David Smith's Recognizable Patterns of Human Malformation* [67] is an excellent resource. An appendix is included in which various physical and metabolic findings are cross-referenced with the numerous syndromes in which they occur. For instance, if an adolescent, retarded boy with behavior problems is examined and found to have hypogenitalism, long auricles, and large teeth, a perusal of the appendix shows that the only syndrome listed under all three of these physical findings is XXY, which is the genotype of Klinefelter's syndrome. One is referred to the page on which Klinefelter's syndrome is described and the further physical findings of long legs and gynecomastia can be confirmed. If a buccal smear shows a single Barr body, a karyotype (chromosome assay) can be performed and confirm the diagnosis of Klinefelter's syndrome. Features of some of the more easily recognized dysmorphic conditions are listed in table IV. If the use of table IV and one of the catalogues of mental retardation syndromes has not enabled one to identify the syndrome, consultation with a geneticist is advisable. This is suggested because identification of an inherited condition may enable one to counsel the parents regarding both the chances of having a subsequent affected child and the prognosis for the current child.

Neurological Examination

A brief review of the neurological examination is provided below. For a more comprehensive discussion of the exam, the reader is referred to *Dodge* [18]. In addition to the mental status, a complete neurological examination should include assessment of the cranial nerves, especially funduscopic exam, eye movements, vision, and hearing; motor system, including strength, tone and reflexes; sensation; cerebellar function and gait. The findings of abnormal movements, distorted posture (dystonia), or myoclonic jerks should raise the suspicion of an organic illness.

The mental status, depending on the age of the child, is assessed with regard to alertness, curiosity, obsessional habits, memory, affect, orientation, speech, intelligence and judgment. Mathematical skill can be tested with simple problems. Reading from either graded readers or such sources as the comics, front page, or editorial sections of the newspaper can be utilized, while making note of reading skill, articulation, and comprehension. Copying of the Gesell figures can be utilized to assess perceptual-motor skills (fig. 4).

Cranial nerves 2 through 12 should be examined. Funduscopic exam can be helpful in identifying the optic atrophy, pigmentary degeneration, or macular abnormalities of degenerative central nervous system disorders, while chorioretinitis will suggest a prenatal infectious disease such as toxoplasmosis, cytomegalovirus, or rubella. Visual acuity is frequently impaired

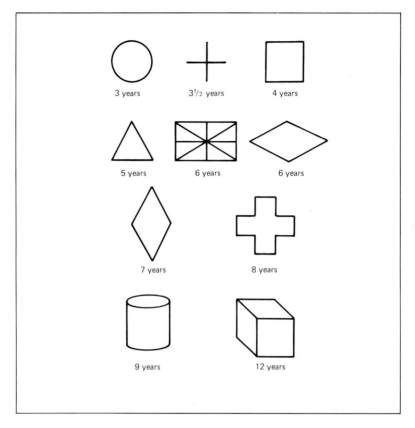

Fig. 4. Age norms for figure copying [from 1].

in degenerative processes. A visual field abnormality will suggest a mass lesion, while papilledema and eye movement abnormalities may result from hydrocephalus or increased intracranial pressure secondary to a mass lesion. Nystagmus suggests a brainstem or cerebellar disorder but may also represent congenital nystagmus or be secondary to a visual defect. An absent corneal reflex or asymmetrical face also suggests a mass lesion or, in the correct clinical context a stroke. Impaired hearing may represent the conductive hearing loss of otitis media or the sensorineural hearing loss of prenatal cytomegalovirus [32] or rubella infections. There are numerous inherited syndromes associated with hearing loss and they are catalogued by *Konigsmark and Gorlin* [42].

Hyperactive gag, brisk jaw jerk reflex, and emotional lability may represent the pseudobulbar palsy of a degenerative disease. The term 'pseudobulbar palsy' implies lower cranial nerve involvement due to a more rostral lesion, i.e. supranuclear. In contrast, lower cranial nerve palsies due to a brainstem process can be identified by absent jaw jerk reflex (may also be absent in normal people), and weak or atrophic tongue with or without tongue fasciculations.

Dysarthria (abnormal speech due to poor articulation) may result from pseudobulbar or bulbar cranial nerve dysfunction as well as developmental delay, cerebellar dysfunction, and intraoral structural abnormalities such as cleft palate.

The motor system is examined by observing the movements and spontaneous postures of the patient and by testing strength, tone, and reflexes. Asymmetry of muscle bulk, tone, or deep tendon reflexes is abnormal. In testing strength, it is useful to have the patient extend his arms in front of himself and close his eyes. A subtle weakness may be identified by watching for downward drift of the arm. This is also a good time to observe for tremor or other involuntary movements. One can assess the strength and symmetry of the shoulder girdle by having the child make 'wings', and test biceps strength by having the child 'make a muscle'. Strength of the grip should be tested. Coordination in performing fine motor movements can be assessed. The muscles of the legs can be tested while evaluating gait by having the child run, arise from a squatting position without holding on, hop on one foot, walk on the toes and heels, and perform tandem gait. The plantar response should always be symmetrical and is normally flexor. In a child that is old enough to walk, plantar extension responses indicate corticospinal tract damage. Below this age, plantar extension responses may be normal.

Sensory testing can be frustrating in a child, but breaking the stick of a cotton swab in half and testing pain sensation with the relatively nonthreatening stick (in lieu of a pin) and 'tickling' the child with the cotton swab can be fairly successful. In older children, graphesthesia, stereognosis, vibratory and position senses and also the presence or absence of sensory extinction on double simultaneous stimulation can be tested.

Cerebellar dysfunction may be manifest as finger-to-nose or heel-to-knee ataxia or dysmetria, intention tremor, dysarthria, nystagmus, truncal titubations, and imbalance or veering to the side when turning. Many of these findings are not specific for cerebellar dysfunction since tremor and unsteady movements can reflect weakness; nystagmus may be secondary to brainstem lesions; dysarthria occurs with cleft palate, etc. As a group, however, these

Table V. Soft signs [11]

Sign	Age of attainment years
Ability to extend the arms without pronation of the arms or spooning of the fingers	6
Balancing on one leg for 10 s	5–6
Forward tandem gait	5
Backward tandem gait	6
Serial apposition of thumb and fingers, slowly with little or no rhythm	3
Serial apposition of thumb and fingers with slow rhythm	5
Absence of mirror movements (synkinesis)	9 or less

findings are associated with dysfunction of the cerebellum or its pathways. Gait has already been mentioned above.

A group of findings relating to immaturity of the central nervous system have been termed 'soft signs' because presence of these signs is not localizable to dysfunction or pathology of a specific structure. Examples are given in table V. These signs may be found in children with learning disabilities, but it should be noted that these signs reflect sensory and motor abilities and may have no relation to the child's cognitive functioning. The clinical value of these signs has been questioned [2, 7, 72].

Psychological Testing

Any child with evidence of mental deficiency should have psychological testing. The most-used tests for measuring IQ include the Stanford-Binet test in the younger child and the Wechsler Intelligence Scale for Children (Revised) in the older child. Serial IQ testing may be helpful in confirming progressive intellectual deficit when this is suspected clinically. Most importantly, the psychological evaluation should focus on and elucidate the particular assets and deficiencies of the individual child, thereby aiding rational remediation, i.e. one should focus less on the actual IQ score. In general, the teacher can make the most constructive use of such an evaluation.

Laboratory Studies

Table VI lists various tests and the indications for them. Hearing and vision tests are indicated in all children with mental handicaps. A blood lead level, serological test for syphilis, and a plasma or urine screening test for phenylketonuria should also be given strong consideration.

Table VI. Indications for the use of various tests in the evaluation of a mentally retarded child

Tests	Indication
1. Hearing and vision tests	any mental handicap
2. Lead level	history of pica exposure to peeling paint iron deficiency anemia minimal cerebral dysfunction
3. Serological test for syphilis	hallucination stigmata of congenital syphilis any psychiatric disease
4. Metabolic studies (urine and plasma amino acids, urinary nitroprusside test, urinary mucopolysaccharides excretion, urinary ketones, ferric chloride, urinary pH and arylsulfatase A)	degeneration family history of degeneration coarsening of features unexplained hepatosplenomegaly episodic nausea or vomiting (acidosis) features of phenylketonuria (or inability to exclude phenylketonura): fair complexion, blue eyes, eczema, seizures, autistic behavior, incoordination, hyperactivity impaired consciousness, hypoglycemia, ataxia abnormal odor of skin or urine features of homocystinuria: ectopia lentis, malar flush, marfanoid habitus, etc.
5. Chromatin studies (buccal smear)	mental retardation or behavioral disorder associated with hypogenitalism mentally retarded girl with minor abnormalities (clinodactyly, hypertelorism, epicanthal folds, etc.)
6. Chromosomal studies	abnormal buccal smear (normal male has no Barr bodies and normal female has one Barr body) multiple malformations, espcially with IQ less than 50 family history of miscarriages macroorchidism in a boy and family history of retarded boys
7. Skull X-rays	evidence of prenatal infectious disease skin lesions of tuberous sclerosis or Sturge-Weber anomaly craniosynostosis

Table VI (cont.)

Tests	Indication
8. Head CAT scan	focal findings on neurological examination (other than those clearly referable to the peripheral nervous system) degeneration increasing head circumference (crossing percentiles) evidence of increased intracranial pressure some cases of severe or profound mental retardation of unknown etiology
9. EEG	clinical seizures degeneration
10. Serum glucose (fasting)	intermittent tachycardia, anxiety, diaphoresis, seizures, drowsiness
11. Serum chemistries	rarely indicated
12. Slit-lamp examination of eyes for Kaiser-Fleischer ring	movement disorder hepatic dysfunction – currently or by history hemolytic anemia – currently or by history
13. Toxicology screen	suspicion of drug ingestion
14. Anticonvulsant drug levels	change of mental status in an epileptic undergoing drug treatment
15. Maternal phenylketonuria test	multiple retarded children with normal or retarded mother
16. Serum thyroxine	features of hypothyroidism: growth deficiency, osseous immaturity, coarse face, constipation, thickened upper eyelids and large tongue, dry skin, hoarse speech, ankle edema
17. Serum uric acid	self-mutilating male
18. Studies for prenatal infectious disease (TORCH titers, IgM – these may be helpful only when the child is less than 1 year old, viral cultures and urine cytology)	microcephaly chorioretinitis intrauterine growth retardation deafness neonatal petechiae, jaundice, hepatosplenomegaly febrile maternal illness during first trimester

Otherwise, the laboratory investigation of the mildly retarded or borderline intelligence child with an otherwise normal physical examination and history should be quite limited. Moderately to severely retarded children, or those children with a degenerative disorder should have a more thorough laboratory evaluation. With two, or possibly three exceptions, even among those with an IQ below 50–54, enzyme deficiency disorders or chromosomal disorders are rare. These exceptions are trisomy 21 (Down's syndrome) and phenylketonuria [26] and perhaps the fragile-X syndrome [27]. Further workup of undiagnosed children with moderate or severe mental retardation should include urinary and plasma amino acid assays, metabolic urinalysis, and, in many cases, a karyotype.

In the past, phenylketonuria was the most common metabolic abnormality associated with mental deficiency [39]. Since phenylketonuria is treatable when detected early, even the slightest suspicion of this condition should be evaluated with a urine ferric chloride test or plasma phenylalanine determination.

Serum electrolytes, complete blood count, and routine urinalysis are probably not helpful in the child with uncomplicated mental retardation, especially those that can be allotted to the categories of prenatal onset of a problem in morphogenesis or perinatal onset of an insult to the brain.

Needleman et al. [53] have shown that neuropsychologic deficits can be found in otherwise asymptomatic children with elevated dentine lead levels. Although dentine lead levels are not generally available, serum lead levels can be obtained to screen children with pica, exposure to peeling paint, or features suggestive of the attentional deficit disorder. The features of this disorder have been discussed by *Shaywitz* et al. [66].

Chromosome determination (karyotype) should be performed in a child with multiple malformations that cannot be identified as specific for a known, nonchromosomal, dysmorphic condition. A family history of frequent miscarriages or stillbirth, especially in a child with an IQ of less than 50 is also an indication for a karyotype. With recognition of the fragile-X syndrome [27], it may be reasonable to obtain chromosome analyses on mentally retarded boys with macroorchidism and family histories of retarded boys. *Turner* et al. [74] have recommended chromosomal analysis, using approrpiate folic acid-deficient media (routine media fails to detect the fragile-X), for all boys with mental retardation of unknown etiology. However, prevalence of this abnormal X chromosome in the normal population has not been determined, therefore, the validity of the above recommendation is not established.

An electroencephalogram (EEG) is not routine in the evaluation of either mental retardation or attentional deficit disorder [46]. In contrast, an EEG should be obtained in any child that has a degenerative process (see 'Differential Diagnosis').

With regard to seizures, an EEG is not used to diagnose epilepsy, an some epileptics have normal interictal EEGs [46]. At the other end of the spectrum, status epilepticus recorded on the EEG has been associated with only minimal behavioral changes [23]. Loss of speech has been reported as a manifestation of epilepsy and the EEG in the cases with loss of speech often shows bitemporal spikes [16, 43, 49, 61]. Although children usually have clinical seizures in addition to the loss of speech, *Hamilton* et al. [31] have reported aphasia as the sole manifestation of focal status epilepticus in an adult.

It is certainly reasonable to obtain an EEG, in a child with intermittent staring spells or lapses of consciousness, especially when associated with stereotyped mannerisms such as lip smacking or eye blinking, or when followed by drowsiness. If one has diagnosed epilepsy clinically, an EEG can be used to classify the seizure disorder as generalized or focal. An EEG pattern of 3/s spike and wave is characteristic of petit mal epilepsy.

A skull X-ray may demonstrate the intracranial calcifications associated with tuberous sclerosis, prenatal infections, or Sturge-Weber syndrome. Since a computerized axial tomographic (CAT) scan of the head is more sensitive in detecting intracranial calcifications, a skull X-ray is superfluous if a CAT scan is planned. In any event, if there are no features of tuberous sclerosis, prenatal infectious disease, or Sturge-Weber syndrome, a skull X-ray is unlikely to contribute any useful information in uncomplicated mental retardation. If the head is obviously malformed, however, a skull X-ray will be helpful in defining craniostenosis (premature fusion of sutures). Specific syndromes of craniostenosis, such as Apert's syndrome (a type of acrocephalosyndactyly), are associated with mental retardation (table IV).

A CAT scan of the head is invaluable in a child with a progressive neurological disease. It will define focal or gross structural intracranial disease. The characteristic appearance of a demyelinating disease with decreased density of the cerebral white matter in the centrum semiovale and/or periventricular areas can be noted. Decreased density or cavitation of the putamen may be apparent in patients with neurological or psychiatric manifestations of hepatolenticular degeneration [55]. Increased ventricular size will diagnose hydrocephalus. A frontal, temporal, or parietal tumor with no manifestations other than progressive intellectual decline can be delineated, as can a posterior fossa tumor causing secondary hydrocephalus. Enlarging porencephalic cysts [44] or intracranial hematomas may be associated with progressive neurological deficits and are easily identified by CAT scan.

In contrast, the role of head CAT scanning in children with static mental deficiency is less clear. *Naheedy and Schnur* [52] studied 35 institutionalized retarded patients with various etiologies for the retardation, including 51.3% with idiopathic mental retardation. These individuals came from the Fernald State School where the great majority of residents have an IQ of less than 50 [35]. Of the individuals with idiopathic mental retardation, 39% had normal CAT scans, and 61% had abnormal CAT scans. In the abnormal CAT scans, the only findings were enlarged ventricles, with or without wide sulci. Even in mentally retarded children who also have seizures, the CAT scan is unlikely to show abnormalities of therapeutic significance [6]. Although the number of children is not specified, *Yang* et al. [78] found that 49% of children with both seizures and mental retardation had abnormal CAT scans. However, if mental retardation was the only neurological abnormality other than seizures, the abnormal CAT scans showed only generalized atrophy, usually mild. Hence, in a child with severe or profound mental retardation of unknown etiology, a CAT scan is probably not of direct therapeutic importance, but, by defining a static lesion, may reassure both the family and the physician.

Features suggestive of hypothyroidism (discussed in the 'Physical Examination' section and in table VI) mandate a serum thyroxine determination. In the absence of these features, thyroid function tests are not helpful outside of the neonatal period (during which time the characteristic features may not be apparent).

Differential Diagnosis

Reference should be made to table VII. Exclusion of a correctable disorder or a disorder mimicking mental handicap is of paramount importance. Family, social, and other environmental influences such as hunger, poor teaching, and overcrowded classrooms should be considered as either contributory or causative factors [71]. Overmedication for treatment of seizures or other conditions is a prime example of a correctable cause of mental handicap and should be evaluated by means of a careful history with consideration of obtaining appropriate drug blood levels or a blood and urine toxicology screen. Vision or hearing disorders may or may not be correctable but must always be excluded. Children with hearing disorders may have delayed speech, stylized mannerisms, poor social interaction, and other autistic-like features [8].

Subclinical epilepsy, or at least previously unrecognized epilepsy, will be suggested by lapses of consciousness or attention, with or without lip-smacking, eye blinking, or other repetitive movements, and these lapses may be referred to as 'staring spells'. In contrast to a poor attention span or daydreaming, these seizures are always associated with diminished consciousness [20]. Calling the child's name or shaking the child will not terminate a seizure immediately, as such a maneuver generally will when the child is daydreaming. Hyperventilating a child with petit mal epilepsy for 3 min will very frequently precipitate an epileptic staring spell [20].

Table VII. Categorization of degenerative and pseudodegenerative processes

I.	Subclinical epilepsy

II. Focal or gross structural intracranial disease
  A. Temporal, parietal, and frontal tumors
  B. Hydrocephalus secondary to tumors of the third or fourth ventricle
  C. Decompensated, low-grade, congenital hydrocephalus
  D. Porencephaly
  E. Hematoma

III. Endocrine disorders
  A. Thyroid disease
  B. Adrenoleukodystrophy (also in category VIII)
  C. Hypoglycemia

IV. Chronic infections
  A. Subacute sclerosing panencephalitis
  B. Rubella panencephalitis
  C. Congenital syphilis

V. Toxin ingestion or exposure
  A. Alcohol
  B. Anticonvulsants
  C. Illicit drugs
  D. Lead
  E. Others, depending on history

VI. Environmental factors
  A. Hunger
  B. Emotional stress
  C. Poor teaching and overcrowded classrooms
  D. Child abuse

VII. Sensory dysfunction (may be a manifestation of a cerebral degenerative disorder)
  A. Deafness
  B. Blindness

VIII. Other degenerative disorders
  A. Gray matter affected primarily (neuronal storage diseases)
  B. White matter affected primarily (leukodystrophies)
  C. Other metabolic degenerative disorders, such as hepatolenticular degeneration (Wilson's disease) or hyperuricemia with choreoathetosis (Lesch-Nyhan disease)
  D. Unclassificed degenerative disorders

IX. Psychopathology
  A. Infantile autism and psychosis
  B. Disintegrative psychosis in childhood
  C. Childhood schizophrenia
  D. Childhood hysteria

There are other types of severe childhood epilepsy such as the Lennox-Gastaut syndrome [50, 56], petit mal status [19], and minor motor epilepsy [47]. These epilepsies are commonly associated with mental retardation or even progressive intellectual deterioration [19, 58]. Characteristically, the seizures are easily recognized by the common occurrence of head-nodding or falling spells and various combinations of myoclonus and atypical absence episodes [3]. Some of these children will have episodes of confusion lasting for several days and accompanied by an EEG showing generalized spike-wave activity. This has given rise to the term 'spike-wave stupor'. Such patients generally have grand mal convulsions in addition to these twilight states [57].

Psychopathological states such as infantile autism and disintegrative psychosis of childhood should be considered. Because of unusual scatter skills such as rote memory, children with autism were often felt to have normal intelligence [40]. It is now recognized that autistic features such as aloneness, bizarre and repetitive mannerisms, etc. increase as the IQ decreases [8]. As noted previously, autistic features are common in children with hearing disorders [8].

In autistic children, the prognosis depends primarily on the child's basic intelligence [40]. Appropriate educational placement has been found to be more important than psychotherapy in the outcome of autistic children [40]. Hence, psychological and educational testing, as well as hearing testing, must be an integral part of the evaluation of these children. Disintegrative psychosis is characterized by severe deterioration in children that were normal or nearly normal prior to the age of 2.5 years [21]. The label 'disintegrative psychosis' should be reserved only for those children in whom thorough clinical and laboratory neurological investigation has failed to reveal an etiology. Numerous neurological disorders (table VIII) have presented with the clinical picture of disintegrative psychosis or other progressive, *apparently psychiatric disorders* [9, 12, 21, 60, 63]. Childhood conversion hysteria may present with almost any neurological symptom or sign, including intellectual deterioration [64]. Helpful positive findings may include a family or prior personal history of psychiatric disease, a current affective disorder, or a history of a suicide attempt [62]. Childhood schizophrenia will have features similar to adult schizophrenia. Table IX lists features which should cast doubt on a primary psychiatric diagnosis. The most important of these is deterioration either in intellectual or motor performance. While it is obvious that environmental stress may manifest itself by somatic complaints and neurological signs, if the child shows atypical features such as those in table IX, concurrent evaluation by a pediatric neurologist may be indicated.

The diagnosis of mental retardation requires that the mental deficiency be static. In some instances, the mental retardation will be associated with a nonchromosomal dysmorphic condition (table IV) or a chromosomal abnormality. Other cases may have dysmorphic features suggesting a prenatal onset of the mental deficiency but may not represent any recognizable condition. One must exclude the conditions previously discussed in this section (e.g. overmedication, environmental stress, sensory dysfunction, etc.) before mak-

Table VIII. Childhood neurological diseases that may present primarily as psychiatric diseases

Disease	Helpful distinguishing features
Hepatolenticular degeneration (Wilson's disease)	Kaiser-Fleischer ring, abnormal movements or posturing, current or previous liver dysfunction or hemolytic anemia
Neuronal ceroid lipofuscinosis (Batten's disease, juvenile amaurotic familial idiocy)	progressive visual loss, seizures
Subacute sclerosing panencephalitis	myoclonus; EEG pattern of 'suppression-burst', elevated cerebrospinal-fluid IgG
Congenital syphilis [37, 60, 75]	hallucinations, positive serological test for syphilis, interstitial keratitis, Hutchinson's teeth, perforation of the palate, dilated and fixed pupils, catatonia
Klinefelter's syndrome (XXY)	male sex, hypogonadism, gynecomastia, positive buccal smear in a male, behavior problems
Hyperuricemia with choreoathetosis (Lesch-Nyhan disease)	male sex, self-mutilation and aggressive behavior, hyperuricemia, choreoathetosis, mental retardation
Psychomotor epilepsy	lapses of consciousness associated with stereotyped behavior, postictal drowsiness
Juvenile metachromatic leukodystrophy [12]	gait disturbance and incoordination, diminished tendon reflexes, extensor plantar responses, decreased nerve conduction velocity, low to absent arylsulfatase A in urine or leukocytes, prominent emotional lability and euphoria, elevated cerebrospinal-fluid protein
Juvenile Gaucher's disease [54]	incoordination with jerky movements, ocular abduction deficits, current or prior hepatosplenomegaly, pancytopenia, erosion of the cortices of the long bones, psychoses
Adrenoleukodystrophy [63]	abnormal behavior in a boy with a disturbance of vision or gait

Table IX. Features increasing the risk for organic disease among patients with psychiatric complaints

Deterioration of school work	'Progressive' cerebral palsy
Visual dysfunction	Seizures
Increasing weakness or paralysis or clumsiness	Posturing (torticollis, dystonia, etc.)
	Neuropathy
Ataxia	Prepubertal age-group

ing the diagnosis of mental retardation. In contrast to learning disorders or the attentional deficit disorder, in which the child has normal intelligence but specific areas of deficit, the child with mental retardation has a global impairment of intellect. The child with a specific learning disability or attentional deficit disorder will often present with a behavior problem associated with school underachievement, but a normal full-scale IQ with intrasubtest scatter. In most studies, the diagnosis of attentional deficit disorder is excluded if the child has obvious neurologic disease, severe emotional disturbance, or psychosis [77].

If pseudodegenerative disorders such as childhood alcoholism, child abuse, etc. (see table VII) have been excluded, the presence of a degenerative central nervous system disorder requires full evaluation. Referral to a neurologist is usually necessary.

In addition to causing seizures, hypoglycemia may be the cause of intermittent mental dysfunction in children. Probably the most common type of hypoglycemia in children is ketotic hypoglycemia. The child is usually between the ages of 2 and 7 years and may be hyperactive. If the child has had a decreased intake of food, the child will often become drowsy with dysconjugate eye movements. A seizure may occur. During the episodes, the child has ketonuria and a low blood sugar [65]. Hypoglycemia due to other causes is frequently associated with signs and symptoms of epinephrine release such as diaphoresis, anxiety, and tachycardia.

Treatment

Treatment leading to a cure is possible in only a few conditions associated with mental impairment. Hepatolenticular degeneration (Wilson's disease) is such a disease that can be cured with appropriate *D*-penicillamine therapy [9]. Details of treatment have been published by *Milne* et al. [51]. Hearing and speech disorders may often be partially or completely remediated. Chelation therapy for lead poisoning is generally successful. Certain structural lesions of the brain, such as hydrocephalus, can be treated effectively with surgery. Early therapy of congenital hypothyroidism improves the outcome while treatment of acquired hypothyroidism is also very successful [48, 68]. Recognition of an inherited syndrome or the association of multiple retarded children and a phenylketonuric mother achieves the potential for the most effective treatment known, i.e. prevention. Elimination of a toxin or manipulation of drug doses to avoid toxic levels is a very satisfying way of curing a pseudodegeneration.

Seizures are treated with the appropriate anticonvulsants [59] while monitoring the clinical response and following the drug blood levels. It is axiomatic that a single anticonvulsant be increased to the level at which it is effective or until maximal blood levels without toxicity are reached before adding a second anticonvulsant. Phenobarbital frequently causes hyperactivity or worsening of a prior behavior problem. Hence, it is definitely not the drug of choice for epileptic children with behavior problems.

Most commonly, there is no specific treatment for mental handicap. Of great benefit to the child is a compassionate physician who treats the child while supporting the family and helping to enlist community resources. Explanation of the underlying disorder to the family and teacher and identifying the child's abilities can lead to formulation of appropriate goals and teaching techniques. Allowing the child to succeed by tailoring the tasks to the child's level often decreases the secondary emotional difficulties, improves the child's self-image, and discourages use of terms such as 'bad child'. Instructions should always be simple. Rules should be kept to a minimum, but all rules should be consistently and completely enforced. Praise for good behavior, e.g. chores, will reinforce that behavior, and parents should be reminded of this. When punishment is necessary, isolation in the child's room for a short period of time, no more than 5–10 min, is quite effective. The impression should always be given that the punishment was for the bad behavior, not a bad child, i.e., a 'good' child did something wrong, for which the child was punished and then forgiven.

In order to function optimally, mentally retarded children require a structured environment without surprises. When change in routine is needed, it should be simply explained to the child beforehand. Complex explanations are useless and are confusing to the child.

If medication such as methylphenidate (Ritalin) or dextroamphetamine (Dexedrine) is used, the child should be given credit for any
improvement which occurs. It would seem that such medication would be
most useful for children with constitutional hyperactivity, short attention
span, and distractibility rather than those children in whom such behavior
is due to environmental influences such as emotional stress or inappropriate school or parental expectations. However, if there is a question as to
whether or not stimulant medication will be useful, a careful trial of medication may be helpful. Specifically, the doctor and parent should arrange a
trial lasting several weeks in which different dosages of the medication are
given for weekly periods. The behaviors that will hopefully improve must
be specified prior to the trial. The teacher should assess (in written form) the
resultant behavior while being kept *unaware* of the presence, absence, or
dosage of the medication. Following the trial, the teacher's assessments of
behavior can be correlated with the presence (and dosage) or absence of
medication. Then, a rational decision regarding future medication use can
be made. Either drug is generally started at a dose of 5–10 mg in the morning prior to school with an additional dose at lunchtime if needed. The dose
may be gradually increased to 20 or 30 mg per dose of dextroamphetamine
or methylphenidate, respectively. No long-term benefits from stimulant
medication have been proven [77].

Secondary emotional problems are a major complicating factor in children with mental handicaps. Their ability to cope with a stressful environment is impaired, and subsequent intolerable anxiety and depression may
occur. In this context, psychiatric care may mean the difference between
later institutionalization and a semi-independent or independent life in the
community [71]. Numerous factors in the mentally handicapped child's life
are amenable to psychiatric intervention, including: presence in a special
class, rejection by peers, family dynamics relative to the child's handicap,
pressure to be 'normal', mourning reactions by the parents, and others. In
addition to their susceptibility to emotional problems, retarded children
also have the same psychiatric diagnostic entities as normal children and
can be good candidates for psychiatric treatment [71].

References

1   Accardo, P.J.; Capute, A.J.: The pediatrician and the developmentally delayed child,
    p. 121 (University Park Press, Baltimore 1979).
2   Adams, R.M.; Kocsis, J.J.; Estes, R.E.: Soft neurological signs in learning disabled
    children and controls. Am. J. Dis. Child. *128:* 614–618 (1974).

3   Aicardi, J.: The problem of the Lennox syndrome. Devl Med. Child Neur. *15:* 77–81 (1973).

4   American Psychiatric Association Task Force on Nomenclature and Statistics: Diagnostic and Statistical manual of mental disorders; 3rd ed. (DSM III) (American Psychiatric Association, Washington, D.C. 1980).

5   American Academy of Pediatrics: Committee on drugs. Anticonvulsants and pregnancy. Pediatrics *63:* 331–333 (1979).

6   Bachman, D.S.; Hodges, F.J.; Freeman, J.M.: Computerized axial tomography in chronic seizure disorders of childhood. Pediatrics *58:* 828–832 (1976).

7   Barlow, C.F.: 'Soft signs' in children with learning disorders. Am. J. Dis. Child. *128:* 605–606 (1974).

8   Capute, A.J.; Derivan, A.T.; Chauvel, P.J.; Rodriguez, A.: Infantile autism. I. A prospective study of the diagnosis. Devl Med. Child Neur. *17:* 58–62 (1975).

9   Cartwright, G.E.: Diagnosis of treatable Wilson's disease. New Engl. J. Med. *298.* 1347–1350 (1978).

10   Caudle, H.F.: Phenylketonuria without mental retardation. Pediatrics *26:* 502 (1960).

11   Chamberlin, H.R.: Mental retardation; in Farmer, Pediatric neurology; 2nd ed., p. 104 (Harper & Row, Hagerstown 1975).

12   Clark, J.R.; Miller, R.G.; Vodgoff, J.M.: Juvenile onset metachromatic leukodystrophy with biochemical and electrophysiologic studies. Neurology *29:* 346–353 (1979).

13   Clarren, S.K.; Smith, D.W.: The fetal alcohol syndrome. New Engl. J. Med. *298:* 1063–1067 (1978).

14   Coleman, M.: Down's syndrome. Pediat. Annls *7:* 36–63 (1978).

15   Crandall, B.F.: Genetic disorders and mental retardation. J. Am. Acad. Child Psychiat. *16:* 89–108 (1977).

16   Deuel, R.K.; Lenn, N.J.: Treatment of acquired epileptic aphasia. J. Pediat. *90:* 959–961 (1977).

17   Dobyns, W.; Goldstein, N.P.; Gordon, H.: Clinical spectrum of Wilson's disease (hepatolenticular degeneration). Mayo Clin. Proc. *54:* 34–42 (1979).

18   Dodge, P.R.: Neurologic history and examination; in Farmer, Pediatric neurology; 2nd ed., pp. 1–43 (Harper & Row, Hagerstown 1975).

19   Doose, H.; Volzke, E.: Petit mal status in early childhood. Neuropädiatrie *10:* 10–14 (1979).

20   Dreifuss, F.E.: The differential diagnosis of partial seizures with complex symptomatology; in Penry, Daly, Adv. neurol., vol. 11, pp. 187–199 (Raven Press, New York 1975).

21   Evans-Jones, L.G.; Rosenbloom, L.: Disintegrative psychosis in childhood. Devl Med. Child Neur. *20:* 462–470 (1978).

22   Farmer, T.W. (ed.): Pediatric neurology; 2nd ed., p. 112 (Lippincott/Harper & Row, Philadelphia 1975).

23   Fincham, R.W.; Yamada, T.; Schottelius, D.D.; Hayreh, S.M.S.; Damasio, A.: Electroencephalo-graphic absence status with minimal behavioral change. Archs Neurol. *36:* 176–178 (1979).

24   Fisher, D.A.; Klein, A.H.: Thyroid development and disorders of thyroid function in the newborn. New Engl. J. Med. *304:* 702–712 (1981).

25   Frankenburg, W.K.; Duncan, B.R.; Coffelt, R.W.; Koch, R.; Coldwell, J.G.; Son, C.D.:

Maternal phenylketonuria: implications for growth and development. J. Pediat. *73:* 560–570 (1968).

26   Garrard, S.D.: On the diagnosis of syndromes in mental retardation. Pediat. Clins N. Am. *15:* 925–942 (1968).

27   Gerald, P.S.: X-linked mental retardation and an X-chromosome marker. New Engl. J. Med. *303:* 696–697 (1980).

28   Gomez, M.R. (ed.): Tuberous sclerosis (Raven Press, New York 1979).

29   Grossman, H.J. (ed.): Manual on terminology and classification in mental retardation; 1977 revision (American Association on Mental Deficiency, Baltimore, Garamond/Pridemark 1977).

30   Gustavson, K.-H.; Holmgren, G.; Blomquist, H.K.; Mikkelsen, M.; Nordenson, I.; Poulsen, H.; Tommerup, N.: Familial X-linked mental retardation and fragile X chromsomes in two Swedish families. Clin. Genet. *19:* 101–110 (1981).

31   Hamilton, N.G.; Matthews, T.: Aphasia: the sole manifestation of focal status epilepticus. Neurology, Minneap. *29:* 745–748 (1979).

32   Hanshaw, J.B.; Schreiner, A.P.; Moxley, A.W.; Gaer, L.; Abel, V.; Scheiner, B.: School failure and deafness after 'silent' congenital cytomegalovirus infection. New Engl. J. Med. *295:* 468–470 (1976).

33   Hart, H.; Bax, M.; Jenkins, S.: The value of a developmental history. Devl Med. Child Neur. *20:* 442–452 (1978).

34   Heilman, K.M.; Watson, R.T.; Greer, M.: Differential diagnosis of neurologic signs and symptoms, p. 221 (Appleton Century Crofts, New York 1977).

35   Holmes, L.; Moser, H.; Halldorsson, S.; Mack, C.; Pants, S.S.; Matzilevich, N.B.: Mental retardation, an atlas of disease with associated physical abnormalities (Macmillan, New York 1971).

36   Illingworth, R.S.: The development of the infant and young child: normal and abnormal; 7th ed. (Churchill Livingstone, New York 1980).

37   Joffe, R.; Black, M.M.; Floyd, M.: Changing clinical picture of neurosyphilis: report of seven unusual cases. Br. med. J. *i:* 211–212 (1968).

38   Kandt, R.S.; D'Souza, B.J.: Cerebral gigantism (on-line with The Computerized Birth Defects Information Center, 1980).

39   Kaveggia, E.G.; Durkin, M.V.; Pendleton, E.; et al.: Diagnostic genetic studies on 1,224 patients with severe mental retardation. 3rd Congr. Int. Asso. for Scient. Study Mental Defic. The Hague 1973; cited by Smith and Simons [70].

40   Knobloch, H.; Pasamanick, B.: Some etiologic and prognostic factors in early infantile autism and psychosis. Pediatrics *55:* 182–191 (1975).

41   Koch, R.; Blaskovics, M.; Wenz, E.; Fishler, K.; Schaeffler, G.: Phenylalaninemia and phenylketonuria; in Nyhan, Heritable disorders of amino acid metabolism: patterns of clinical expression and genetic variation, pp. 109–140 (Wiley & Sons, New York 1974).

42   Konigsmark, B.W.; Gorlin, R.J.: Genetic and metabolic deafness (Saunders, Philadelphia 1976).

43   Landau, W.M.; Kleffner, F.R.: Syndrome of acquired aphasia with convulsive disorders in children. Neurology *7:* 523–530 (1957).

44   Leahy, W.R.; Singer, H.S.: Progressive focal deficit with porencephaly. Archs Neurol. *34:* 154–156 (1977).

45   Lenke, R.R.; Levy, H.L.: Maternal phenylketonuria and hyperphenylalaninemia: an

international survey of the outcome of untreated and treated pregnancies. New Engl. J. Med. *303:* 1202–1208 (1980).

46 Lewis, D.V.; Freeman, J.M.: The electroencephalogram in pediatric practice: its use and abuse. Pediatrics *60:* 324–330 (1977).

47 Livingston, S.; Eisner, V.; Pauli, L.: Minor motor epilepsy. Pediatrics *21:* 916–928 (1958).

48 Macfaul, R.; Dorner, S.; Brett, E.M.; Grant, D.B.: Neurological abnormalities in patients treated for hypothyroidism from early life. Archs Dis. Childh. *53:*611–619(1978).

49 Mantovani, J.F.; Landau, W.M.: Acquired aphasia with convulsive disorder: course and prognosis. Neurology *30:* 524–529 (1980).

50 Markand, O.N.: Slow spike-wave activity in EEG and associated clinical features: often called 'Lennox' or 'Lennox-Gastaut' syndrome. Neurology *27:* 746–757 (1977).

51 Milne, M.C.; Lewiss, A.E.; Lyle, W.H. (eds): Penicillamine. Post-grad. med. J., suppl. (1968).

52 Naheedy, M.H.; Schnur, J.A.: Value of computerized tomography scanning in syndromes associated with mental retardation; preliminary report. Comput. Tomogr. *3:* 1–8 (1979).

53 Needleman, H.L.; Gunnoe, C.; Leviton, A.; Reed, R.; Peresie, H.; Maher, C.; Barrett, P.: Deficits in psychologic and classroom performance of children with elevated dentine lead levels. New Engl. J. Med. *300:* 689–795 (1979).

54 Neil, J.F.; Glew, R.H.; Peters, S.P.: Familial psychosis and diverse neurologic abnormalities in adult-onset Gaucher's disease. Archs Neurol. *36:* 95–99 (1979).

55 Nelson, R.F.; Guzman, D.A.; Grahovac, S.; Howse, D.C.N.: Computerized cranial tomography in Wilson's disease. Neurology *29:* 866–868 (1979).

56 Niedermeyer, E.: The Lennox-Gastaut syndrome: a severe type of childhood epilepsy. Dt. Z. NervHeilk. *195:* 263–282 (1969).

57 Niedermeyer, E.; Khalifeh, R.: Petit mal status ('spike-wave stupor'). Epilepsia *6:* 250–262 (1965).

58 Patvy, G.; Lyagoubi, S.; Tassinari, C.A.: Subclinical status epilepticus induced by sleep in children. Archs Neurol. *24:* 242–252 (1971).

59 Penry, J.K.; Newmark, M.E.: The use of antiepileptic drugs. Ann. intern. Med. *90:* 207–218 (1979).

60 Rivinus, T.M.; Jamison, D.L.; Graham, P.J.: Childhood organic neurological disease presenting as psychiatric disorder. Archs Dis. Childh *50:* 115–119 (1975).

61 Rapin, I.; Mattis, S.; Rowan, A.J.; Golden, G.G.: Verbal auditory agnosia in children. Devl Med. Child Neur. *19:* 192–207 (1977).

62 Roy, A.: Hysterical seizures. Archs Neurol. *36:* 447 (1979).

63 Schaumberg, H.H.; Powers, J.M.; Raine, C.S.; Suzuki, K.; Richardson, E.P.: Adrenoleukodystrophy. A clinical and pathological study of 17 cases. Archs Neurol. *32:* 577–591 (1975).

64 Schneider, S.; Rice, D.R.: Neurologic manifestations of childhood hysteria. J. Pediat. *94:* 153–156 (1979).

65 Senior, B.: Ketotic hypoglycemia. J. Pediat. *82:* 555–556 (1973).

66 Shaywitz, B.A.; Cohen, D.J.; Shaywitz, S.E.: New diagnostic terminology for minimal brain dysfunction. J. Pediat. *95:* 734–736 (1979).

67 Smith, D.W.; Recognizable patterns of human malformation: genetic embryologic clinical aspects (Saunders, Philadelphia 1976).

68   Smith, D.W.; Blizzard, R.M.; Wilkins, L.: The mental prognosis in hypothyroidism of infancy and childhood. Pediatrics *19:* 1011–1022 (1957).

69   Smith, D.W.; Bostian, K.E.: Congenital anomalies associated with idiopathic mental retardation. J. Pediat. *65:* 189–196 (1964).

70   Smith, D.W.; Simons, F.E.R.: Rational diagnostic evaluation of the child with mental deficiency. Am. J. Dis. Child. *129:* 1285–1290 (1975).

71   Szymanski, L.S.: Psychiatric diagnostic evaluation of mentally retarded individuals. J. Am. Acad. Child Psychiat. *16:* 19–27; 67–82 (1977).

72   Touwen, B.C.L.; Sporrel, T.: Soft signs and MBD. Devl Med. Child Neur. *21:* 528–538 (1979).

73   Turner, G.; Brookwell, R.; Daniel, A.; Selikowitz, M.; Zilibowitz, M.: Heterozygous expression of X-linked mental retardation and X-chromosome marker fra(X) (q27). New Engl. J. Med. *303:* 662–664 (1980).

74   Turner, G.; Daniel, A.; Frost, M.: X-linked mental retardation, macroorichidism, and the Xq27 fragile site. J. Pediat. *96:* 837–841 (1980).

75   US Department of Health, Education and Welfare: Syphilis: a synopsis. Public Health Service Publication No. 1660, pp. 88–93 (US Government Printing Office, Washington 1968).

76   Werlin, S.L.; Grand, R.J.; Perman, J.A.; Watkins, J.B.: Diagnostic dilemmas of Wilson's disease: diagnosis and treatment. Pediatrics *62:* 47–51 (1978).

77   Wolraich, M.L.: Stimulant drug therapy in hyperactive children: research and clinical implications. Pediatrics *60:* 512–518 (1977).

78   Yang, P.J.; Berger, P.E.; Cohen, M.E.; Duffner, P.K.: Computed tomography and childhood seizure disorders. Neurology *29:* 1084–1088 (1979).

9 The Epilepsies

Ernst Niedermeyer

Epileptic manifestations are abnormal reactions of the brain caused by a large number of diseases. These reactions either involve the brain in an almost global manner or the disturbance is confined to certain cerebral regions. The basic disorder may be located within the brain or the failure of other organs may give rise to secondary encephalopathies. In all these epileptic conditions, the role of genetic factors and individual predisposition to seizures may play a certain part. Epileptic phenomena cut across vast areas of the entire domain of medicine and, for this reason, the physician should be familiar with various facets of seizure disorders.

For the investigator of mental retardation and its wide variety of causes, familiarity with the seizure disorders is a necessity. There is reason to presume that approximately 50% of children and older patients in institutions for the mentally retarded are suffering from epileptic seizures.

Basic Considerations of Epileptic Mechanisms

1. Neurobiochemistry

(a) Disease-Specific Chemical Changes Creating a Predisposition to Seizures. A long list of hereditary *inborn errors of metabolism* is growing longer every year.

(b) Chemical Changes Occurring in Focal Epileptogenic Lesions. Acetylcholine may render membranes hyperexcitable. Increased influx of sodium and depletion of intracellular potassium also enhance excitability of membrane. Failure of inhibitory action of GABA is of dubious significance. Role of calcium recently emphasized.

(c) Facilitation and Precipitation of Seizures due to Chemical Changes. Consider again the role of acetylcholine, sodium and potassium. Intrinsic instability of the membrane may be another factor.

(d) Chemical Changes during Epileptic Seizures. Steep rise of cerebral blood flow, oxygen consumption, glucose consumption, CO_2 production and lactate concentration.

(e) Chemical Changes Related to Termination of Seizures. Active neuronal inhibition appears to be more important than gradual increase of neuronal hypoxia ('brain running out of fuel during seizure').

2. Electrophysiology

(a) The EEG. 'Macro'-electroencephalogram represents the 'noise' of the brain in which minute 'clicks' of individual neuronal responses merge into the rhythmical oscillations generated by huge cellular contingents. Epileptic activity is characterized by unusually abrupt EEG discharges: spikes or sharp waves.

(b) Micro-Electrophysiological Events. The all-or-nothing axosomatic 'spike' of the single neuron contributes but very little to the macro-EEG. Slower potentials of graded character are apparently of much greater significance.

(c) Electrical Characteristics of Epileptic Neurons. Behavior of single cells in epileptogenic foci has been the object of numerous micro-electrode studies in recent years, especially by *Prince* [6]. Abnormal synchronization of neuronal activity is an important factor. Most recently, the role of glial cell has been intensively studied. *Ward* [8] has emphasized the role of hypersensitivity and potential epileptogenicity of de-afferented neurons deprived of dendritic synapses.

(d) Propagation of Epileptic Activity. Mechanisms of propagation: (a) intracortical diffusion; (b) volume conduction and (c) along conducting pathways ('synaptic conduction' – probably most important mechanism). Spread involves preferentially 'low threshold areas' of greater susceptibility to bombardment with epileptic activity (such as amygdala, hippocampus). *Secondary epileptogenic foci* may develop in this manner. Contralateral secondary foci in homologous area may evolve due to firing via commissural pathways.

(e) Generalization of Epileptic Activity. Generalization is often the result of progressive propagation. In human epileptology, *primary generalization* may also occur and is exemplified by the *petit mal absence* (generalized-synchronous 3/s spike waves) and also by *grand mal seizures without focal initiation.*

(f) Inhibitory Mechanisms and Termination of Seizures. Modern experimental work has de-emphasized the role of the subcortex in primary general-

ization [2, 3]. Several inhibitory neuronal mechanisms have been demonstrated. The most important type of inhibition (from the epileptological viewpoint) seems to involve cerebellar structures and their output. These concepts have promoted the recent technique of chronic cerebellar stimulation in recalcitrant epileptics; its practial value, however, is still unproven.

Types of Epileptic Seizures

The variety of epileptic seizures is determined by the following principal factors: (a) localization of involved cerebral area; (b) age of patient, and (c) basic epileptic condition (such as hypsarrhythmia – see 'Age-determined epileptic conditions').

1. Grand Mal
Tonic-clonic seizure in profound coma, lasting mainly 40–90 s. The most common type of seizures, occurring at any age except for the first 6 months of life.

Grand mal seizures may be *initiated by focal seizure activity* (motor, sensory, psychomotor, etc., often experiences as '*aura*'). In other epileptic conditions, grand mal may occur in *primary generalization.*

2. Petit Mal Absences
Short-lasting mild *absence,* duration 5–30 s, often with slight myoclonic activity. Onset never before age of 3 years, occurs mainly between age 4 and 16 years, then gradual decline of incidence and prevalence, rare after age 25.

Impressive EEG correlate: 3/s spike waves in generalized synchrony; no cortical focus. Occurs usually in the condition called 'primary generalized epilepsy' (see 'Age-determined epileptic conditions').

3. Psychomotor Seizure (Complex Partial Seizures)
A complex form of seizure with a variety of subgroups, originating from the temporal lobe and discussed under 'Special types of epilepsy according to site of focus'.

4. Myoclonic Seizures
Frequently repetitive brief attacks of bilateral-synchronous mass movements, mostly in flexion, involving extremities more commonly than

face or trunk. There is a wide variety of etiologies and epileptic conditions leading to myoclonus (essential myoclonus epilepsy, hypsarrhythmia, Lennox-Gastaut syndrome, etc.).

5. Focal Motor and Other Focal Seizures
Will be discussed under 'Special types of epilepsy according to site of focus'.

6. Hemiconvulsions
To be separated from focal motor seizures. No Jacksonian march. Limited to infancy and early childhood.

7. Atonic Seizures
Characterized by sudden vehement fall, often traumatizing. Requires *protective headgear.* Occurs mostly in children between age 2 and 10 years. These seizures are almost completely limited to the *Lennox-Gastaut syndrome* (see 'Age-determined epileptic conditions'). Many synonymous terms are used for these seizures (akinetic, petit mal, static seizures, drop attacks, etc.).

8. Tonic Seizures
Divided into axial (longitudinal spinal muscles) and rhizomelic type (shoulder, hip muscles). Very common in Lennox-Gastaut syndrome (see 'Age-determined epileptic conditions') but also as focal manifestation of supplementary motor region ('mesiofrontal epilepsy', see 'Special types of epilepsy according to site of focus').

9. Akinetic Seizures
A more prolonged type of absence with complete loss of motility, seen only in the Lennox-Gastaut syndrome (see 'Age-determined epileptic conditions').

10. Head-Nodding Attacks
A special type of myoclonus, limited to infantile spasms (hypsarrhythmia, see 'Age-determined epileptic conditions').

11. Jackknifing and Salaam Attacks
Only in infantile spasms (hypsarrhythmia, see 'Age-determined epileptic conditions).

Etiologies of Epileptic Conditions

Every type of cerebral pathology or insult to the brain could give rise to epileptic seizures, either acutely or after some delay due to the epileptogenic effects of secondary scar formation.

1. The Role of Genetic Factors

A very complex issue because of the presumed existence of numerous genes involved in epileptic conditions. 'Threshold genes' [*Metrakos and Metrakos*] may create a certain predisposition to seizures which renders one person more susceptible to epileptic manifestations after a cerebral insult.

There is still some controversy as to whether there is an *epilepsy as a disease entity* in the absence of any other plausible cerebral disturbance or pathology. This will be discussed under 'Primary generalized epilepsy' (see 'Age-determined epileptic conditions').

2. Inborn Errors of Metabolism

(a) Tay-Sachs Disease. Tonic convulsions and spasms are typical manifestations, usually induced by auditory startle.

(b) Other Forms of Cerebral Lipidosis (Cerebromacular Degeneration). Convulsive manifestations, frequently with myoclonus.

(c) Aminoacidurias. Epileptic manifestations and especially myoclonus are very common in phenylketonuria. Seizures are not as frequently observed in most of the other forms of aminoaciduria.

(d) Pyridoxin Dependency. Severe and even fatal convulsions in neonates and infants on a genetic basis, responsive to pyridoxin. May also occur as a nutritional deficiency *(pyridoxin deficiency).* Very rare.

3. Essential Hereditary Myoclonus Epilepsy
(Lafora-Unverricht-Lundberg)

A progressive encephalopathy due to an autosomal recessive gene, occurring as a variety of subentities according to the severity of the clinical picture.

Onset usually between age 6 and 16 years. *Progressive myoclonic twitching and jerking,* grand mal seizures, cerebellar symptomatology (intentional tremor, dysmetria) and dementia are the main characteristics.

4. Prenatal, Perinatal and Postnatal Infantile Brain Damage

This is a highly heterogeneous group of traumatic, hypoxic, ischemic, metabolic and infectious disorders; even genetic syndromes (tuberous sclerosis, Sturge-Weber's syndrome) are included. This variety of causes reflects the heterogeneous nature of the various *forms of cerebral palsy* which are very frequently associated with epileptic seizures; this is particularly true for the hemiplegic form.

5. Infectious Disease (Encephalitis)

Acutely epileptogenic in neonates; in viral disease (especially herpes simplex, contracted from herpes simplex genitalis of the mother) or most commonly of bacterial origin (*H. influenzae, E. coli,* etc.). Postmeningitic subdural collections may lead to a recrudescence of the seizures.

During infancy and childhood, infectious causes of acute convulsions are: exanthem subitum (innocuous), *measles* (may be followed by a chronic postencephalitic seizure disorder), *smallpox vaccination* and others.

6. Craniocerebral Trauma

An important distinction must be made between immediate, early (24–48 h) and delayed posttraumatic forms of epilepsy which are due to secondary cerebral scar formation with an onset of seizures between 3 months and 2 years after the injury.

The most common substratum of posttraumatic epilepsy is the *laceration of the brain due to open gunshot wounds;* for this reason, posttraumatic epilepsy is more commonly seen during and after periods of war.

7. Intracranial Tumors

About one third of the cases of intracranial tumors are associated with epileptic seizures; this figure rises to around 50% when tumors of the cerebral hemispheres are considered separately.

The role of a tumor as the cause of seizures must be considered mainly in *patients with onset of seizures in adult life.* Epileptic children are most likely to have seizures from causes other than tumors; moreover, most of the intracranial tumors of childhood are located in the posterior fossa or along the brain stem.

8. Brain Abscess

Brain abscess may be *highly epileptogenic.* In infants and children with *congenital heart disease,* the occurrence of seizures in association with lethargy and neurological deficits is very suspect. Penetrating cerebral wounds, *chronic infection of the ear* and the paranasal sinuses and particularly *chronic purulent diseases located in the chest* (pleural empyema, lung abscess, bronchiectasy, endocarditis) are further common causes of brain abscesses.

9. Cerebrovascular Disorders

Seizures occurring during acute cerebrovascular accidents are most commonly of focal motor character: a *focal-motor status* may occur for some hours or days.

Recurrent seizures of late onset due to progressive *cerebral arteriosclerosis* most commonly originate from hippocampic structures and manifest themselves either as psychomotor automatisms or, more commonly, as grand mal.

Systemic lupus erythematosus often involves the CNS and grand mal seizures may be the first manifestation. One must keep in mind that lupus erythematosus may also develop as a reaction to anticonvulsive therapy.

Arteriovenous malformations may be the cause of grand mal as well as focal seizures with a most common age of onset between age 10 and 35 years.

10. Metabolic Disorders

Renal insufficiency may give rise to seizures in acute as well as in chronic states. Myoclonus and grand mal attacks are common in such uremic conditions. Peritoneal dialysis may temporarily activate the seizures.

Hypoglycemic states may be the cause of seizures, especially grand mal. *Hypocalcemia* and other electrolyte imbalances may give rise to seizures especially in neonates.

Withdrawal from chronic use of barbiturates (especially in addiction to short acting barbiturates) gives rise to grand mal seizures, usually on the third day. Some nonbarbituric sedatives and hypnotics have similar withdrawal effects (Doriden, Placidyl, Valium). *Long-term psychiatric treatments with phenothiazines* may lead to major convulsions; this is also true for prolonged treatment with *electroconvulsions*.

Acute states of *intermittent porphyria* and *chronic lead poisoning* are further toxic-metabolic causes of seizures.

11. Chronic Alcoholism (Alcohol-Withdrawal Seizures)

These seizures of the grand mal type are caused by transient metabolic disturbances due to sudden alcohol withdrawal or sudden discontinuation of alcohol intake. The seizures usually occur 6–30 h after the last drink and are most often observed on Mondays. Transient lowering of the magnesium level and a pH shift to the alkaline range have been described. A delirium tremens may follow 1–3 days later.

This is a self-inflicted seizure disorder in basically nonepileptic individuals. EEG tracings taken in the interval are almost invariably within normal limits. Anticonvulsants are of little or no use.

This condition must be distinguished from the seizures of epileptics who happen to become alcoholics.

Age-Determined Epileptic Conditions

These conditions are characterized by (a) distinct age range; (b) certain types of seizures; (c) certain EEG patterns, and (d) certain characteristics of course and prognosis. The etiology is usually of secondary or little importance and often remains obscure (a notable exception are neonatal seizures; their eventual outcome is often determined by the causative disorder).

1. Neonatal Convulsions

Seizures occurring in the first 3 months of life, mostly of an *irregularly mixed tonic and clonic character* (without the orderly sequence of a tonic and a clinic state as in grand mal). Some atonic, autonomic and automatism-like manifestations may also occur. Seizures may be relatively mild (and not always easily distinguishable from normal neonatal motor activity) but tend to be rather prolonged. More common etiologies are listed in table I.

Table I. The most common causes of epileptic seizures according to age of onset of seizures (listed in order of importance)

1st week
1. Perinatal trauma
2. Perinatal anoxia
3. Cerebral malformations (atrophy, porencephaly, etc.)
4. Hypocalcemia
5. Hypoglycemia
2nd week
1. Hypocalcemia
2. Cerebral malformations

Table I (cont.)

---

   3. Early CNS infection (*E. coli,* Staph., Herpes simplex virus)
   4. Extracranial infection (pneumonia, gastro-enteritis)
   5. Perinatal trauma
   6. Perinatal anoxia
   7. Kernicterus

3rd week to 3 months
   1. CNS infection (*H. influenzae,* and others)
   2. Cerebral malformations
   3. Subdural collection following CNS infection
   4. Inborn errors of metabolism (Tay-Sachs and others)

4 months to 2 years
   1. *Febrile convulsions* (triggered by upper respiratory disease; predominantly genetic)
   2. CNS infection
   3. Cerebrovascular disorder (arterial occlusion, venous thrombosis)
   4. Residual scars of earliest CNS insults (mostly with cerebral palsy)
   5. Inborn errors of metabolism (phenylketonuria, Tay-Sachs and others)
     Note: Minor seizures at this age tend to occur as infantile spasms (hypsarrhythmia)

3–10 years
   1. Residual scars of early CNS insults (in severe cases; Lennox-Gastaut syndrome)
   2. Genetic: common generalized epilepsy (presenting as petit mal)
   3. CNS infection
   4. Trauma
   5. Lead poisoning (residual, ingestion around age 2)
   6. Inborn errors of metabolism (brain tumor uncommon)

11–20 years
   1. Genetic: common generalized epilepsy (petit mal plus grand mal)
   2. Trauma
   3. Residual scars of early CNS insults (in severe cases: Lennox-Gastaut syndrome)
   4. A-V malformation
   5. Brain tumor (in general, onset of seizures not very common in this decade)

21–40 years
   1. Trauma   4. A-V malformaiton
   2. Brain tumor   5. Residual scars of early CNS insults
   3. Chronic alcoholism   6. Vasculitis (systemic lupus erythematosus)

41–60 years
   1. Brain tumor   4. Cerebral arteriosclerosis
   2. Chronic alcoholism   5. Neurosyphilis
   3. Trauma

Above age 60
   1. Cerebral arteriosclerosis   2. Brain tumor (primary or metastatic)

At all ages: *cause frequently remains unknown.* In subtropical and tropical countries: always consider intracranial parasites. Even malaria may be followed by epileptic seizures.

---

2. Infantile Spasms (Hypsarrhythmia)

These seizures occur between age 4 months and about 2½ years: also known as West's syndrome. *Infantile spasms have unmistakable ictal-clinical and EEG characteristics.* Salaam spasm (anteroflexion of upper part of the body) and '*jackknifing*' are essentially identical brief ictal phenomena. *Massive myoclonic jerking* and especially head nodding are also noted.

The EEG shows the typical 'hypsarrhythmic' character with very high voltage, frequent, widespread bursts of single and multiple spikes and stretches of suddenly depressed voltage, especially during sleep. —

Infants with originally normal milestones show arrest of their mental development resulting in progressive intellectual deficit (starting with the onset of the seizures). Many infants, however, had first neonatal seizures and signs of brain damage. These children usually show only temporary response to therapy which is based on ACTH and steroids whereas the usual anticonvulsants are useless. Some benzodiazepines are helpful, especially Nitrazepam (Mogadon®) which, however, is not marketed in the United States.

3. Febrile Convulsions

Convulsions triggered exclusively by fever usually occur at an age from 6 months to 3 years; they very seldom present earlier but are not so rare between 3 and 5 years of age. *Febrile convulsions are the most common and also the most benign type of all epileptic conditions.* The prevalence has been thought to exceed 5% of the total population (compared with an overall prevalence of 0.5% 'hard core' epilepsies in the total population).

The convulsions are tonic-clonic and represent an early form of grand mal. Trivial *upper respiratory tract infections* are the most common cause; the seizures tend to occur at the very beginning of the temperature rise. Febrile convulsions must be strictly separated from seizures due to febrile brain disease (encephalitis, acute cortical venous thrombosis; see table II). A genetic predisposition to febrile convulsions is likely.

The EEG of the inter-seizure interval is normal in about 80–95% of the cases. The presence of seizure discharges is suggestive of a more complex type of epilepsy which is likely to change to febrile convulsions. The vast majority of children with febrile convulsions (about 85–95%) have an *excellent prognosis.*

There is no cogent reason for anticonvulsive treatment (usually phenobarbital) but the physician is well advised not to resist parental pressure.

Table II. Differences between febrile convulsions and seizures due to febrile brain disease

	Febrile convulsions	Seizures in febrile brain disease
Typical age range	6 months to 3 years (seldom 5 years)	mainly 0 to 3 years
Genetic predisposition to seizures	may be strong	mostly minor or insignificant
Type of seizure	tonic-clonic (modified or attenuated grand mal)	tonic-clinic (grand mal-like) or hemiconvulsions
Duration of seizure	mostly 1–3 min, seldom prolonged	often prolonged, 10 min to hours, status-like or in rapid succession
Clinical setting in which seizures occur	at the onset of a febrile disease, mostly upper respiratory illness, often coinciding with the first sharp rise of temperature	in a variety of CNS infections (encephalitis, meningo-encephalitis), intracranial venous thrombosis, cerebro-vascular accidents of infancy; also in exanthema subitum and after vaccination (smallpox) but usually less severe
Type of underlying cerebral pathology	none	various types of inflammatory and vascular changes, in milder cases limited to edema
Post-ictal neurological deficit (Todd's paralysis)	very uncommon	common and often mixed with pathology-determined neurological defect
EEG	rapidly normalizes after convulsion, normal interval tracings in 80–90%	abnormal throughout febrile episode, abnormal in interval (except for mild encephalitis)
Anticonvulsive medication	not necessary (either for acute convulsions or for prevention of further seizures)	Acutely needed (preferably diazepam, phenobarbital), long-term treatment required afterwards (except for mild encephalitis)
Prognosis	excellent in the vast majority (especially those with normal interval EEGs)	guarded; neurological defects and further seizures common

4. The Lennox-Gastaut Syndrome

A severe and mostly therapy-resistant epileptic condition, developing mainly between ages 1 and 10 years, more seldom during the second decade. *Mental retardation is almost always present in children with early onset.*

The EEG has been helpful in the delineation of this syndrome (*slow spike-wave complexes,* multiple spikes, runs of rapid spikes). Almost all types of seizures may occur but some of them are diagnostically highly suggestive, especially the *atonic-akinetic type* associated with sudden fall and often with head injuries (necessitates wearing protective headgear). *Myoclonus,* more prolonged attacks, *brief tonic attacks* (mainly in sleep) are also very common. Psychomotor automatisms, adversive and focal motor seizures may be abundant. Grand mal may be limited to the period of the onset of seizures; petit mal-like absences are sometimes noted. Many children have more than 2 or 3 types of seizures.

The cause remains often unknown. Some children have a history of cerebral palsy, others may have evidence of an inborn error of metabolism. About 20% of the children pass through a period of hypsarrhythmia (infantile spasms) before showing the EEG and ictal signs of the Lennox-Gastaut syndrome.

Therapeutic attempts are mostly quite unsatisfactory; benzodiazepines have been used with temporary success. Surgery is not indicated. Some children have prolonged seizure-free periods of spontaneous remission. Many children will eventually require institutionalization.

5. Primary Generalized Epilepsy
(also Called Centrencephalic or Idiopathic)

This form is presumed to be determined by a *genetic predisposition* in addition to the factor of age. A history of earlier brain disease, the presence of neurological deficits, focal EEG signs or focal-cortical types of seizure would be incompatible with primary generalized epilepsy.

The maximally involved age ranges from 4 to 20 years; the seizures tend to disappear in early adulthood.

Most typical type of seizures is the classical petit mal absence. The generalized synchronous character of the 3/s spike-wave discharge reflects primary generalization. Petit mal is most common between age 4 and 12 years; about 30–50% of the children will have grand mal in the second decade. Myoclonus may occur, sometimes in the morning as a warning sign of an imminent grand mal attack (especially after a night of poor sleep). The waking-sleeping cycle plays an important role ('dyshormia concept' of deviant arousal responses [4]). *Sensitivity to flickering light is a feature* in a subgroup of primary generalized epilepsy.

The treatment of petit mal requires special anticonvulsants (suximides, diones. Ethosuximide (Zarontin®) is highly effective in most cases; sodium valproate (Depakene®) is also very useful. Trimethadione (Tridione®) is very potent but beset with undesirable side effects.

6. Benign Rolandic Epilepsy

Many epileptic children between age 3 and 12 years show well-defined focal spikes. The central, mid-temporal and parietal regions are most often affected. These children have grand mal as well as focal motor attacks. The seizures occur almost always during nocturnal sleep.

The prognosis of these forms of epilepsy is excellent; most of these children will 'grow out' of their seizures in early adolescence. The prognosis is guarded, however, when the spikes are multifocal and also in children with evidence of cerebral palsy.

Special Types of Epilepsy according to Site of Focus

The local origin of epileptic seizure disorders may reveal itself by the focal character of the seizures. Well-documented clinical details of a seizure in combination with EEG findings and also the reproduction of ictal phenomena by local cortical stimulation [5] have enormously contributed to (a) deeper knowledge of epileptology, and (b) better comprehension of cortical functions.

1. Temporal Lobe Epilepsy

The *temporal lobe* is by far *the most common seat of cerebral epileptogeni foci.* This is due to intrinsic proclivity to epileptic responses of mesio-temporal limbic structures such as amygdala and hippocampus ('low threshold areas' [7]) and also to the vulnerability of the hippocampic region because of a relatively poor blood supply.

The classical temporal lobe type of seizure is the *psychomotor seizure* (complex partial seizures, according to a more recent terminology). The ictal symptomatology consists of (a) psychical; (b) motor; (c) autonomic, and (d) sensory symptoms. Psychomotor seizures should be basically divided into (a) *psychomotor automatisms,* and (b) *experienced psychomotor seizures.*

Automatisms occur in a state of *impaired consciousness;* the automatic behavior expresses itself in (a) uncoordinated-purposeless; (b) coordinated-purposeless; (c) uncoordinated-purposeful, and (d) coordinated-purposeful movements. This sequence indicates a continuum from the most primitive to the highest type of psychomotor automatisms. Postural reflexes remain intact even in the lowest types and the patient does not fall.

Movements are often *stereotyped-repetitive* (fumbling with clothes or various objects, picking and searching hand movements). An *oral component* is very common: swallowing, lip licking, smacking, grunting, drooling. Staring and sniffing is frequently noted. *The duration range from about 30 s to 5 min.*

Experienced seizures (psychical and sensory symptoms) are usually shorter and sometimes reduced strange 'flash'-like sensations. Strange and weird thoughts or emotions are experienced. Most common is the *'déjà vu'-experience* consisting of an *extreme familiarity* of the present situation (the present is experienced as though it always had been this way); this is due to abnormal epileptic neuronal circuitry in pathways subserving memory mechanisms.

There are also complex misperceptions (pseudo-hallucinations) involving all senses: strange sceneries, micropsia with Liliputian illusions, Alice-in-Wonderland-type experiences. Dreamy states and twilight states may result. *Olfactory sensations* (usually bad odors) are especially common in psychomotor seizures due to temporal lobe tumors.

Autonomic symptoms are multifold but are most commonly of abdominal character with gastrointestinal hypermotility and especially with a *'rising epigastric sensation'.*

In children, psychomotor seizures are less common than in adulthood and are not as readily diagnosed; *sudden fear* is one of the most important manifestations in childhood.

The *EEG* shows a wide variety of ictal changes; the inter-ictal EEG, however, shows very clearly anterior temporal spikes or sharp waves, often becoming more prominent in sleep. This typical finding is often absent in children with psychomotor seizures.

The *prevalence* is high, especially in adults, probably second to grand mal but more common than grand mal in populations of institutionalized epileptics.

Most temporal lobe epileptics also have grand mal seizures; sometimes, a psychomotor automatism or experience may be the aura-like prelude of a grand mal.

Personality changes are particularly common in temporal lobe epileptics, especially *irritability,* strangely associated with marked *hyposexuality* (often with complete lack of sexual response). Acts of aggression may occur, mainly in the interval, seldom in a seizure. The aggressiveness of temporal lobe epileptics has been badly overrated [*Rodin*].

The *most common cause is a residual epileptogenic lesion (gliosis),* mostly due to infantile damage with markedly delayed onset of seizures. There are many other forms of pathology; tumors of the temporal lobe are frequently noted in patients with onset of seizures in adulthood.

The prognosis is mostly guarded and often quite gloomy. There are, of course, numerous cases with good response to anticonvulsants but poor responses are very common. These patients should be considered candidates for temporal lobectomy (see section 'Anticonvulsive treatment'). Carbamazepine (Tegretol®) and Primidone (Mysoline®) are more effective than diphenylhydantoin and phenobarbital.

2. Frontal Lobe Epilepsy

Seizures arising from the frontal lobe have a strong tendency to become generalized; prior to the grand mal attack, an aura-like focal phase is often present. The most important focal manifestations are:

Adversive seizures (turning eyes, head and body, usually to opposite side), either with unconsciousness (closer to frontal pole) or in a conscious state (closer to motor cortex).

Autonomic-visceral sensations, mainly rising epigastric aura. The same sensations may occur in temporal lobe epilepsy.

Aphasic and dysphasic seizures or *ictal vocalization,* from Broca or upper frontal region. Similar aphasic attacks may occur in temporal lobe epilepsy.

Ictal thought disturbances, especially forced thinking. Usually regarded as a temporal lobe phenomenon but may also originate from frontal lobes.

Less well known but epileptologically very important are the manifestations of *supplementary motor region (mesiofrontal epilepsy)* with predominant *tonic seizures* and occasionally very poor response to anticonvulsants.

3. Focal-Motor (Rolandic, Jacksonian) Seizures

Clonic twitching of contralateral limbs and facial (seldom trunkal) muscles, often starting in one muscle and then gradually spreading *(Jacksonian march),* may result in a grand mal. Often caused by tumors over or within the Rolandic region but also by AV malformations, arteriosclerosis and syphilis. EEG localization often unsatisfactory. In children, these attacks are most commonly associated with benign Rolandic epilepsy (see above).

Epilepsia partialis continua (Koshevnikov syndrome) consists of virtually continuous twitching of a small muscle segment, lasting for months and years. The truly continuous cases are almost confined to the effect of the Siberian spring-summer encephalitis (postencephalitic manifestation).

4. Parietal Lobe Epilepsy: Focal Sensory Epilepsy

Rather uncommon. Paroxysmal paresthesias of the contralateral half of the body are typical manifestations of seizures arising from the postcentral gyrus. Ictal pain is quite rare.

Sudden violent vertigo, epigastric sensations and visual illusions may occur in seizure activity of other regions of the parietal lobe.

5. Occipital Lobe Epilepsy

Characterized mainly by *elementary visual sensations* (gross light, ball of fire, sparks). Blurring of vision, darkness and complete transient blindness may occur as ictal symptoms. *Epileptic nystagmus (oculo-clonic seizures)* represents a motor seizure manifestation of the occipital lobe and is not uncommon. The possibility of a tumor as the cause of the seizures must be carefully ruled out.

6. Epilepsies of Deep Origin

Basal ganglia and thalamic diseases are only exceptionally associated with epilepsy. *Hypothalamic lesions* may occasionally give rise to grand mal attacks and even to classical petit mal absences (usually in association with diencephalic-autonomic and endocrine disturbances).

Paroxysmal manifestations in the pontine and oblongata level are customarily not regarded as epileptic (for instances trigeminal neuralgia). 'Cerebellar fits' is a misleading term and denotes tonic posturing in decerebrate states. The glosso-oro-pharyngeal myorhythmias do not belong to the domain of epilepsy. Spinal epilepsy is a controversial term and is limited to segmental myoclonus.

Rare Special Forms of Epilepsy
(Unusual Triggering Mechanisms)

(a) Reading Epilepsy
Convulsions precipitated by reading. Preceded by strange laryngeal sensations and 'jaw clicking'. Precise neurophysiological mechanisms are poorly understood.

(b) Various Types of Visually Induced Epilepsies
Sensitivity to flickering light, usually an important segment of 'primary generalized epilepsy' (see section 'Age-determined epileptic conditions'), easily triggered in the EEG laboratory by flashes of the strobe lamp, especially at rates of 14–18 flashes/s. Manifested mainly by myoclonus, absences and grand mal. May occur under certain natural conditions (play of light through foliage of trees, etc.). Self-induced seizures by rapidly moving hands in front of eyes in bright sunshine are sometimes observed in mentally retarded flicker-sensitive epileptics.
Pattern vision sensitivity and *television-induced* seizures are based on the very rare epileptogenic effect of geometrical patterns. Other forms of photosensitivity are seizures induced by *visual exploration* and by eye *closure.*

(c) Musicogenic Epilepsy
Seizures (mostly psychomotor automatisms) induced by listening to music; very rare, not consistently reproducible.

(d) Startle Epilepsy
Produced by unexpected strong stimuli, especially by loud noise. Very typical in *infants with Tay-Sachs disease.* Occasionally noted in patients with hemiplegic form of cerebral palsy in the paretic limbs (tonic spasm).

(e) Tapping Epilepsy
Very rare; myoclonic phenomena produced by somatosensory stimuli, especially by tapping (examination of deep tendon reflexes).

(f) Arithmetic-Induced Epilepsy
Extremely rare; triggered by calculation. Decision-making (playing chess) may trigger seizures.

(g) Movement-Induced Epilepsy
Observed in connection with *paroxysmal choreo-athetosis* and with *tonic seizures.*

(h) 'Reflex Epilepsy'
Based on experimental work of Italian and Russian schools, essentially comprising all peripheral mechanisms in the precipitation of epileptic seizures.

Status epilepticus

Status epilepticus is a state of prolonged or continuous seizure activity or a state of recurrent seizures in rapid succession with no recovery of consciousness between the attacks. It is not simply a cluster of seizures.

1. Grand Mal Status epilepticus

A serious condition associated with *profound coma* between attacks, hyperthermia (of central nature and without apparent infectious cause), blood leucocytosis (with no evidence of infection) and sometimes with albuminuria. One major convulsion follows another in intervals of a few minutes.

The status is thought to be due to the breakdown of inhibitory (seizure-terminating) mechanisms, probably of cerebellar origin and possibly damaged by seizure-induced cerebellar hypoxia.

Therapeutically, the use of *intravenous diazepam (Valium)* or *intravenous paraldehyde* or intravenous diphenylhydantoin (Dilantin) in combination with *intramuscular phenobarbital* is the treatment of choice; its effectiveness decreases if the status does not respond during the first 2 days. *Intensive care unit treatment* with *intubation,* artificial respiration and muscular relaxation are life saving in the most serious forms of status. Some cases are determined by the cause of the seizures, for instance terminal status in an undiagnosed advanced brain tumor.

Sudden withdrawal of anticonvulsants, haphazard intake of medication or a trivial gastrointestinal infection (giving rise to poor absorption of medication) may be the cause of status in chronic epileptics.

2. Petit Mal Status
(Ictal Stupor, Spike-Wave Stupor, Absence Status)

Mostly consisting of *prolonged twilight states* with *stuporous behavior* (but no severe impairment of consciousness), occurring at any age (except for infancy). These episodes usually last from 6 to 48 h; the behavior is strange, speech is slurred, subtle myoclonic twitching is common; a few grand mal attacks may occur at the height of the episode. The EEG shows constantly recurrent long runs of generalized spike waves, mostly 3–4 complexes/s. The episodes stop abruptly and the patient is himself again (with sudden normalization of the EEG).

Some of these patients have a history of petit mal absences in childhood and grand mal in adolescence (common generalized epilepsy; see

'Age-determined' epileptic conditions); others have no history of any previous seizure disorder. In contrast with typical petit mal absences (usually in childhood and early adolescence), petit mal status may occasionally start in old age.

3. Temporal Lobe (Psychomotor) Status
Prolonged states of rapidly repetitive psychomotor automatisms for hours or days are extremely rare.

4. Adversive, Focal-Motor and Other Types of Status epilepticus
A prolonged status-like sequence of *adversive seizures* is not very uncommon. The status-form of focal motor seizures is *epilepsia partialis continua* (Koshevnikov's syndrome), discussed under 'Special types of epilepsy according to site of focus'.

'Borderland of Epilepsy' and Differential Diagnosis of Seizures

1. Migraine, Abdominal Pain and Vertigo: 'Borderland of Epilepsy'
Classical migraine (with scintillating scotoma preceding unilateral headache, nausea, vomiting) and *ordinary migraine* without initiating visual disturbances are very common ictal syndromes. Their physiopathogenesis is still controversial and their relationship to the epilepsies is rather remote.

Paroxysmal abdominal pain is particularly common in children and may frequently represent a forerunner of migraine. Abdominal pain is an epileptic manifestation and especially as an autonomic symptom of temporal lobe epilepsy is quite rare (compared with epigastric sensations and intestinal hypermotility as fairly common, true epileptic signs of short duration).

Vertigo and *dizziness* are most commonly due to non-epileptic disorders such as labyrinthine or eighth nerve disease; true epileptic vertigo is very rare.

2. Syncopal Attacks
Syncopal loss of consciousness (fainting) is a manifestation of acute generalized *insufficiency of the cerebral circulation* and may be due to a variety of disorders:

(a) Syncope with peripheral circulatory inadequacy
     Vasodepressor syncope
     Postural hypotension
(b) Syncope with cardiac disorders
     Heat block (Adams-Stokes syndrome)
     Paroxysmal tachycardia
     Coronary insufficiency and myocardial infarction
     Aortic stenosis and insufficiency
     Congenital heart disease
(c) Syncope with respiratory and pulmonary disorders
     Hyperventilation
     Breath holding
     Laryngeal syncope
     Cough syncope
     Sneezing
     Valsalva
     Pulmonary hypertension, pulmonary embolism
(d) Syncope with cerebrovascular disorders
     Chiefly due to vertebro-basilar artery insufficiency
(e) Fainting of primary psychic origin
     Conversion hysteria
     Acute stress
     Neuroses and psychoses

The *vasodepressor type of syncope* has also been termed *vasovagal* because of prominent vagotonic mechanisms. It may be triggered by venipuncture, sight of blood, minor painful injuries or the receipt of frightening news. A *convulsive type of syncope* with a few clinic movements or brief tonic spasm *is quite common but should not be diagnosed as epilepsy.*

Important forms of syncope are: *hypersensitivity of the carotid sinus, micturition* syncope (nocturnal urination in the male) and *breath-holding attacks* in older infants and small children (divided into pale and cyanotic forms).

3. Attacks Caused by Sudden Changes of Blood Chemistry

All forms of *hypoglycemia* fall into this category. A hypoglycemic state may occasionally trigger a grand mal seizure. *Tetanic* attacks with *hypocalcemia* and *carpopedal spasm* are of non-epileptic nature but true epileptic seizure may occur on the basis of severe hypocalcemia.

4. Psychogenic Seizures

Divided into *classical or major hysterical attacks* (arching of back, wild and disorderly sequence of tonic and clonic movements) and *minor types of psychogenic spells* (fainting, trembling, shaking, stuporous behavior).

5. *Faked Epileptic Seizures*
Willfully initiated and with artful imitation of grand mal or other seizures (in contrast with the subconscious-neurotic governing mechanisms in
psychogenic seizures).

Anticonvulsive Treatment

The modern era of anticonvulsive treatment began in 1857 with the
introduction of the bromides. Phenobarbital was introduced 1911, diphenylhydantoin 1938, the diones (Tridione) 1945, primidone (Mysoline)
1952. The suximides were developed in the 1950s; their most effective
derivative, ethosuximide (Zarontin), was introduced 1958. In the same
year, the efficacy of ACTH in infants with hypsarrhythmia was reported.
Carbamazepine (Tegretol) was introduced 1962 and the anticonvulsive
action of diazepam (Valium) was reported in 1965. Sodium valproate was
introduced in 1970.

1. Barbiturates
a) Phenobarbital. One of the most widely used anticonvulsants,
essentially safe and quite inexpensive. Most effective in grand mal and focal
seizures. *Neural action* thought to be multiple and nonselective. *Absorption*
in GI tract is slow. *Maximal brain concentration* reached after 10–15 h,
maximal serum levels after 10–12 h. *Slowly metabolized,* excreted in urine.
Half-life of 53–140 h.
Dosage. 1–3 mg/kg/day, common starting dose for adults 100 mg/day
(usually 32 mg three times daily). A total of 300 mg/day should not be
exceeded. Infants receive 15–30 mg/day, children 30–60 mg/day (initial
amounts). The *intramuscular route* is safe, the intravenous route, in general,
not advisable. Therapeutic *serum concentration levels* lie between 10 and
40 mg/1,000 ml with a safe average range of 10–20 mg/1,000 ml. These
levels are usually obtained after 2–3 weeks.
Side Effects. After long-term use, side effects consist mainly of
drowsiness. In children, *hyperactivity* is a very common undesirable side
effect.
b) Mephobarbital (Mebaral®). Less sedative than phenobarbital and
also less potent as anticonvulsant. Offers no advantage but is generally safe.
Daily *dosage* for adults: 200–600 mg.

c) Primidone (Mysoline®). A desoxybarbiturate, effective mainly in grand mal but also in psychomotor seizures. The *absorption rate* is fast. The *metabolism* is quite complex. Primidone itself is quickly metabolized; it is then broken down into PEMA (phenylethyl-malonamide) and phenobarbital.

Dosage. Average dosage for an adult is about 10 mg/kg/day, mostly 750 mg given in 3 single doses of 250 mg. Children receive 150–250 mg/day. The therapeutic levels of *serum concentration* lie between 5 and 15 mg/1,000 ml, but a therapeutic serum concentration of phenobarbital will also be obtained.

Side Effects. These are more serious than in phenobarbital; occasionally, the very first tablet may give rise to severe hypersomnia. Dizziness, diplopia and ataxia may develop. GI disturbances, skin rashes, impotence and hemopoietic responses have been described.

2. Hydantoins

(a) Diphenylhydantoin, Phenytoin, DPH (Dilantin®). A potent anticonvulsant with very little sedative effect. Most effective against grand mal. *Neural action* consists mainly in stabilization of excitable membranes; the effect on the cellular turnover of sodium results in a decrease of intracellular sodium. *Absorption* in the non-ionized form is rapid but limited by its extremely slow solubility in GI fluids. The *metabolism* of DPH is based mainly on parahydroxylation; the product of this process is excreted into the bile but mostly eliminated through the kidneys.

Dosage. Usually 4–8 mg/kg/day; an adult of average weight receives 300 mg/day, preferably divided into 3 doses. Amounts of more than 400 mg/day are usually poorly tolerated. Daily amounts of 100–200 mg are usually given in children. The *intramuscular route* is surprisingly slow (poor water solubility); the *intravenous route* has to be used with caution. Clinically effective *serum concentration* obtained within 1 week and range from 10 to 20 mg/1,000 ml.

Side Effects. Side effects of long-term use are common (table III).

(b) Mephenytoin (Mesantoin®). Very effective in grand mal seizures. The dosage is higher than that of DPH, maximal dosage in children is 600 mg/day, in adults 1,200 mg/day. Neurotoxicity and gum hyperplasia are much less common than in DPH treatment but *serious hematological changes* (bone marrow toxicity) are a formidable drawback.

(c) Ethotoin (Peganone®). Effective mainly against grand mal. Weak anticonvulsive potency; for this reason, large amounts are required. *Average*

Table III. Diphenylhydantoin toxicity

A Effects of overdosage
   Acute effects
      CNS (cerebello-vestibular, delirium), gastric distress
   Chronic effects
      Cerebello-vestibular syndrome
      Encephalography with increased seizures, severe EEG changes, mental
         changes
      Peripheral neuropathy

B Probable hypersensitivity, 'allergic' effects
   Febrile responses with various dermatoses
   Erythema multiform, Stevens-Johnson syndrome
   Lymphadenopathy, pseudolymphoma (? lymphoma)
   Acute systemic collagen disorder reactions (lupus erythematosus)
   Hepatitis
   Certain blood dyscrasias (neutropenia, agranulocytosis, aplastic anemia)

C Other effects
   Gum hyperplasia (effects in connective tissue)
   Megaloblastic anemia (folate deficiency)
   Endocrine effects (role in toxicity unclear)
      Adreno-cortical, pituitary
      Hirsutism in young females

---

dosages are 1,500–2,500 mg/day in adults and 500–1,500 mg/day in children. It is a relatively safe drug; it does not give rise to gingival hyperplasia and hypertrichosis; neurotoxic and hematological effects are rare and usually not severe.

3. Acetlyurea

(a) Phenacemide (Phenurone®). A very effective anticonvulsant, especially against psychomotor seizures. *The toxic effects outweigh its anticonvulsive usefulness* and the drug must be used with greatest precaution. Fatalities have been reported from hepatic, renal and hemopoietic disturbances. The *dosage* ranges from 1,000 to 6,000 mg/day in adults and from 500 to 3,000 mg/day in children.

4. Diones (Oxazolidinediones)

(a) Trimethadione (Tridione). Very effective against *petit mal absences.* Therapeutic dosage range from 600 to 1,800 mg/day in adults and older

children and from 300 to 900 mg/day in children under age 6 years. *Undesirable side effects are common and sometimes serious.* Photophobia is a mild and early side effect; hiccups are also noted. Severe renal complications and, above all, severe bone marrow toxicity may lead to fatal outcome. Blood count controls are mandatory.

(b) Paramethadione (Paradione). Its effect against petit mal seizures and its toxic side effects are similar to Tridione.

5. Succinimides (Suximides).

(a) Phensuximide (Milortin). Was used for the treatment of petit mal absences but its use has been all but abandoned. Side effects are very common.

(b) Methsuximide (Celontin). Effective against petit mal and probably also against psychomotor seizures. Serious side effects are rare; drowsiness, personality change, nausea and vomiting have been reported.

(c) Ethosuximide (Zarotonin). Very effective against *petit mal absences* and presently considered the *treatment of choice* against this type of seizure. *Absorption* is rapid, peak serum concentrations are reached within 1–3 h after ingestion. The *metabolism* is poorly understood. The optimum *dosage* is determined empirically since there are no specific signs of overdosage. The range lies between 750 and 2,000 mg/day for adults and children above 6, and 500–1,000 mg/day for children below 6 years. The *serum concentration* levels range from 10 to 55 mg/1,000 ml. *Side effects* consists of drowsiness, hiccups, nausea, headaches, dizziness and gastric distress and may necessitate permanent withdrawal. Severe bone marrow depression is very rare.

6. Sulfonamides

(a) Sulthiame (Ospolot). Not marketed in the USA. Considered to be effective against psychomotor seizures. Average *dosage* lies between 300 and 600 mg/day for adults. *Side effects* are not serious (hyperpnea, tachypnea, occasional renal disturbances).

(b) Acetazolamide (Diamox). An adjunct of anticonvulsive therapy rather than an anticonvulsant; a carbonic anhydrase inhibitor and found to be useful in female patients with *clusters of grand mal in the premenstrual phase.*

7. Iminostilbenes

(a) Carbamazepine (Tegretol). Effective against grand mal and psychomotor seizures; probably the *treatment of choice for psychomotor attacks.* The

dosage lies between 400 and 800 mg/day for adults and 100 and 400 mg/day for children. Side effects are fairly common: diplopia, 'heavy feeling in the eyes', abnormal liver function tests, leucopenia and rashes; many of these reactions are considered dosage-related and thus avoidable. Therapeutic *serum* concentration levels lie in the range of 3–14 mg/1,000 ml.

8. Bromides

Effective against grand mal and focal motor seizures. Sodium and potassium have been mostly used. In general, this form of treatment offers no advantage over any other anticonvulsant; *side effects* (bromism) are common and often serious.

9. Benzodiazepines

(a) Diazepam (Valium). Originally introduced as a tranquilizer; *its anticonvulsive effect is essentially limited to status epilepticus* (intravenous route). The effect is very short-lasting. The *serum* concentration level lies around 0.2 mg/1,000 ml determined 1 h after administration of 10 mg.

(b) Nitrazepam (Mogadon). Not marketed in the USA. Effective against infantile spasms (hypsarrhythmia) although not quite as effective as ACTH. Drowsiness is a common side effect.

(c) Clonazepam (Clonopin®). Used mainly in the treatment of status epilepticus (intravenous route); the effect is thought to be more prolonged than the effect of Valium. Clonopin may be (at least temporarily) helpful in children with Lennox-Gastaut syndrome and in patients with myoclonus. Small dosages are recommended at the beginning (about 0.02 mg/kg/day) with gradual increase. Drowsiness is a common side effect.

(d) Clorazepate (Tranxene®). Not specifically recommended as an anticonvulsant.

10. ACTH and Steroids

The *treatment of choice for infantile spasms* (hypsarrhythmia). The anticonvulsive action is completely enigmatic.

Treatment must be started as soon as the first seizures are observed. A course of treatment consists of daily intramuscular injections of 25–30 units of respiratory corticotropin for 4–6 weeks. If no clinical and no EEG improvement is seen, the infant is placed on cortisone or prednisone for at least 2 months.

11. Sodium Valproate (Depakene)

Available in Europe around 1970, marketed in the USA in 1977. Excellent medication in cases of *primary generalized epilepsy* with *petit mal absences* and myoclonus. Usually well tolerated. Dosage lies around 750–1,500 mg/day (older children, adults) and therapeutic serum concentration levels are found above 50 mg/1,000 ml or in the range of 100–300 μmol/100 ml. The toxicity threshold appears to be very high (probably above 60 mg/kg). Sodium valproate has been also recommended as an adjunct in poorly responsive temporal lobe seizures. Sodium valproate may enhance the sedative effect of other anticonvulsants if given at the same time.

12. Possible Teratogenic Effects of Anticonvulsants when Taken during Pregnancy

The evidence has been rather tenuous, more research in this field will be needed. Seizure surgery is limited to a small group of drug refractory patients but has an important place in the therapeutic armamentarium of the epilepsies.

Neurosurgical Treatment

1. Temporal Lobectomy

This is *the most commonly used surgical procedure in the treatment of seizures.* Clinical evidence of temporal lobe epilepsy with typical psychomotor seizures (with or without additional grand mal) must be substantiated by corresponding EEG findings (classically: anterior temporal sharp waves or spikes). The seizure discharges should be predominantly unilateral. The insertion of depth electrodes is helpful in the delineation of the focus. Diffuse or consistently bilateral EEG abnormalities usually represent a contraindication for surgery.

The surgical procedure must be limited to one side; bilateral temporal lobectomy would lead to crippling personality changes (Klüver-Bucy syndrome). The superior temporal gyrus is usually spared (especially when the operation is performed on the dominant hemisphere); the anterior 55–70 mm of the temporal lobe are removed together with amygdala and hippocampus; the insula is left intact.

Postoperative complications are uncommon and usually not severe; the mortality lies below 1%. Quadrantic hemianopsia and memory deficits are undesirable sequelae of temporal lobectomy.

The *results* are excellent (seizure-freedom for many years) in at least 50%, with good patient selection probably in about 70%.

2. Other Major Procedures

Partial frontal, parietal and occipital lobectomies are much less frequently performed than temporal lobectomies. *Hemispherectomy* has its place in the treatment of recalcitrant seizures in children with the *hemiplegic form of cerebral palsy.*

3. Stereotaxic Surgery for Seizures Disorders

Seldom performed; amygdalotomies and fornicotomies have been done with questionable results in temporal lobe epileptics.

4. Cerebellar Implantation of a Stimulating Device

Electrical stimulation of the cerebellar cortex has been thought to exert an inhibitory effect on cerebral seizure activity. *Cooper* et al. [1] have recently begun to insert a stimulating device in contact with the cerebellar cortex. The stimulation is carried out from an outside stimulator (in a radio-frequency envelop without connecting wires). Initially reported good results have not been reproducible at other institutions. It is still too early to judge the value of this type of treatment.

References

1   Cooper, I.S.; Amin, I.; Riklan, M.; Waltz, J.M.; Poon, T.P.: Chronic cerebellar stimulation in epilepsy. Archs Neurol., Chicago *33:* 559–570 (1976).

2   Gloor, P.: Evolution of the concept of the mechanisms of generalized epilepsy with spike and wave discharge; in Wada, Modern perspectives in epilepsy, pp. 99–137 (Eden Press, St. Albans 1978).

3   Naquet, P.: Perspective on epilepsy; in Wada, Penry, Advances in epileptology, pp. 1–11 (Raven Press, New York 1980).

4   Niedermeyer, E.: The generalized epileptics (Thomas, Springfield 1972).

5   Penfield, W.; Jasper, H.: Epilepsy and the functional anatomy of the human brain (Little, Brown, Boston 1954).

6   Prince, D.A.: Neuronal correlates of epileptiform discharges and cortical DC potentials; in Rémond, Handbook of electroencephalography and clinical neurophysiology, vol. 2C, pp. 56–70 (Elsevier, Amsterdam 1974).

7   Walker, A.E.: The propagation of epileptic discharge; in Niedermeyer, Epilepsy: recent views on theory, diagnosis and therapy of epilepsy, pp. 13–28 (Karger, Basel 1970).

8   Ward, A.A., Jr.: The epileptic neuron: chronic foci in animals and man; in Pope, Jasper,
     Ward, Jr., Basic mechanisms of the epilepsies, pp. 263–288 (Little, Brown, Boston
     1959).

Suggested Reading

1   Charlton, M.H.: Myoclonic seizures (Excerpta Medica, Amsterdam 1975).
2   Janz, D.: Epileptology (Thieme, Stuttgart 1975).
3   Lacy, J.R.; Penry, J.K.: Infantile spasms (Raven Press, New York 1976).
4   Lennox-Buchthal, M.A.: Febrile convulsions. A reappraisal (Elsevier, Amsterdam
     1973).
5   Niedermeyer, E.: Compendium of the epilepsies (Thomas, Springfield 1974).
6   Penry, J.K.: Epilepsy (Raven Press, New York 1977).
7   Penry, J.K.; Daly, D.D.: Complex partial seizures and their treatment (Raven Press,
     New York 1975).

10 An Overview of Ego Psychology and Developmental Theory
Correlates in Child Psychiatric Diagnosis of Retardation Syndromes
Peter B. Henderson

Introduction

1. History

During the 18th Century many leading biologists were convinced that the human existed completely preformed within the ovum as a microscopic homunculus. A number of eminent scientists disagreed. They insisted that the animalcule resided in the spermatozoa and not in the ovum. The inordinately intricate step-by-step differentiation of the organism from the fertilized germ cell could not be grasped, or even observed, because of rationalistic and religious judgments of 'what made sense'. The understanding of personality development and integration has been deterred by similar preconceptions. An individual's personality traits were long ascribed primarily to his or her ancestry. Aberrant behavior could readily be attributed to inheritance, for it clearly runs in families. 'Constitutional psychopathic inferiority' was still a proper diagnosis only a few decades ago – when delinquents were born, not made! At present, most psychiatrists accept axiomatically that persons suffering from schizophrenic disorders are genetically blighted, or in some other way constitutionally maldeveloped from the beginning, though research findings are still quite a way from a solid substantiation of that hypothesis.

An appreciation of the complexity of personality development has emerged slowly. Even the most dynamic of students of personality functioning tended to assume that the infant human would develop into a well-integrated and highly adaptable individual, unless an inherent defect, a childhood emotional trauma, or gross maternal neglect, induced a fixation of libidinal investment during childhood. The many factors that enter into personality development and the many requirements that must be supplied by the nurturing process and the enveloping social system(s), could be overlooked because all viable societies must provide for the essential needs of their off-spring and because the family is so essential that it is universal, many of its functions were taken for granted.

In a relatively brief overview it is hardly possible to consider in rich detail each phase of the individual's life cycle that occurs with the inevitability of the passage of time. It is important to instill the concept, though, that each developmental phase in an individual's life is not simply an end in itself, but is directed toward the attainment of a cohesive identity and a workable integration by the end of adolescence and the entry into young adulthood. The person, as an individual, should be studied therefore, not as an isolate, but within the interpersonal, social and cultural settings in which he or she lives and gains support and direction.

Any developmental study of the individual must appreciate and give serious consideration to the unique nature of the human's adaptive capacities – that is, ways of coping with the environment and surviving its hazards. The emergence of the human individual depended upon the evolution of a brain and a neuromuscular system capable of using tools, and especially that most supreme of all instrument – *language*. Human development emphasizes the central position of language and of thought, as eloquently expressed in Meyerian psychobiology, as well as Freudian psychoanalytic observation and theories. *Adolf Meyer* taught that man can be properly understood only as integrated at a symbolic level, because what the individual thinks and feels influences functioning down to the cellular and biochemical levels of human integration.

Some aspects of personality development are common to all humans, reflecting the basic similarities in their biological structure and functioning. The prolonged period of helplessness and dependency of the human infant and young child, late puberty, the dependence upon language and learning adaptive techniques, the need to provide prolonged care for offspring, and many other such factors, tend to lead to common features in all humans, and also to set a sequential pattern of the phases of the life cycle.

2. Developmental Knowledge as a Professional Instrument
Individuals who are in the care-taking profession of medicine should find it increasingly important during their lifetimes to come to consider the human factors intrinsic in the daily life-functioning of their patients, many of whom will be seen over the lifetime of the physician if he/she remains fairly settled in one community. Overviews, and even intensive study courses, that present developmental phenomenology can only scratch the surface of what needs to be understood about human function and adaptation. What is important to grasp is that the individuals as a total person, with his or her own life history, and with relationships that provide mean-

ing to existence, should be seen behind every individual who presents themself for patienthood. With children, this concept becomes even more poignant, for it is generally the child's parents who bring them for care, so that there may be several generations of intangible, yet important, material that the physician must not overlook in proper consultation. The tangible elements in the consultation relate more to the physical and physiologic maturation of the person's biologic equipment. The intangible matters of thoughts and feelings evolving over time requires an even more facile and mature knowledge. One must study the individual's development from a helpless animal infant into a specific person with relationships to self and others, and to events that influence individual physical make-up, physiologic responses, and state of overall health.

Medical education itself does not always assist the beginning physician in becoming aware of the nuances of human development. The medical student enters medical school to learn 'to treat people'. He is immediately confronted by a person – but, a dead person; and one that must be dissected, taken apart bit by bit. For added variety, the student peers at very thin slices of yet another human body through the microscope. The student then progresses to the study of human pathology – the subject is no less dead, simply more recently alive! This process, necessary as it is to assist in the incorporation of the vast number of facts relevant to the human organism, does run the risk of enhancing the belief that an ideally treatable patient is a very passive one indeed, devoid of a human history, and unrelated to any current human relationships beyond the medical consultation room.

There is no proper standard of human normality, no proper way of life – but rather, different types of workable integrations. Everyone has defects, weaknesses, problems. But we are all more human than otherwise, and these deficits are usually offset, if not at least balanced, by assets. Tolerance of the more negative, perplexing, or anxiety-producing characteristics of patients can be developed through the knowledge and understanding of the same individual's cultural, social, familial and general psychological makeup. This needs to start early in the career of care-giving others, and should continue to flourish throughout the lifetime of that person, as he or she is allowed into the human dilemmas that routinely present in physicians' offices throughout their years of practice.

Theoretical Frameworks in Developmental Theory

1. A Developmental Model

A detailed outline of a psychiatric examination of the child is given in table I.

The development of the human personality, and the course of the life cycle, unfold in phases – not at a steady pace. It depends not only upon the

Table I. Outline of a psychiatric examination of the child

---

1 Identifying information
   Name
   Age
   Gender
   Color
   Ordinal position in sibship
   Number of times examined in current consultation
   Referral source(s)

---

2 Reason for present referral
   Cover in brief detail the referral problem(s)
   Include pertinent information from referral source(s) that have bearing on this examination

---

3 General appearance
   Body build and habitus (estimate of growth and development percentile?)
   Characteristic facial expression(s) during contact(s)
   Self-care characteristics and clothing
   Defects in general physical health
   Sensory apparatus, i.e. hearing, vision, etc.
   Striking personality traits
   Mannerisms and rituals
   Other significant data

---

4 Interpersonal relations
   a   Interactions(s) with parent(s) or other caretaker(s)
       1   Waiting room or ward/classroom behavior
       2   Degree and type of emotional response manifest upon separation
       3   Ability (or not) to respond to reassurance
       4   Reaction(s) of child (and, where appropriate, parental response) upon reunion
   b   Interaction(s) with examiner
       1   General attitude: cooperative, fearful, arrogant, suspicious, etc.
       2   Capacity to relate to examiner
       3   Type of relationship with examiner: controlling, trusting, erotic, etc.
       4   Role taken by examiner, in contrast with role assigned by examinee
       5   Response engendered by interaction with examinee, i.e. sympathy, anxiety, anger, curiosity, etc.
       6   Beginning compared with end of time spent with patient
       7   Initial interview compared with subsequent one(s)

---

5 Capacities
   a   Intelligence
       1   Clinical estimate of intellectual level of current functioning
       2   Fund of general knowledge
       3   Imagination
       4   Grasp of situation of examination
       5   Estimate of potential capacity (especially pertinent if greater than current estimate of function)

Table I (cont.)

---

  b Affects
     1 Mobility (smoothness vs. lability vs. fixed affect)
     2 Appropriateness to given, and described, situations
     3 Predominant (cheerfulness, solemn, sadness, etc.)
     4 Described affect(s) i.e. anger, depression, anxiety, etc. (especially significant if can be verbalized by child)
     5 Shifts in tension level(s) during examination
     6 Somatic expression(s) of affect, i.e. sweating, blushing, pallor, etc.
  c Motor skills
     1 Coordination (gross and fine motor)
     2 Station and gait
     3 Muscular bulk and symmetry
     4 Use of hands and handedness
     5 Body activity pattern (restricted motions, hyperactive)
     6 Maturity of body movements related to age of child
  d Speech
     1 Clarity of speech
     2 Articulation abilities (stuttering, stammering, word blockages or word finding difficulties)
     3 Expressive abilities (descriptions of ideas, use of words as abstract tools, general spontaneity)
     4 Vocabulary (paucity of words known or understood, unusually large number of words used, etc.)
     5 Voice quality
     6 Aberrations: echolalia, perseveration, etc.

---

6 Content and trends of thought
  a Attitude toward clinical examination
     1 Reaction to play techniques and other exam procedures
     2 Grasp of purpose of examination
     3 Awareness of own difficulties
     4 Reaction to behavioral or physical abnormalities
     5 Ability to become constructively involved in examination
  b Attitudes toward self
     1 Thoughts displayed (in play) or verbalized about body image, sex, intellect, etc. (example: does child describe self as 'stupid', 'dumb', etc.)
     2 Expressed worries, fears, preoccupations (or displayed)
     3 Somatic expressions, i.e. hypochondrical ruminations, other evidences of somatization
  c Attitudes and feelings toward other (object relations)
     1 Toward parents
     2 Toward sibling(s)
     3 Toward extended family members
     4 Toward peers

Table I (cont.)

---

     5 Toward teachers
     6 Toward other important persons
  d Attidutes and feelings toward physical objects
     1 Hobbies
     2 Personal possessions (and those of others)
     3 Money (steals it, meaningless, unable to comprehend, etc.)
     4 Food (hoards it, anorectic, etc.)
     5 Schools, camps, activity equipment, etc.

---

7 Play and fantasy
  a Play
     1 Approach to and interest in toys
     2 Type(s) of toys utilized in play
     3 Mode of play most consistently observed (incorporative, extrusive, intrusive, etc.)
     4 Manner of child's play (constructive, destructive, disorganized, nurturant, etc.)
     5 Distractibility during play sequences
     6 Play disruptions and regressions
  b Fantasy content
     1 Wishes ('If you had three wishes, what would they be?')
     2 Dreams remembered and recounted
     3 Daydreams
     4 Fantasies child will share
     5 Expressions portrayed in drawings, clay, sand, etc.
     6 Ambitions and thoughts about his/her future

---

8 Clinical impression(s)
  a Summary of pertinent life experience, current and past
  b Important developmental data related to earlier developmental difficulties, delays, arrests, fixations, etc.
  c Describe as clearly as possible the genesis of any evident emotional and/or mental disorder(s)
  d Descriptive and phenomenologic diagnosis
  e Dynamic formulation(s) of important
     1 Include major area(s) of conflict, chronic or intermittent
     2 Note any precipitating event(s)
     3 Summary of nature and adequacy of ego's defensive organization and ego strength of child
     4 Current degree of psychologic homeostasis (with self and important others)
     5 Estimate of psychologic general health, i.e. the positive adaptive mechanisms the patient current uses

Table I (cont.)

9	Statistical diagnosis
a	Diagnostic and Statistical Manual (DSM-II)
b	Group of Advancement of Psychiatry Descriptive Diagnosis (GAP Manual, including categories and subcategories of behavioral diagnosis)
10	Estimate of prognosis
a	Benign, progressive, acute, chronic, etc.
b	With treatment, without treatment
11	Dispositional decision(s)
a	Further diagnostic studies (specifiy)
b	Need for treatment
c	Treatability (including parents, where indicated)
d	Environmental changes needed ('social engineering')
e	Other factors relevant
12	Treatment(s) recommended
a	Individual – investigative, relationship-oriented, supportive, art therapy, etc.
b	Group activity, social skills acquisition, etc.
c	Collaborative approach (specify collaboration with whom: parents, another agency, etc.)
d	Consultative (to another specialist? institution?)
e	Qualitative aspects of treatment
1	Frequency and estimated duration of therapy
2	Treatment goals and limitations
3	Family management or family therapy
4	General approach to total case

biological unfoldings and physical growth (maturation), but upon the evolution of personality functions. The developmental model here described considers human development not only on an internal processes model, but strongly considers the transaction and interpersonal processes that may be impacting on a human organism at any given point in time. The internal individual developmental framework is necessary for any student of this subject. That study exclusively will contribute to a one-sided view of human function and development, and exclude rich knowledge of the complex human transactions, which includes various interpersonal parameters, i.e. social, cultural, economic, health systems, education, and so forth.

An interesting simile drawn by *Lidz*, expanding upon a conceptualization of a developmental-interactional model, likens the developmental process to the evolution of a mountain-climbing expedition. In that example, camps must be made at varying levels of altitude, guides and other help found, the terrain at each level explored, new skills acquired repeatedly, rests taken before moving up to the next level. The descent process is similar, also made in gradual and appropriate stages. The human goes through periods of relative quiescence, and then undergoes another marked change, as movement to a new phase of life occurs, which opens new potentialities, provides new areas to explore, and poses new challenges and problems for mastery that require the learning of new sets of skills and abilities.

Thus, when the infant learns to crawl and can move toward objects that attract him, a new world opens that enables him to channel his energies in a new way, permitting a new zest to become manifest, and opening up opportunities for yet new learning. But, it also alters the mother's life, and the mother-child relationship. Because of this he will also have to learn to relate to her differently, expect rewards for different types of performance, and gain greater control of his behavior before achieving a new relative equilibrium, both within self, and in his various external important relationships.

It is this constant changing from an equilibrium to disequilibrium as new developments occur, with then a pressure toward establishing a new equilibrium (or, with less fortunate circumstances, falling backward, regressing in the process, to earlier, simpler systems of homeostatic equilibrium), that has led some developmental theorists to formulate a variation of an *input-output systems model* to understand the complex strategies of human development in an international field. This same conceptualization might apply to a phenomenon as presumably simple as a unicellular organism, with the input mainly the chemical substrate of its milieu, and the output its cellular metabolites and its waste products. Or, this same understanding can be applied to something as large as a major industrial complex, focusing on the myriad of human and material inputs into a conversion process that may have massive interlocking human and mechanical interconnections, which, in turn, leads to the production of various outputs that further extend the complexity of circular types of conversion processes.

Figure 1 has been more specifically filled in with details that would represent an interactional model of human development. The human organism in this theoretical model is understood to be an open system, responding to environmental input, as well as equally influencing the surrounding environment by the various signals and other outputs of which the human system is capable. The highly unique capability of the human is the capacity to develop highly complex feedback loops between individual output and input. From studying figure 1, it can be seen that as the human child

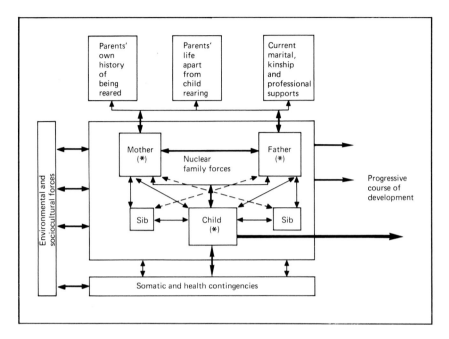

Fig. 1. An interactional model of development. * = Nature of behavior and degree of investment of primary caretakers in rearing this child; + = idiosyncratic nature of child's endowments.

acquires specific skills (be they social, cognitive, or motor skills) these will then directly and indirectly influence further effects of input (stimulation, approval, affection, other rewards). In the earlier example of the infant developing the capacity to crawl and reach for new objects, one cannot dismiss the impact this new development has upon that infant's caretaking environment, most especially the mother. She may react to this developmental progress in a number of different, idiosyncratic fashions. Many of her reactions will be influenced by her own current, past, and expected future supporting systems. To take that example further, if she is aware that her husband has developed a new affectionate relationship outside of their marriage, it may cause her to react to the developing capacities for greater autonomy on the part of her infant, as a further experience of personal abandonment, therefore causing her to react to that development in a quite different fashion than if she conceived her marital supports to be more stable.

In the Cohen and Rose developmental model, a great deal of focus is initially on the supporting systems of the mother during the pregnancy period. These supporting systems are seen as the key in understanding the relative high and low risk factors of the pregnancy with any individual child. Figure 2 is derived, though in a simpler fashion, from figure 1. It is meant to further represent the complex of interacting variables that relate to individual (mother-father and husband-wife, in this example) and nuclear family supporting systems. This further expands upon the idea of reverberating human systems and subsystems within the nuclear family and the psychosocial field of the extended family, community, cultural and health regulators. Through an understanding of the vectors, which are two-directional, one can see how an individual may come to acquire the biological, social and psychological identity that will become the end product of the first two decades of an individual's life, i.e. so-called adult identity formation.

2. Divisions of the Life Cycle

The division of the human life cycle into developmental stages follows a fairly clear set of lines of demarcation. *Infancy* approximates the first 15 months of life when the baby can neither properly walk nor talk, and requires almost total nurturant care, both for survival and for the stimulation necessary for emotional and cognitive development.[1] The *toddler* stage begins with the ability to ambulate and take initiative, which outruns the child's capacities to comprehend, speak and delimit him or herself. In this period the ensuing essential control by parental figures leads to critical conflicts over control and initiative. In the *preschool* (or *oedipal*) period the child finds a place as a boy or girl within the nuclear family. The child must rescind eroticized attachments to the parent of the opposite sex, as well as reduce an egocentric view of mother and father, while internalizing parental directives sufficiently to move from the close circle of the family out into age-appropriate peer groups. The *juvenile* (or *preadolescent*) moves further from the family and into various peer groups, as well as the continuation in a school environment, where acceptance and recognition further follow from his or her achievements and characteristic attributes. Personality

---

[1] Many developmental specialists, including *Benedek, Anthony, Cohen, Rose,* et al. include pregnancy as the initial developmental period in an individual's life history. Refer to the previous section for further information on that position.

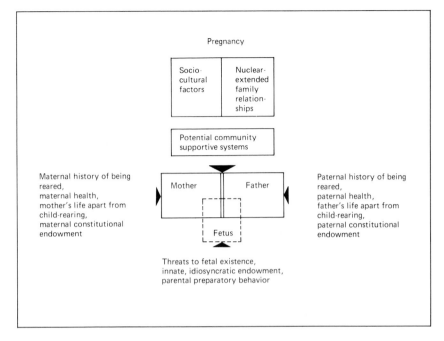

Fig. 2. An interactional model of the nuclear family.

structure gains new coherence and further organization through the impacts of how outside others (extrafamilial others, most especially, at this time) relate to, and help, him or her in the further definition of an individualized sense of self. *Adolescence* involves the discrepancy between sexual maturation and incomplete physical maturity, and between the upsurge of sexual impulses and the unpreparedness for adult responsibilities and parenthood.

Since development is dynamic, and not static (even during periods of apparent quiescence), it is important to not think of developmental phases and phase-specific accomplishments only in the childhood and adolescent periods of life. In the *young adult* the personality undergoes marked modifications through the choice of an occupation, in relation to marital choice (or not) and marital adjustment, and the reorientations necessarily required by emerging parenthood and its attendant responsibilities.

Middle age concerns the changes that follow upon the person's moving toward, and ultimately later away from, the peak generative years of the live cycle – when children usually are no longer a central preoccupation, professional accomplishments have been acquired to varying degrees of satisfaction, and declining physical capacities often lead the individual to a later-life reevaluation of him- or herself. In *old age* the physical abilities become increasingly limited: employed people retire, mental abilities are subject to much greater potential decline, and persons again (as in the early years of the life cycle) become more dependent upon various others for the provision of their essential life needs.

`The descriptions above, and the study of the important features of these developmental stages, evolve from three rather different approaches to understanding the phasic emergence of the essential attributes of the human personality, i.e. the *psychosexual phases,* the *psychosocial stages,* and the processes of *cognitive development.* Familiarity with these approaches is essential to the understanding of the literature and language of personality development and psychopathology. A brief review of each perspective follows.

(a) Phases of Psychosexual Development

In his epoch-making studies of childhood sexuality, although based primarily upon historical reconstruction of childhood histories of his adult patients, *Sigmund Freud* outlined five phases of psychosexual development between birth and adult maturity.

Oral phase: Virtually equivalent to infancy; the child's needs and energies focus upon nursing and close relatedness to the mothering other. The lips and mouth are highly invested, and a primary source of sensuous gratification. Either too much or too little oral gratification *or* some inate or constitutional predisposition to orality, can supposedly cause fixation in this phase, and cause unpreparedness to move to the subsequent phase(s).

Anal phase: Bowel training was considered a primary developmental task of the second year of life, and the anal zone a primary source of erotic gratification during that period. Fixations at the anal phase have been related to various character traits such as obsessiveness, stubbornness, miserliness, a perduring sense of shame, and many other related characteristics, as well as varying degrees of lasting erotization of the anal zone.

Phallic-oedipal phase: In this period the primary erogenous zone has been considered to shift to the penis in the boy and the clitoris in the girl, with an upsurge of sexual feelings toward the parent of the opposite sex. The boy's wish to possess the mother and be rid of the rival father, and the girl's desire for the father and jealousy of the mother – 'the oedipal situation' –

comes in conflict with reality, creates a fear of retribution from the rival-hated parent, and leads the child to repress his or her sexual feelings and possessiveness toward the incestuously desired parent. Instead, the boy pursues the more realistic goal of ultimately becoming a person like his father, who can possess a person like his mother. The reverse occurs in the girl. The child gains ego strength by identifying with the previously hated and feared opposite-sex parent, internalizes general parental controls, and increasingly becomes more related to reality.

Latency: A period, roughly correlating with the school-age period, when sexual impulses are supposedly latent, either because of a biological subsidence of libido, or because of the repression of the sexual impulses that seemed to the child to be dangerous during the earlier oedipal phase.

Genital phase: Starts with the upsurge of biologic puberty, with an erogenous reinvestment of the phallus in the male, but supposedly with a shift from clitoris to the vagina in the female. The capacity for genital sexuality was originally equated with the achievement of emotional maturity as the second decade of the life cycle occurred.

Freud's *epigenetic principle* has served as a major guide to personality dynamic studies and theories of personality functioning since his discovery of the psychosexual stages. This principle maintains that proper development progress requires the meeting and surmounting of the distinctive developmental tasks of each phase at the proper time, and in the proper sequence. This concept was derived from embryology, in which the proper unfolding of the embryo depends upon each organ's arising out of its anlage in the proper sequence and with proper timing, with each development depending upon the correct unfolding of the preceding phase(s). Personality development is not, however, so rigidly set as embryonic maturation; and it is apparent that even though developmental difficulties might occur, compensations are possible, and deficiencies can even be turned into strengths, which is not the case with embryologic development.

(b) Stages of Psychosocial Development

Erik Erikson also opened new approaches by superimposing an epigenesis of psychosocial development upon the psychosexual phases, and then designated the critical psychosocial task of each phase that the individual must surmount in order to be prepared for the next stage. This is outlined in table II. He has formulated *eight stages of psychosocial development,* focusing upon the specific developmental tasks of each stage and how society meets the needs of that stage by providing essential care, promoting inde-

Table II. Eight ages of man (Erikson)

Adaptive ego functioning		Maladaptive ego functioning (character pathology)
1 Basic trust	vs.	basic mistrust
2 Autonomy	vs.	shame and doubt
3 Initiative	vs.	guilt
4 Industry	vs.	inferiority
5 Identity	vs.	role confusion
6 Intimacy	vs.	isolation
7 Generativity	vs.	stagnation
8 Ego integrity	vs.	despair

pendence, offering roles, and having institutionalized ways of assuring the child's survival, proper socialization and emotional health. These different tasks are handled differently in each culture, so that one can understand the much heavier anthropologic influence of Erikson's studies than the more specifically individually oriented studies of Freud. An example of Erikson's paradigms might relate to the psychosocial task of 'basic trust' superimposed upon the oral phase of psychosexual development. In this regard, the task concerns the achievement of *basic trust,* both in self and others. Failures in this task attainment during this stage leads to varying degrees of *basic mistrust.* The other stages deal with other important phenomena as the development of *individual autonomy, initiative, industry,* resulting in the adolescent stage of a sense of *developed ego identity.* Failure in these stages (one or more) leads to enduring difficulties in the area(s) of the developmental psychosocial tasks, throughout the subsequent phases of the life cycle (see right hand column, table II).

(c) Cognitive Development

Jean Piaget has sought, in his monumental studies of the development of cognition, to trace and conceptualize how each new capacity develops through the reorganization and expansion of prior capacities by means of the assimilation of new experiences and skills. Briefly stated, the input *(aliment)* is *assimilated* by the cognitive processes insofar as they are then currently prepared to do so, and the cognitive processes *accommodate* to include what has been newly assimilated, reorganizing and expanding in this process. Cognitive experiences are assimilated into a *schema*, which reorganize in the process. The organism seeks to repeat schemata that produce new experiences, thereby setting up series of *circular reactions* in order to gain the reward of new input, until the input is thoroughly assimilated into the schema in the cognitive apparatus that has accommodated to it.

Piaget has described four major periods in his formulations:

Sensorimotor period (birth through first 18–24 months of life) – essentially covers preverbal intellectual development. Development is tracted from the most primitive reflex sucking, hand movements, and random eye movements, to the stage when the child uses internalized visual and motor symbols to invent new means of solving problems.

Preoperational period (from 2 until approximately 6 years) – the child becomes capable of using symbols and language. He moves away from an egocentric orientation and static ways of thinking as he gains experience, and as words becomes symbols of categories (i.e. classifications systems emerge defining categories of reality).

Period of concrete operations (from 6 to 12 years) – the child has acquired a coherent cognitive system with which he can understand his world and work upon and within it, and into which he can now increasingly fit new experiences.

Period of formal operations – starts early in adolescence when the youth becomes capable of conceptualizing, or thinking propositionally, deductively and inductively, and of using (and eventually generating) hypotheses about the world of reality. Not all individuals achieve this stage, which is the one most highly dependent upon the extent of the individual's formal education.

(d) Other Factors in Ego Development

The student of ego psychology should seriously note the emergence of what is usefully termed the ego, a construct used to designate the decision-making, self-directing aspects of the self, or of the personality. Ego functions (such as *reality testing, control of impulse, object relationships,* etc.) depend upon the use of language to construct an internalized representation of the world which may be manipulated in a trial-and-error fashion to weigh potential outcomes and to contain gratification of wish, drive and impulse in order to cope with 'reality' and the pursuit of personal objectives. The ego has been conceived as mediating between *id* impulses (the pressures of the basic drives and their pleasure-seeking or tension-releasing derivatives) and the *superego* (a construct that designates the internalized parental directives and controls and, to some extent, also the internalized parental figures who continue to seem somewhat outside of the self).

It is important to note that in the ever-broadening field of ego psychology, the whole concept of ego development is now being heavily influenced by the theories of Mahler, Winnicott, and others. Their theories relate well to the several approaches to development outlined in the paragraphs above (a–c), particularly as these theories relate to the psychological development of a stable sense of self, as the child passes through a series of internal processes of reorganization. Currently, this differentiation and structuralization process is referred to more frequently, using terms from the predominantly psychoanalytic literature, though *separation-individuation,* as a process of the first 36–48 months of life, has received increasing attention. The separation-individuation process that is enacted between any child and his/her mother has received critical evaluation and current study, as it relates to an eventual attainment (most theorists agree, by the 36th to 44th month of life) of internal libidinal object constancy. This important milestone is correlated with the 'in tandem' process of self-constancy, i.e. as the important outside object becomes variously invested with positive and negative attributes, so does the self. This attainment of a sense of constancy of self, as well as relevant important other(s), must have reached adequate attainment for the child to proceed developmentally with some of the important other crises of normal development, and must be well-refined in order for a child to adequately complete the important tasks of oedipal mastery and resolution.

In each of the four areas of developmental theory (psychosexual, psychosocial, cognitive, and objective relationships) a separate portion of individual function and/or structure has been noted and studied. It should be evident, though, that a synthesis of these (as well as others that can be ascertained from a wide reading in the developmental literature: see bibliography) viewpoints is necessary in the understanding of the individual in a holistic sense. The completion of the first two decades of life should see the completion of the developmental process from the helpless state of the fetus in utero, to the adult, autonomous and self-regulating, individual. Every person presents with a rich panoply of possibilities of inner and outer identity characteristics. It is hoped that the lines above will lend to a useful fundamental background for understanding ego factors in development, and be applicable in assessments and evaluation of various individual studies of typical, and atypical, function.

Assessments of Ego Disturbance in Organic Syndromes

Interest in the concept of dysfunctional states related to organic factors within individuals, has led to major efforts to identify the characteristics of the syndrome(s). The use of the so-called medical model has resulted in an emphasis on diagnosis as the initial logical step in planning effective management. The neurologic emphasis of this model has been less than satisfactory, probably because patterns of behavior and learning are determined by the complex interaction of numerous factors: genetic, neurological, psychosocial, and environmental. A unitary approach, that is, neurological and psychosocial, may be practical only in the extreme cases where clear etiologies are demonstrable. Such examples would more realistically constitute neurologic dysfunction, or emotional disturbance as a diagnosis, rather than a diagnosis of mental retardation, minimal brain dysfunction, etc., which implies often less obvious clinical findings. The frequent inability to replicate or correlate minimal clinical characteristics of one of these more elusive syndromes stresses the present need for a broader approach to the understanding of these important, and often interrelated, dysfunctions.

There is an increasingly predominant viewpoint that the identification of retardation is essentially a phenomenological diagnosis based on observable impairments of ego functions, rather than relying exclusively on assumptions concerning dynamic structure, or other causative criteria. The ultimate goal of an ego-disturbance approach to psychopathology is to establish normative procedures for the diagnosis of ego strengths and weaknesses, and significant patterns of variation. Certain ego functions and patterns may be regularly or more crucially involved in the various diagnostic syndromes. The diagnostic issue, from the ego frame of reference, is the degree to which a specific ego function is impaired – in the context of impairment, or lack of impairment, of *other* ego functions. Such an approach allows one to clearly specify and understand the deficit in relation to other forms of ego disturbance, without the necessity of a (very often) presumption about etiology.

What follows is an attempt to present the retardation syndrome(s) from an ego-disturbance frame of reference, describing those ego functions that may be regularly or characteristically involved. In this fashion, an attempt will be made to define syndrome(s) in a clear and less diffuse way, to distinguish, on the basis of both history and behavior, between retardation syndrome(s) and other clinical entities.

For assessment purposes, it is useful to divide the functions of the ego into the following five categories (understanding that advanced theorists may subdivide these even further, but keeping to five major subdivisions for purposes of this exercise): (1) Autonomous functions – those intellectual skills that are a function of language and perceptual-motor organization, and the corresponding skill that reflects language and perceptual motor organization – learning. (2) Relation to reality – a perceptual process with two major components (a) the capacity to test reality, and (b) the capacity to maintain an adequate sense of reality. (3) Thought processes – consist primarily of cognitive focusing, reasoning, and concept formation. (4) Object relations and defenses – the major mode of handling impulses, social skills and interpersonal relations. (5) Synthetic functions – the ability to synthesize experience and integrate functioning effectively.

Previously efforts to conceptualize retardation syndrome(s) have resulted in systems that contain many features of these five ego functions. The lack of focus on an ego model, however, resulted in an emphasis of one or two functions, without clearly attempting to integrate all five considerations. This also led to a lack of clarity in considering, as well as differentiating, the interrelationships of retardation and other childhood disorders.

Many important investigators agree about disturbances in areas related to 'autonomous functioning' and all agree (to varying degrees) on a normal 'relation to reality'. In areas of thought processes, all agree about a deficit in cognitive focusing and potential difficulty in area(s) of reasoning. There is no clear consensus about effects on concept formation. Object relationships are usually affected, but in a variable manner. Synthetic functions, as a separate entity, have been rarely considered in previous reports.

To facilitate a differential diagnosis based on an ego model, these areas of dysfunction should be contrasted with other types of childhood behavior or organic disorders. Considering the distinct probability of a continuum of causality ranging from severe organic impairment to serious emotional disturbances, retardation may represent a variable point between these two poles. The point in the continuum can fluctuate depending on which of the ego function(s) is involved. One might, for instance, compare and contrast ego disturbances in relation to extremes in organic, learning disorders and in schizophrenia.

1. Autonomous Function

Autonomous functioning impairment is a primary dysfunction experienced by the retarded subject. Autonomous ego functioning impairment will be evidenced in three interrelated modalities: (a) Deficiencies in those global intellectual functions that reflect learning, such as fund of general knowledge, word knowledge, memory, sequencing skills, and imitative skills. (b) Deficiencies in specific academic areas, such as in reading, spelling, arithmetic. (c) Specific impairment in perceptual motor organization and language processes. It is suggested that impairment in these three modalities is a necessary and sufficient condition for the phenomenological diagnosis of retardation with minimal cerebral dysfunction.

An intellectual evaluation is necessary to rule in or out, for surety, retardation, and, if present, its degree. If a subject's overall intellectual functioning is low average (80 FSIQ), it is expected that autonomous ego functioning should reflect a corresponding level of skill. It is the discrepancy between overall functioning and autonomous areas that suggests learning disability, without other etiological implications.

Besides indications of impairment in global intellectual functioning – and general impairment in academic skills and performance – specific impairment(s) in perceptual-motor and/or language functioning may indicate impairment in autonomous functioning.

A final criteria related to autonomous functioning relates to a failure to learn in an optimal educational environment with adequate educational input. In the face of this environmental contingency, underperformance and underachievement may indicate a significant abnormality in the crucial area(s) of autonomous function.

2. Relation to Reality

Reality testing consists of accurate perceptions of the environment, and its impairment is identified by autistic (highly personalized, and usually inappropriate) perceptions, poor judgment, and inability to recognize conventional modes of social response. A 'sense of reality' is based upon a person's perception of his own body and perceptual apparatus (visual, auditory, tactile, etc.), and its disturbance is reflected in indefinite ego boundaries and often distorted body image.

A review of the retardation syndromes suggests that subjects who experience autonomous functioning impairment(s) may still have quite intact reality testing, and a stable sense of reality. To the degree that a retarded subject's percepts are not determined by reality stimuli that elicit them, there is the possibility that the subject has moved toward a schizophrenic or quite severe organic impairment.

3. Thought Processes

The terms of thought processes, the retarded subject may demonstrate reasoning impairment, related to the extent of the impairment of the other processes considered above. If truly disturbed thinking is demonstrated, one should consider that the child may be experiencing a schizoid, or even schizophrenic dysfunction.

The failure to establish and maintain focus indicates that an individual is having difficulty selecting the most relevant aspects of a stimulus field, as well as adjusting appropriately his/her attention to changes in the external situation to which he/she is responding.

Clinical experience indicates that severe focusing disturbances – such as unusual location choices, or figure-ground blurring on unstructured tasks (such as the Rorschach projective test), is indicative of extensive organic and/or schizophrenic dysfunction. However, perseveration and figure ground deficiency on more structure tasks (such as the Bender-Gestalt) would suggest cognitive deficiency, more primarily.

Behavioral distractibility and hyperactivity are reflective of cognitive focusing difficulties. Support of this hypothesis is found in the positive focusing effects of stimulant medication. The impulse difficulties associated with certain brain-injured subjects are not specifically a problem of controlling primitive aggressive and sexual impulses, but an indication of difficulty organizing and experiencing stimuli in a focused manner. The impulse problem that seems to be associated with retardates with known brain damage is a non-primitive, non-id-imbued quality, and is not a question of weak ego defense. The specific impulse problem of the brain-damaged subject is phenomenologically a problem of focusing and is reflected behaviorally as distractibility and hyperactivity. It depends on a child's defensive style whether primitive asocial characteristics predominate.

Concept formation in the typically functioning person is marked by the capacity to interpret experience at appropriate levels of abstraction. At one time concrete thought was deemed to be characteristic of both brain-damaged children and many retarded children. Work by Birch and co-workers does not support this simple dichotomy as characteristic, but suggests great variability among these children in concept formation. In terms of phenomenological diagnosis, it is not necessary that there be a clear manifestation of concrete concept formation, though its presence should be carefully considered, when found in the course of assessment.

4. Object Relations and Defenses

The psychologically healthy individual is able to establish and maintain satisfactory relationships with people, which in terms of ego functioning indicates generally satisfactory development of object relations. Object relations in retardation syndromes differ from schizophrenic ego disturbances, in that basic object relations are present, but dysfunction(s) occur in the more developed and sophisticated levels of object relations, i.e. the secondary level. Indicators of problems with secondary object relationship development includes excessive dependency, lack of flexibility, lack of reflectivity, and lack of capacity to inhibit impulsive behavior. A review of the literature *(Wender)* suggests that these children show various and divergent types of secondary object impairment. In looking at object relations theory in assessments of character strength, or pathology, it is important to note passive-dependent type(s) of adjustment (in which objects are experienced in a passive, overwhelming way) and general adaptation in interpersonal experience (where the diagnostician may note that objects are avoided, or pathologically manipulated; the latter suggesting possible delinquent character development).

The differentiation between pathological characterological adaptation and neurotic adaptation is a question related to ego defensive organization and level of refinement in development. The neurotic is seen as utilizing a developmentally higher level of defense, in the tendency to use either repression (hysterical phenomena) or intellectualization (obsessive-compulsive phenomena). The use of avoidance, either into fantasy or into activity, is considered more primitive and shows less delay and reflective ability of the subject. It should be noted that the difference between retardates' character styles is often reflected in their defensive use of avoidance; the extent to which this is characterologic pathology needs to be assessed within the context of that individual's social situation. In extreme cases, the avoidance may be manifest by retreat into fantasy or into impulsive activity!

5. Synthetic Function

The final ego function to be assessed is synthetic function. The typical person is able to organize and integrate his/her thought processes, relation to reality, interpersonal skills, defensive resources, and intellectual capacities in the service of a stable and rewarding life pattern. Such integrative and organizing activity constitutes the synthetic function of the ego, i.e. the synthesis and integration of the other major ego functions into a 'workable apparatus'. Schizophrenia involves severe impairment(s) of synthetic functioning, while the retarded subject need not reflect nearly the similar degree of this ego impairment. If a person with many clinical indicators of retardation does experience such deterioration of the synthetic function, then that individual might be considered at that time to have phenomenologically regressed into a schizophrenic state; so much so that the latter condition might become the primary diagnosis.

Conclusion

The degree of impairment in each function raises the possibility of the type of disorder a child may be experiencing. In this approach to phenomenologic diagnosis, the disorder can be understood by the particular pattern(s) of ego strengths and impairments. From this, an appropriate therapeutic program might then concentrate on the areas of specific defect, while supporting and enriching the area(s) of asset. This would seem to be a more generally effective and potentially more successful way of planning intervention(s) with this clinical population.

Suggested Reading

Abelson, G.; Paluszny, M.: Gender identity in a group of related children. J. Autism dev. Disorders 8: 403–411 (1978).

Bauer, R.; Kenny, T.: An ego disturbance model of MBD. Child Psychiat. hum. Dev. 4: 238–245 (1974).

Brody, S.; Axelrad, S.: Anxiety and ego formation in infancy. Structure and events in earliest ego formation, chap. 1–7, pp. 3–78 (International Universities Press, New York 1970).

Chess, S.: Emotional problems of mentally retarded children; in Menolascino, Psychiatric approaches to mental retardation, pp. 55–67. (Basic Books, New York 1970).

Drucker, J.: Development from one to two years: ego development; in Nosphitz et al., Basic handbook of child psychiatry, pp. 157–163 (Basic Books, New York 1979).

Erikson, E.H.: Childhood and society; 2nd ed. Eight ages of man and epigenetic chart, chap. 7; pp. 247–274 (Norton, New York 1963).

Galenson, E.: Development from one to two years: object relations and psychosexual development; in Nosphitz et al., Basic handbook of child psychiatry, pp 144–156 (Basic Books, New York 1979).

Goldings, H.: Development from ten to thirteen years; in Nosphitz et al., Basic handbook of child psychiatry, pp. 199–204 (Basic Books, New York 1979).

Hartman, H.: Essays on ego psychology: selected problems in psychoanalytic theory. Psychoanalysis and developmental psychology, chap. 6, pp. 99–112 (International Universities Press, New York 1964).

Heinicke, C.M.: Development from two and one-half to four years; in Nosphitz et al., Basic handbook of child psychiatry, pp. 167–178 (Basic Books, New York 1979).

Lidz, T.: The person: his development throughout the life cycle. Childhood integration, chap. 8, pp. 238–263 (Basic Books, New York 1968).

Mahler, M.S.: On human symbiosis and the vicissitudes of individuation, vol. 1. On the concepts of symbiosis and separation-individuation, chap. 1, pp. 7–31 (International Universities Press, New York 1968).

Mahler, M.S.: On the first three subphases of the separation-individuation process. Selected papers of Margaret S. Mahler, vol. 2, pp. 119–130 (Jason Aronson, New York 1979).

Mahler, M.S.; Pine, F.; Bergman, A.: The psychological birth of the human infant: symbiosis and individuation, chap. 4-7, pp. 52–120 (Basic Books, New York 1975).

Mannoni, M.: The backward child and his mother: a psychoanalytic study. Cases of organic origin, Mental deficiency, chap. 1/chap. 2, (Random House, New York 1972).

Meers, D.R.: Psychoanalytic research and intellectual functioning of ghetto-reared, black children. The psychoanalytic study of the child, vol. 22, pp. 395–418 (Yale University Press, New Haven 1973).

Ottenbacher, K.: An investigation of self-concept and body-image in the mentally retarded. J. clin. Psychol. *37:* 415–418 (1981).

Parish, T.S.; Baker, S.K.; Arheart, K.L.; Adamchak, P.G.: Normal and exceptional children's attitudes toward themselves and one another. J. Psychol. *104:* 249–253 (1980).

Powell, G.J.: Psychosocial development: eight to ten years; in Nosphitz et al. Basic handbook of child psychiatry, pp. 190–199 (Basic Books, New York 1979).

Shapiro, C.B.: Development from one to two years: normal coping mechanisms; in Nosphitz et al., Basic handbook of child psychiatry, (pp. 164–167) (Basic Books, New York 1979).

Shapiro, M.: The psychatric examination of the child. Handbook of child psychiatry techniques. (University of Pittsburgh, Pittsburgh, 1968).

Solnit, A.J.: Psychosexual development: three to five years; in Nosphitz et al., Basic handbook of child psychiatry, pp. 178–184 (Basic Books, New York 1979).

Solnit, A.J.: Psychosexual development: five to ten years; in Nosphitz et al., Basic handbook of child psychiatry, pp. 184–190 (Basic Books, New York 1979).

Uno, T.; Leonardson, G.: Creativity and self-concept of mentally retarded adolescents. J. creative Behav. *3:* 294 (1980).

Wender, P.H.: Minimal brain dysfunction in children (Wiley-Interscience, New York 1971).

Woodward, K.F.: Early psychiatric intervention for young mentally retarded children; in Menolascino, Psychiatric approaches to mental retardation, pp. 276–293 (Basic Books, New York 1970).

Zisfein, L.; Rosen, M.: Self-concept and mental retardation: theory, measurement, and clinical utility. Ment. Retard. dev. Disabil. *19:* 15–19 (1974).

11 A Developmental Frame for the Care of Normal and Handicapped Infants

Magda Gerber

In the last decade a growing number of infant programs have been established in the United States. Some are designed to provide alternative care environments to the home, while others, referred to as early intervention programs, are geared to stimulate and educate the handicapped, the retarded, or otherwise disadvantaged infants.

Preceding the development of these centers, an increased number of scientific publications including books, articles, and journals for professionals and the public at large have popularized new research findings on infancy. Most reports have emphasized that infants are capable of a wider range of activities and learning than was previously believed. In one single volume, entitled *The Competent Infant,* more than 200 studies are published in an abbreviated form dealing only with the first 15 months of infancy, in 1,314 pages [*Stone and Smith, 1973*].

These studies convinced many that if infants can learn, we must teach them. Thus, many current projects emphasize 'cognitive development' and are often specific-achievement oriented. Their curricula are based on levels of performance as defined by various infant studies and tests [*Bayley, 1969; Gesell, 1940; Piaget, 1963*] and their goals are to enhance achievement. Specific methods are also designed to teach, drill, and help to facilitate the development of certain milestone acquisitions. In addition, there are home teaching programs which are intended to educate mothers and families in areas of infant stimulation [*Gordon, 1970; Painter, 1971*].

Generally the program staff have preconceived ideas as to when, how, why, and for how long infants should be stimulated. Many times the principle of 'the more the better' is carried out.

While it is assumed that all infants would benefit from early sensory stimulation, it is a 'must' for handicapped infants to prevent or lessen retardation. It is generally believed that left alone the infant would not master the tasks parents and/or professionals consider necessary. This may reflect the parents' anxiety that their children will not 'make it'. Those caring for handicapped children experience even greater anxiety and therefore are more eager to provide early stimulation.

A large number of books, packaged programs and infant curricula are available and used as prescriptions in many infant programs. These often serve as guidelines or crutches to caregivers who may be inadequately prepared in the field of infancy or the needs of the 'special' child. Following instructions the caregiver tries to elicit a desired response to a prescribed stimulus in the areas of gross motor, fine motor, social-emotional, and language. New skills are introduced to the infants, skills one step ahead of their development, skills they themselves cannot master yet. The adult's attention is focused on teaching, rather than observing the whole child's reactions to his environment and his carer.

I am proposing a different view of how infants learn and of how we can facilitate learning during infancy. In the past 10 years I have been a consultant to infant programs, initiated and directed model infant programs, and organized Resources for Infant Educarers, RIE (a nonprofit membership organization of infant educarers, parents and professionals concerned with improving the care and education of infants). Based on my experiences and my work as a child therapist, all programs are guided by a humanistic-therapeutic approach to young children. They are not child care facilities but teaching, training, and demonstration programs. As preventive mental health programs they are designed to actually demonstrate our theories of caring for 'normal' as well as 'high risk' infants. The overall therapeutic goal is twofold: (1) To help parents to develop, from the very beginning, sound patterns of living with their babies whether 'normal' or 'handicapped'. Some early high risk signs: hypo- or hypertonia, limpness, rigidity, high pitched or poor cry, absence of progressive orientation to light and sound, apathy, restlessness, irritability, hyperkinesis, lack of eye contact, body resistance to physical contact with mother, lack of response to stimuli, feeding problems, sleeping problems or impaired developmental level with no apparent physical cause. (2) To train 'infant carers', professionals who provide group care for infants in different environments (e.g., centers, or family homes) [*Gerber*, 1971, 1979]. The designation of 'carer' is preferred by the author, to care-giver or caretaker because of the emphasis on caring, rather than on giving or taking. It will be used for the caring person whether parent or professional. An Educarer is trained in our method.

Our programs in Los Angeles (Pilot Infant Program, Dubnoff Center, North Hollywood) and Palo Alto (Demonstration Infant Program, directed with *Tom Forrest,* MD, The Children's Health Council of the Mid-Peninsula). California varied considerably from the types of programs described earlier. Our approach was essentially based on the experience of more than a quarter century of research and clinical work with infants who were reared at the National Methodological Institute of Residential Nurseries in Budapest, Hungary (popularly called 'Loczy'), a residence for normal infants from birth to 3 years of age with a capacity to serve 70 infants, founded in 1946 by *Emmi Pikler,* MD.

The following outline defines the principles and philosophy of Loczy: (1) While all infants derive security from a *predictable environment,* and the opportunity for *anticipation* and *making choices,* this is absolutely essential for the infant living in an institution. (2) An infant needs an *intimate, stable relationship* with one constant person (a mother figure). This relationship can best be developed during *individualized caregiving activities.* (3) *Respect* is shown by treating the infant as an active participant rather than as a passive recipient in all interactions. (4) The infant *does not need direct teaching or help* to achieve natural stages of gross motor and sensory-motor development [*Pikler,* 1971].

The approach to infants at Loczy is based on achieving a balance between adult stimulation and independent exploration by the infant. Infants are exposed to adult stimulation by the infant carers during all caregiving activities (e.g., feeding, bathing, dressing, etc.). These are unhurried pleasurable times for both adults and infants. Because these activities occur during the necessary daily routines of infant care, stimulation is constant and consistent. In contrast, in the areas of gross motor and fine motor development, the staff of Loczy does not interfere or promote but rather relies on maturation and development at the infant's own pace. Detailed description of the philosophy, methodology and the actual care of the infants at Loczy is provided by [*David and Appel,* 1973].

In our California programs the emphasis is similarly on *observation, anticipation* and *selective intervention.* Observing her child helps the mother or carer to learn about individual characteristics of her child and to realize what she can reasonably expect of him (him or her – for simplicity's sake the infant is referred to as he, the caregiver as she) at any given developmental level. This in turn helps the mother synchronize her behavior with the child's needs, tempo and style. Anticipating each others' reactions fosters mutual understanding, acceptance and basic trust for both mother and child; thus, anticipation becomes the forerunner of communication. Selective intervention means knowing when *not* to intervene, and this is more difficult than intervening indiscriminately.

Our study was designed on the assumption that there are certain conditions under which a healthy, normal infant can develop his potentials. They are as follows: (1) availability of a mother figure who responds to physical and emotional needs; (2) mother's correct perception and basic acceptance of the child, seeing and accepting him for what he is; (3) synchronization of his inner rhythm (sleep, hunger, etc.) with the family's daily routine: mutual adaptation (to plan the day's activities in such a way that there should be as little conflict as possible between the infant's and family's needs); (4) availability of space (to facilitate locomotion); (5) availability of objects (to facilitate manipulation), and (6) availability of other children within the same age range (to observe and imitate, and with whom to interact and socialize) – this condition is optional.

In sum, our goals are influenced by our concept of an ideal human being as one who has some or many of the following characteristics: realistic *trust* in himself and his environment, perceptions of his *inner needs* and an ability to communicate them, the ability to make *choices* for himself, which includes knowing and accepting the consequences of his choices, *flexibility* and the capacity to learn from past experiences, ability to deal actively with the present and plan for the future, *free access to his creative talents and resources,* and is goal-oriented and also *enjoys the process of problem-solving,* whether physical, emotional, or cognitive. Identification with these ideals implies that we have to critically examine child-rearing practices in order to determine which would facilitate and/or hinder the emergence of the desired characteristics in infancy as follows:

Trust develops when the primary *carers* allow the child to anticipate what is going to happen to him. They must relate their trust in the infant and view him as an initiator of activities.

Case 1. Danny provides an example of an extreme case of an infant who could not develop trust. Danny's parents described him as a constant screamer from birth. No matter what they did, Danny's high pitched wails continued, even throughout each night. All attempts to soothe him – rocking, holding – were to no avail. I met Danny at 6 months when he entered a family day care home. As a consultant to this day care home, I observed that Danny's screams were accompanied by a facial expression of utter terror. He was at this time experiencing intermittent calmness when sitting right next to his carer, Ann, but her slightest movement triggered a new crying spell. Following my suggestion, Ann spent time sitting with Danny and then would tell him what to expect: 'Danny, I'm going to stand up now.' Once standing, she would tell him: 'Danny, I'm going to sit down again.' Following many repetitions of this procedure Ann could eventually move across the room and then even out of Danny's sight. After 2 months, Danny was able to tolerate Ann's normal activity around the home and began napping with the other children. After a few more months Danny began noticing the rest of his environment and interacting with the other children.

Infants are absorbed by their *inner feelings* of satisfaction/dissatisfaction and they try to communicate their needs. Carers, however, when not sensitively observing the infant, do not respond to his communications, but rather to their own interpretations of the infant's needs. For example, a mother who is cold may cover the crying infant without trying to find out whether *he* is warm or cold, a hungry caregiver would offer a bottle to the crying infant without finding out whether *he* is hungry or not.

It is not unusual to find withdrawn apathetic infants in group homes. This author has seen many such children while visiting different group homes. Johnny's case is typical of the impact of a multiple and random caregiving system.

Case 2. In one center Johnny awakes from his nap. He is diapered and placed in a high chair by one adult. After giving him a bowl of food she leaves him to diaper the next child. Another caregiver arrives and notices that Johnny looks sleepy. Removing his food, she returns him to a crib. Johnny does not protest during these changes for he has become accustomed to it. Johnny is quite apathetic due to the lack of bonding, since he had missed all his life the opportunity of having a stable caregiver. He has no expectations and no frustrations, he learned to live as an object in people's hands. Johnny is at risk of becoming an autistic child.

Making appropriate choices in life is a learning process lasting from birth to death. Few people realize at what early age infants are able to make proper choices if given the opportunity. The carer has to differentiate between situations according to whether the infant has a real choice or not. If there is a real choice (e.g., 'Do you want to be picked up now?'), and the child responds negatively or with disinterest, he is left alone. If no choice is involved, the carer does not ask but states the intended action (e.g., 'I am going to pick you up now. It is time to go.') The child is then picked up.

Flexibility of the body and mind develops throughout repeated exploratory exercises of infants in free play. Infants who are restricted by mechanical devices such as infant seats, bouncers, walkers and swings, or encouraged to assume positions which they are not yet ready for, are not moving freely. Propping up an infant into a sitting position before he can sit up or lie down by himself will not accelerate his motor development, help him to become flexible or make him autonomous.

While some research both in the United States and in Africa indicates that children may sometimes walk earlier if they are given 'practice' in walking, there is no evidence that the child who walks a few weeks earlier than he might otherwise have done, gains any benefit. On the other hand, there is evidence that premature 'practice' can be harmful both physically and emotionally.

Critically describing commonly used interventions such as helping, teaching, exercising, which supposedly are needed to promote the progression of gross motor skills, *Pikler* [1971] gives us new insight into this process: 'When the mother considers it timely (according to schedules) she introduces a new posture to the child.' Obviously, the infant feels uncomfortable, is unbalanced, unfree and fully dependent on the adult to rescue him from his predicament.

Next the infant is being 'exercised by an adult or with the aid of an apparatus such as special chair, swing, baby-walker, etc., to attain the ability of remaining in the new posture or to move according to the new way'. Eventually, the child becomes less rigid and awkward in the position he is placed. Finally, 'the child learns to take on, abandon and practice new forms of motions and postures, on his own, independently ... Thus, after the child has learned to be prone, he learns to turn prone and back again. After having learned to sit, he learns to sit up and get down; after having learned to stand, he learns to stand up and get down; and after having learned to take some steps independently, he learns to stand up without support and to start and stop walking and to get down ... Only after he has learned these, is the child able to use the advanced motor skills in everyday life on his own initiative. Only after this third period does he really become independent in the more advanced postures and motions' [*Pikler,* 1971, p. 55, 56].

In the rest of the article *Pikler* describes how the children at Loczy attained all stages of motor development independently on their own (self-induced) initiative without any direct interference by adult or aid of supporting equipment.

Let us consider: if indeed children can develop all required motor skills with as well as without adult help (about 2,000 infants have been raised at Loczy) what are the benefits in *not* helping them.

From my personal observations of infants in both situations described, I have found that infants moving on their own are constantly busy moving, exploring, choosing objects, overcoming obstacles with caution, having longer attention spans, being peaceful, and enjoying their autonomy.

During the sensory-motor stage, explorations are optimal learning experiences and should be one of the two most important parts of the curriculum. Independent, self-absorbed infants who need much less adult intervention make the other important part – a special individualized interaction – possible. The infant-carer in charge of a group of peacefully exploring infants can devote her full undivided attention to the one individual infant she is caring for. In this way the infant's basic need for a warm attentive special human relation, as well as his need for autonomy, are met. The adult has more time to just observe, which will make her interventions more appropriate and her knowledge of the children more accurate. Both infants and adults feel more relaxed and fulfilled. A relationship of mutual trust develops. This trusting and respectful approach becomes a pattern of interaction and goes way beyond its effect on gross motor development.

Infants do naturally have *access to their own resources* unless we super-impose tasks which are beyond their capabilities. It is truly fascinating to observe infants *solving their own problems* with concentration, endurance, and good frustration tolerance. This happens if adults are available rather than intrusive, and if they learn to wait and see whether the child could work it out by himself before offering help. A freely exploring child 'selects' his own problems and is internally motivated to solve them in his own way, continuously learning without experiencing failure. Though some individual modifications are necessary when working with high risk children, providing learning experiences without failure is even more important for them than it is for the average child.

While emphasizing the infant's need for *autonomy*, one must keep in mind the utmost importance of the relationship that the infant develops with his primary carer. An intimate trusting relationship is the prerequisite for healthy separation and individuation of the child. Only after he gets 'refueled' during the unhurried times he spends with his carer will he be willing to let go of the carer and explore his environment.

In this paper I have discussed infants' needs and adults' goals for them and suggested how to synchronize them. If our goal is an authentic individual then we should let him be an authentic infant. Meeting the needs of infants is not an easy task for the family, and it becomes increasingly more difficult in various types of infant centers. Even good families find that infants are time and energy consuming and frequently their needs conflict with those of the parents. Constancy – so important to the infant – is threatened by disruption of the family and/or the mother's need or desire to work. Nevertheless, in his own family the infant usually experiences care and closeness from the same primary carers in his life. However, in even the best of institutions infants are exposed to all kinds of inconsistencies, to many different carers and caring styles, and subject to constant change.

Appropriate curriculum for infants should not be special teaching plans added to daily activities, but rather it should be built into the infant's every experience. The types of programs offered as well as curricula should evolve as a joint effort between carers and infants. The carer provides space, objects and loving care; the infant explores the space, manipulates the objects, develops trust and self-confidence. The guidelines for any and all intervention must be based on observation, empathy, sensitivity, and respect for the infant.

References

Bayley, N.: The manual for the Bayley scales of infant development (Psychological Corporation, New York 1969).

David, M.; Appel, G.: Loczy ou le maternage insolite. Loczy an unusual way of caring. Translation by Gerber. (Scarabée/Centres d'entraînement aux méthodes d'éducation active, Paris 1973).

Gerber, M.: Infants expression. The art of becoming; in Jakab, Psychiatry and art, vol. 3, pp. 170–175 (Karger, Basel 1971).

Gerber, M.: Resources for infant educarers (1979).

Gesell, A.: Gesell developmental schedules (Psychological Corporation, New York 1940).

Gordon, I.J.: Baby learning through baby play. A parents guide for the first two years (Griffin Series, Saint Martin 1970).

Painter, G.: Teach your baby (Simon & Schuster, New York 1971).

Piaget, J.: The origins of intelligence in children (Norton, New York 1963).

Pikler, E.: Learning of motor skills on the basis of self-induced movements. Exceptional infant studies in abnormalities, vol. 2 (Brunner Mazel, New York 1971).

Stone, L.J.; Smith, H.: in Murphy, The complete infant (Basic Books, New York 1973).

12 Psychiatric Disorders in Mental Retardation
Recognition, Diagnosis and Treatment
Irene Jakab

Occurrence and Frequency of Psychiatric Disorders in Mental Retardation

The diagnosis of psychiatric disorders in a retarded person requires establishing both the presence of retardation and sufficient data to warrant a psychiatric diagnosis. Deficiencies in adaptive behavior are part of the diagnostic criteria for mental retardation, in addition to subaverage intelligence. Therefore, in order to qualify for a psychiatric disorder, the presenting symptoms of deficient adaptation must be either too intense, too frequent or all together of such a distorted quality that they do not occur at any normal developmental level.

The diagnostic criteria for persons who are both mentally retarded (MR) and emotionally disturbed (ED) (psychosis, personality disorders, hyperactivity, etc.) are still an almost uncharted territory. The excellent diagnostic descriptions for identifying MR/ED children established in 1966 by *Provence and Marsh* [67] for the Joint Committee on Retarded Children with Emotional, Psychotic and Personality Problems, in Connecticut, have unfortunately not received sufficiently broad exposure in the psychiatric literature.

The recognition and diagnosis of these doubly handicapped MR/ED persons requires the skills of more than one specialist (psychiatrist, neurologist, developmental pediatrician, psychologist, educator, etc.). It is not surprising, therefore, that case finding statistics are very sparse. The whereabouts of the doubly handicapped (MR/ED) patients must be searched out by screening school populations, institutions for retardates, mental health facilities and juvenile detention centers. This in itself is a time-consuming and costly proposition which has been only marginally successful in gathering statistical data about the frequency of occurrence of emotional disturbance in the mentally retarded. The above-mentioned task force report [67] yields the following data based on a survey of mental hospitals, training schools for the retarded and correctional facilities: 837 MR/ED children under age 20 were found – 118 in correctional institutes, 39 in MH department facilities and 680 in mental retardation facilities. In addition, a report quoted from the Yale Child Study Center revealed that it accepted 500 MR/ED children for evaluation in 8 years, and more than 100 such children were expected to be recognized each year in Connecticut. Impressive data show 353 (42.7%) MR/ED children among the 827 residents of the Southbury Training School (Connecticut), while 318 (47.2%) among the 670 residents under age 20 at Mansfield (Connecticut) were also found to be MR/ED.

A survey in 1979 by the Department of Mental Retardation in the State of Connecticut [66] presented the following data: 'a small number of mentally retarded clients referred to the Department of Mental Retardation for residential placement each year.' 'According to DMH (Department of Mental Health), they currently have approximately 128 mentally retarded clients in their hospital population.' Nonetheless, the same report acknowledges the 'concern of both departments over the problems of the disturbed/retarded client for a number of years'. 'DMR lacks the psychiatric services these clients need and DMH lacks the appropriate program services.' Although plans have been developed, their implementation was halted by budgetary restraints. This report comes to the surprising conclusion that: 'In summary, it can be anticipated that approximately 25 mentally retarded clients may be referred to DMR during the next five years from these sources' (the sources meaning the Department of Children and Youth Services and the Juvenile Court).

In Massachusetts a study conducted by this author in 1972 at the Community Evaluation and Rehabilitation Center of the Eunice Shreiver Kennedy Center (Waltham, Mass., Director: *Robert Flinn,* MD), yielded the following statistical data: among 595 referrals for evaluation, in the first 5 calendar years of that facility's functioning, 194 mentally retarded children were diagnosed as having psychiatric disorders. Furthermore, 29 of these patients suffered from the additional handicap of perceptual-motor disorder (table I), thus requiring complex multimodality treatment.

Statistical figures from a Pennsylvania survey indicate that early identification of developmentally disabled children at risk for mental health problems is apparently not effective for children aged 0–3 years. During 1980, two agencies of the Allegheny County Mental Health/Mental Retardation Programs served 194 developmentally disabled infants, 0–3 years, and their families (Association for Retarded Citizens (ARC) served 90, and United Cerebral Palsy (UCP) served 104). Statistics of March, 1981, indi-

Table I. Psychiatric syndromes in a retarded population of 595 evaluated at the Community Evaluation and Rehabilitation Center in Waltham, Mass. (1972)

Diagnosis	Without perceptual handicap	With perceptual handicap	Total
Mental retardation + childhood schizophrenia	18	1	19
Mental retardation + psychosis (undefined)	9	0	9
Mental retardation + autism (or autistic behavior)	13	5	18
Mental retardation + depression	14	7	21
Mental retardation + anxiety reaction	14	0	14
Mental retardation + hyperactive behavior	22	3	25
Mental retardation + hyperactive behavior + aggressive behavior	9	1	10
Mental retardation + behavioral reaction	17	1	18
Mental retardation + unsocialized aggressive reaction	46	11	57
Mental retardation + passive aggressive personality disorder	1	0	1
Mental retardation + phobia	1	0	1
Mental retardation + schizoid character	1	0	1
Total	165	29	194

cate that 220 infants (ages 0–3) were enrolled in early intervention services in Allegheny County (Pa.). It is important to note that of these 220 infants only 4 were identified as having mental health diagnoses, while an analysis of preschool programs for developmentally disabled children aged 2–6 years indicated in 1981: 96 mental health preschool enrollments and 492 mental retardation preschool enrollments. The survey also indicates that there were waiting lists for the mental health preschool programs. The obvious conclusions are that the mental health problems were not detected earlier, and that the doubly handicapped MR/ED patient is forced into one or another of the administrative categories, instead of being provided with a special program addressing both his handicaps.[1]

[1] In Pittsburgh, Pa., The John Merck Program, designed in 1975, by this writer at the Department of Psychiatry of the University of Pittsburgh Medical School, provides specialized services to doubly handicapped MR/ED children aged 3–12 years. The census of this program is 20 inpatients and 5 day patients. It carries a lengthy waiting list ever since its opening; showing the need for more services in this area.

In 1978, several journals and NIMH publications [18–20, 53, 71] launched the news about a proposal for the 'most in need' program, by *Hersh and Platt* [36]. The target population of that program of about 1.5– 2 million children 'suffer from a combination of mental health problems and other conditions which impede their growth and development' [36]. According to the proposal, this group of 'most in need' children with mental health problems includes, among others, those with 'Handicaps requiring special education, vocational training, rehabilitation, special recreational programs.' The number or percentage of these children within the target population is not specified, but it covers, no doubt, the emotionally disturbed category of retarded children. These doubly handicapped children who frequently suffer from additional disorders such as brain damage and epilepsy, or physical handicap are truly 'most in need' and deserving appropriate services. However, according to recent information, even that well-designed NIMH program has never reached its expected development, having been curtailed by lack of funds.

In summary, the identification and treatment of MR/ED patients faces difficulties due on the one hand to the inherent problems of diagnosing the psychiatric illness of retardates, and on the other hand to the problems of funding the treatment if the diagnosis has been made. These difficulties are compounded further by a political factor in a very unexpected way. The problem is related to the Education for All Handicapped Children Act, which mandates that each state must provide free services to handicapped children. The states must demonstrate in their 'Annual Program Plans' the estimated number of handicapped children who need special education and related services [23]. Furthermore, the number of children receiving such services, as well as those 'not receiving a free appropriate public education' must also be submitted [24]. The problem of reporting becomes evident if one realizes that statistics showing unserved children would place the reporting State in the condition of violating the Federal law.

Due to lack of funds for the very expensive services required by the doubly handicapped MR/ED children, only a few can be served. However, services are mandatory under the Federal Right to Education law, therefore the self-evident solution is to declare that this category does not exist.

The state statistics on the occurrence and prevalence of emotional disturbance in mental retardation, contrary to data from task force reports, are at best grossly underestimating the number of doubly handicapped MR/ED persons.

The DSM III offers no statistical data on the occurrence of emotional

disturbance in mental retardation. Nonetheless, it is stated under the differential diagnosis of mental retardation that 'mental retardation may, however, coexist with specific developmental disorders, and frequently coexists
with pervasive developmental disorders' [DSM III, p. 49, ref. 3].

Russell and Tanguay [69] found that behavioral disturbance, after the degrees of
intellectual deficiency, constitutes the single most important cause of institutionalization
of the retarded. Other authors are also dealing with the relationship of mental retardation
and emotional disturbance [54, 58, 63, 70]. In a follow-up study of 41 children with
minimal brain damage, as compared to 83 without minimal brain damage who were each
inpatients (1966–1973), *Klicpera and Heyse* [45] found that the MBD groups showed more
immature and disruptive, or too passive and withdrawn behavior, even after discharge.
Supportive data for the greater frequency of emotional disturbance in mentally retarded
than in nonretarded persons are provided in the literature by *Beier* [8] based on 93 cases. A
review of scales suitable for epidemiological and clinical research in the assessment of
psychopathology and behavioral problems in children is provided by *Orvashel* et al. [59].
For additional data in the literature the reader is referred to the following authors whose
works provide extensive bibliographies: *Balthazar and Stevens* [5], *Bellak* [9], *Bernstein*
[11, 12], *Szymanski* [76], and the Proceedings of the 1980 Health Education and Welfare
Conference on the Needs of Emotionally Disturbed/Developmentally Disabled Individuals, which includes 110 bibliographical entries [65].

Etiology

The etiology of the psychiatric disorders associated with mental retardation may be divided into the following categories: organic [17], environmental [1], and mixed organic and environmental causes in the same
patient [for this study, see diagnostic chapter].

Detailed literature on the etiology of mental retardation is provided in
the chapter on diagnosis of mental retardation.

(a) Both the mental retardation and the psychiatric disorder may have
the same organic cause. Any of the following entities: genetic disorder,
intoxication, injury, or infection in infancy or early childhood may each
cause both the arrest (or slowness) of mental development and the disorganized emotional development.

(b) Environmental sociocultural factors may cause both mental retardation and psychiatric disorders (either the mental retardation or the psychiatric disorder being considered to be the primary disability). Sociocultu-
rally deprived children may not develop the intellectual capacities with
which they are born. Their emotional adjustment and social maturity could

also become distorted and inadequate for adapting to the demands of school discipline and to interaction with other children.

(c) Organic brain syndrome causing mental retardation may be complicated by superimposed secondary psychogenic reaction due to causes independent of the retardation; e.g., the co-incidence of Down's syndrome and reactive depression caused by losses in life such as death of a parent, divorce, the moving away of a significant caregiver (sibling, institute staff member, etc.). Similarly, the moving out of the home of the retarded person who is starting an independent life in the community may cause depression. The 'home' lost by the retarded person may be that of the biological family or an institute in which many years of the retarded person's life were spent.

Diagnosis and Differential Diagnosis

The Symptoms

At any given time in history society designs and attempts to enforce both age-related and situation-related 'norms' of behavior. If an individual does not adequately fulfill cultural stereotypes because of slow physical development or genetic and family variations, he may suffer negative feelings about his body [56]. A large percentage of high school students express dissatisfaction with one physical trait or another [25]. The mentally retarded emotionally disturbed person is unable, or unwilling, to act according to the 'norms' of a given environment's social context. The resulting behavioral aberrations and subjective discomfort are indicators of the need for psychiatric intervention and are generally considered 'symptoms' in the medical terminology.

The psychiatric symptoms of the retarded patient are influenced on the one hand by the patient's age and on the other hand by the level of the retardation (IQ).

Symptoms characteristic of specific chronological ages (and related to the mental age) of retardates:

Childhood (1–8 years) – symbiosis; enuresis; encopresis; distorted or delayed language; hyperactivity; unsocialized habits of toileting, eating, dressing; aggression; anxiety states.

Adolescence (8–18 years) – running away; aggression; promiscuity; depression; delinquency; schizophrenia.

Adulthood (18 years and over) – depression; psychosomatic symptoms; regression; conversion hysteria.

Psychiatric symptoms characteristic at different levels of mental retardation (IQ):

Severe mental retardation (IQ 20–34): antisocial-uncensored primitive drives; pervasive developmental disorder.

Severe and moderate mental retardation (IQ 20–49): asocial-'amoral' behavior.

Moderate and mild mental retardation (IQ 35–70): undifferentiated psychosis, conversion hysteria, autism, schizophrenia.

Mild mental retardation (IQ 50–70): depression; neurotic and psychosomatic symptoms.

Special attention must be paid to the concrete thinking, and to the language delay, of retarded individuals [78]. In cases of language delay or aphasia, the only signal of frustration may be a generalized bodily expression, such as a temper tantrum. In the developmentally delayed person, the lack of time concept causes much confusion. In many cases it causes the low frustration tolerance of the brain-damaged retarded person – 'if there is no tomorrow,' all wishes must be fulfilled 'in the present.'

Target Ages and the Reasons for Psychiatric Referral

The psychiatric evaluation of retarded persons is requested more frequently at specific target ages: at 3 years, 6 years, puberty, and at over 50 years of age.

Age 3 Years. The child is mobile enough and strong enough to cause problems if he is aggressive or hyperactive. On the other hand, the language delay by age 3, and withdrawal paired with avoidance of peers and adults as well as lack of appropriate toy play, become of concern, even to parents who do not pay much attention to their infant's and young child's developmental milestones.

At this age the diagnosis will focus on determining the level and the quality of adaptive deficiencies. Conditions most frequently requiring differential diagnostic assessment are infantile autism, childhood onset pervasive developmental disorder, attention deficit disorders with or without hyperactivity, and organic brain disorders with arrested or progressive dementia (genetic-metabolic diseases, perinatal anoxia, trauma, infection, tumors).

Age 6 Years. This marks the time of school entrance when emotional disturbance is detected more readily or even develops under the demands of social adaptation to a new environment including such requirements as sitting in place, paying attention to the teacher, working on assignments and getting along with peers. Last, but not least, coping with the 'leaving of the home' – separation from parents (mother) and siblings – are stresses which may cause, or increase, the symptoms of pathological adaptive deficiencies. Aggressive tendencies, hyperactivity, or withdrawal and depressive reactions, become more marked under stress.

A tabulation of the differential diagnostic criteria of mental retardation and childhood psychiatric disorders is given in table II. Depression is not separately listed in this tabulation since it is not presently recognized in the DSM III as an entity of the childhood psychotic disorders. Depression in childhood reveals itself frequently by atypical symptoms instead of a visibly depressed mood.

In this age group, in addition to the childhood psychiatric disorders, the diagnostician should consider the neuropsychological evaluation of the child for specific localization of multiple developmental disabilities (learning disorders) caused by diffuse organic brain damage (most frequently anoxia). Repeated aggressive, impulsive, behavior requires the ruling out of psychomotor epilepsy, or more generalized pathology of the limbic system. Regression with enuresis and encopresis of a formerly toilet-trained retarded child should be investigated for the possibility of being the first symptoms of progressive organic brain damage caused by viral infection (slow encephalitis) or degenerative CNS disease.

Adolescence: Age 14–18 Years. The teenage years of retarded children are usually the most difficult of their lives. The hormonal and emotional upheaval which besets normally maturing teenagers are compounded by lack of peer support and by realistic difficulties of separating from the family ties. These are the loneliest years of a growing up retarded child. The average teenager finds support in peer groups. As every parent knows, they talk for hours on the phone with their peers, about their problems, their achievements and their rebellions against parental rules. They gradually gain more freedom and independence. On the contrary, retarded teenagers do not have the intellectual and verbal skills to 'discuss' with each other their daily struggles and achievements, and their interests in the opposite sex. They are not accepted socially by the nonretarded teenagers who, at that age, actually have the least patience for a retarded child. Furthermore, the parents, instead of encouraging more freedom and increased independence, tighten the supervision and, in many cases, over-protect the retarded

Table II. Differential diagnosis of mental retardation and psychiatric disorders in children

Diagnostic criteria	Mental retardation	Pervasive developmental disorders	
		early infantile autism	childhood onset pervasive developmental disorder
Age of onset of symptoms	Under age 18 years (by definition)	Before 30 months of age	After 30 months of age and before 12 years
Family history (any or all may occur within the same family)	1% of population Genetic-metabolic disorders 2 boys/1 girl Lower socioeconomic class Mentally retarded parents and siblings Cultural-social deprivation Single parent family	2–4/10,000 upper socio-economic class 3 boys/1 girl Siblings: 50 × more frequent than normal siblings No specific data	Mental retardation Cultural deprivation Psychotic parent Abusing parent Lower socioeconomic class
Etiology	Organic Sociocultural Mixed	Unknown Organicity suspected Maternal 'coolness' suspected	Organic Sociocultural Mixed
Motor (physical) development	Delayed	Generally normal Early peculiarities Toe walking Twirling	May be normal Delayed motor develop ment – frequent
Intellectual development	Low IQ (under 70) Delayed intellectual growth Concrete thinking	Normal or delayed	May have normal poten-tial, but retarded on measured IQ
Emotional development	Dull Infantile-egocentric Low frustration tolerance Temper tantrums	Pervasive lack of responsiveness Autistic withdrawal from earliest infancy 'Too quiet baby'	Profound disturbance of affective responses with bizarre ambivalence Early signs of self-abuse
Social development	Undersocialized Acts like a younger person	Negativism Active avoidance of eye contact and body contact Panic reaction if intruded upon	Gross and sustained impairment of social adaptation Unresponsive to praise or punishment Does not learn from expe-rience Set patterns of behavior
Language development or pathology	May be normal Delayed language develop-ment Echolalia Prolonged babbling Concrete concepts Reading-writing-number concept, deficit	Gross deficit in language development (receptive aphasia differential diagnosis) Immediate and delayed echolalia Sing-song intonation Nonsense speech No gesture language Pronomial reversal	Bizarre intonation or idio-syncratic use of word meanings Resistance to correction by adults Refusal of sign language
Relating to objects	Disinterested Monotonous play Stereotype manipulation May be normal in the use of everyday objects and toys	Peculiar attachments (safety blanket) Bizarre idiosyncratic use of objects Phobias of objects Resistance to newness Interested in mechanical toys	Hypo- or hypersensitivity to stimuli Requires sameness Monotonous play Running around aimlessly Destructive Careless Self-injuries

A Schizoid disorder of childhood B Schizophrenia	Attention deficit disorder (hyperactivity)	Organic brain syndromes (and disorders)
5 years to young adulthood	3–6 years	Any age; may be caused by prenatal or perinatal brain injury
A Higher % in family with identified member; more boys than girls B Schizophrenia %: male = female Pathogenic family interaction Low socioeconomic class	3 % of children before puberty Boys 10 × more than girls Home adjustment may be satisfactory Inability to sit still or concentrate more evident in school	Genetic-metabolic disorders; nutritional deficiencies Any socioeconomic class Vascular disorders in the family or degenerative central nervous system disorders
Unknown Organicity suspected	Unknown Organicity frequently demonstrated	1 Acute or chronic brain damage 2 Functional brain disorder
Generally normal Early bizarre patterns	May be normal Delayed milestones Hyperactivity early in life Clumsiness	May be normal or delayed
Normal or high May be delayed	Frequently delayed May be normal May be gifted	May start as normal and become demented Mentally retarded
Premorbid – aloofness Ambivalence Blunted affect Cruelty to animals	Impulsive Low frustration tolerance Temper tantrums	May start as normal and deteriorate with dementia Premorbid personality traits influence emotional adjustment
Inappropriate reactions to social situations Outbursts of anger Withdrawal Ambivalence Negativism	Unsocialized-aloof Negativistic Absorbed in a hyperactive pattern Stimulus bound	May start as normal and deteriorate with dementia Losing acquired social habits (toilet training, eating habits, sexual habits)
Normal Bizarre Stereotype-logoclonia Incoherent Incomprehensible Echolalia (immediate and delayed) Reversal of pronouns	Often inadequate Sing-song Echolalia Disorganized Changing subject midsentence when new stimulus is perceived Stream of words, continuous 'chatter'	May be deficient from infancy (aphasias), acquired deficit, circumstantial, confabulation *Not* bizarre
Disinterest Perceptual disturbances (illusions) Panic reactions Ambivalence Resistance to change Lack of initiative Destructiveness	Fleeting relations Stimulus bound Attracted to moving objects or parts and to shiny objects Inquisitive Careless Destructive	Monotonous play Stimulus bound Clumsy No symbolic use of toys Panic reaction may occur in spacial agnosia at any age

Table II (continued)

Diagnostic criteria	Mental retardation	Pervasive developmental disorders	
		early infantile autism	childhood onset pervasive developmental disorder
Relating to people	May be normal Infantile-egocentric, clinging-overdependent, stubborn and demanding Primitive sense of humor (laughs if someone falls in an awkward position) Grasp humor in pictures better than in words	Most profoundly disturbed Anxiety reaction at closeness Requires a wide empty zone of comfort around, inside of which intrusion causes panic or aggression Tuning out: people and dolls No sense of humor	Overly clinging or selectively attached Generalized fear of strangers Panic attacks Rage attacks at intrusion No sense of humor
Main symptoms necessary for diagnosis (any or all may be present at a given time)	Subaverage intelligence Deficits in adaptive behavior Acts like a chronologically younger individual Does not show gross deviation of behavioral adaptation May show identifiable cortical function deficits May be associated with epilepsy	Lack of relations with people No eye contact Deficient and bizarre language Ambivalence Negativism Need for sameness in objects and space Stereotype behavior Panic reaction	Lack of affective responsivity Anxiety attacks Resistance to change Bizarre movement patterns Self-mutilation Aggression toward others Bizarre language No hallucinations or delusions Require wide 'comfort zone' Intolerant to intrusion
Behavioral consequences of the illness or condition	Unable to judge physical danger Slow learner; short attention span Poor eating habits Clinging behavior Dull and stubborn Low self-esteem	Hyperalertness or aloofness Negativism Stereotypy Mannerism Noncommunicating speech and gestures May appear hyperactive due to hyperalert defensive avoidance	Isolation from the environment Self-stimulating Monotonous activity Unexpected emotional reactions
Society's reaction to symptoms of the disease or condition	Rejection (battered child) Overprotection Emphais on 'teaching' Distrusting ability of independence	Rejection (battered child) Rescue fantasies High demands 'the hidden genius' with hostility for not getting through	Rejection (battered or 'locked-up' child) Giving up after repeated rejection by child who responds with panic or rage attack if approached
Treatment of choice in order of importance	1 Special education 2 Stable enriched environment 3 Training in self-reliance	1 Psychotropic drugs 2 Psychotherapy 3 Milieu therapy 4 Special education 5 Behavior modification 6 Family therapy	1 Tranquilizers 2 Stable and predictable environment 3 Firm statement of 'rules' 4 Behavior modification

A Schizoid disorder of childhood B Schizophrenia	Attention deficit disorder (hyperactivity)	Organic brain syndromes (and disorders)

Ambivalent
Negativistic
Overly possessive
Jealousy guided by delusions and
  hallucinations
Unpredictable
Sadomasochistic
Repetition compulsion leading to
  constant 'testing of the norms'
Sarcastic sense of humor
Clowning
	Superficial
	Impulsive
	Resisting discipline
	Making the environment hyperactive!
	Aggression
	Self-abuse
	May grasp brief situational humor,
	  but no attention to lengthy jokes
		Variable: dependent, anxious, hostile-
		  aggressive, paranoid, inappropriate
		  sexual advances, stealing, hoarding,
		  inappropriate joking

Duration before diagnosis is
  confirmed:
A at least 3 months
B at least 6 months
Lowering of social level of functioning
Gross thought disorder
  (content and form)
Hallucinations; delusions blunted or
  inappropriate affect, ambivalence,
  agitation, withdrawal, deperson-
  alization, anxiety states
Obsessive-compulsive defenses
Depression
'Premonition of going insane'
Volition impaired
Spontaneous remissions
	Attention deficit
	Hyperactivity
	Frequently associated with: specific
	  cortical deficits (learning disabili-
	  ties), mental retardation, epilepsy
		Variable: specific cortical deficits
		Acute: delirium, post-traumatic
		  agitation
		Chronic: disoriented – memory loss –
		  confabulation, bulimia, pica, enure-
		  sis, encopresis, combativeness,
		  apathy, moria (inappropriate
		  wittiness) emotional dulling, lack of
		  initiative

Mannerism
Stereotypie
Catatonia
Lack of initiative
Agitation
Aggression toward self and others
Suicidal attempts
Seeks danger
	Inability to sit still
	Worse in group situation
	Academic difficulties
	Unable to 'select' from environmental
	  stimuli
		Becomes the 'caricature' of his/her
		  premorbid personality: (euphoric,
		  apathetic, depressed, aggressive,
		  expansive, jubilant, 'the jester')

Bewilderment
Anger, admiration, ambivalence,
  rejection; 'rescue efforts' in spite
  of repeated failure
	People become 'hyperactive'; trying
	  to follow and redirect the child;
	  they use loud voice to 'out shout'
	  him and get his attention
		Care and protectiveness ('the poor
		  dear has lost his faculties')
		Impatience
		Rejection
		Institutionalization

1 Psychotropic drugs 2 Psychotherapy 3 Milieu therapy 4 Behavioral therapy 5 Family therapy	1 Drugs a stimulants or b tranquilizers 2 Stable environment 'Tuned down' stimuli 'Tuned down noise' level	1 Etiological treatment 2 Supportive milieu 3 Tranquilizers 4 Ritalin for the agitated OBS may be useful 5 Institutionalization

youngster to prevent 'their sexual acting out'. This being the most frequent anticipatory apprehension of the parents of retarded children [77].

Reactive depression or severe rebellious aggressive manifestations are the most frequent psychiatric symptoms at this age. We must also keep in mind that retarded teenagers and young adults are not immune to any of the psychiatric disorders occurring in the general population. Therefore, the following clinical entities should be considered in the differential diagnosis: schizophrenia; major affective disorders; psychosomatic disorders; adjustment and conduct disorders; substance abuse (iatrogenic drug intoxication is not rare, since the retarded persons may not complain of drug side effects until they become severe enough to be evident to the family or the prescribing physician). Conduct disorders may be caused by lesions affecting the temporal lobe and the limbic system. Not to be overlooked is the possibility of dissociative phenomena in temporal lobe epilepsy [72]. General paresis in teenage years may be the result of congenital syphilis. Foremost importance must be given to the correct diagnosis of schizophrenia, occurring in a retarded person, since early treatment increases the chances of a successful outcome.

Later Adulthood: Age 50 Years and Over. This is the age when the support system of retarded persons living in the community with their family usually breaks down. The caretaking parents (or aunts and uncles) get old, sick or disabled, or even die. Family members of the younger generation have their own families and are unlikely to take-in the retarded person who needs care. This abandonment is the social stressor which causes depression in many adult and elderly retardates.

The deficits in adaptive behavior of recently deinstitutionalized adult retardates may increase when they have to cope with small group living and other stresses of living in the community, including the tasks of shopping, cooking, paying bills, and transportation to and from work or rehabilitation centers. The greatest deficiency of the new living situation is usually the lack of integration into community recreational activities. This in most cases, leads to a very bleak existence for the retarded persons who are living enclosed within the four walls of their home. At best, they are commuting to their job site, where they spend part of the day without socializing with their co-workers, who generally just tolerate them but do not include them into their social contacts. Under these conditions adult retardates may develop psychiatric symptoms. Chronic depression is frequent.

Of course, any of the psychiatric disorders of adult age, occurring in the

Table III. Outline of the diagnostic process

---

1   Social evaluation, social history, home visit where indicated
2   Medical procedures and history
    a   Presenting problem and reason for referral
    b   Medical and developmental history
    c   Physical examination, neurological examination, laboratory and genetic screening
    d   X-ray (skull, chest and bone age), EEG (and tomography if indicated)
    e   Dental evaluations, nursing and dietary evaluation
    f   Psychiatric evaluation
3   Other professional evaluations
    a   Psychological testing and observation, psychological profile, MA, IQ
    b   Educational testing and observation
    c   Communication skill and speech evaluation, hearing evaluation
    d   Art-diagnostic evaluation
4   Consultants as needed
5   Case conferences
    a   Diagnostic conference of the evaluating specialists
    b   Interagency conference with members of the referring agencies
    c   Family conference

---

general population, may affect the retarded individual, regardless of environmental stress. Therefore, the following entities should be considered in evaluating behavioral adaptation deficits of adult retardates: schizophrenia; affective disorders; organic brain disorders (syphilis, arteriosclerosis); degenerative CNS diseases (presenile and senile dementia); substance abuse (mostly alcohol); somatoform disorders. The diagnostician should be aware of the danger of failing to recognize a real disease like cancer, by not following up the vague complaints of a retarded patient who is not articulate enough in describing the symptoms.

Diagnostic Procedure

The following procedure outline is suggested for the efficient multidisciplinary diagnostic work-up of the MR/ED patient, who frequently suffers from additional organic brain damage and other handicapping conditions.

(a) A brief screening evaluation to establish the chief complaint and to gather available information about previous treatments and evaluations. (b) The diagnostic evaluation itself. This may include some, or all of the items listed in table III. (c) Case conferences and treatment plan prescription.

Jakab 284

Table IV. Diagnostic data and treatment chart sample

Admission data	Assets	Pathology	Short-term goals

Intellectual
Chronological age:
  4 years 5 months
Psychological testing
Stanford-Binet LM
  Mental age:
  2 years 9 months
  IQ = 50
Vineland Social Maturity
  Scale
  Social age:
  4 years 2 months
Leiter International
  Performance Scale
  Mental age:
  4 years 2 months
French's PTI
  Mental age:
  4 years 6 months
	a Good visual
	  discrimination
	b Good basic self-help
	  skills (toilet trained, can
	  dress with minimal
	  help, eats with spoon)
	c Nonverbal reasoning
	  present
		1 Visual motor skill delay
		2 Deficient verbal
		  conceptual thinking
		3 Delayed receptive and
		  expressive language
		4 Noncompliant
		  (negativistic)
		5 No peer relations
		6 No play skills
			Increase assets
			a Expand visual discrimina-
			  tion skills
			b Expand self-help skills
			c Expand nonverbal reason-
			  ing skills
			
			Decrease pathology
			1 Improve visual motor
			  skills
			2 Improve verbal conceptual
			  thinking
			3 Foster language develop-
			  ment
			4 Decrease noncompliance
			5 Facilitate peer relations
			6 Improve play skills

Educational evaluation
Fine motor adaptive
  4 years
Conceptual skills 2.5 years
Language skills 2.5 years
	A Good visual perception
	B Capable to attend to
	  tasks
	C Works independently
	D Talks occasionally in
	  short sentences
		1 Poor conceptual skills
		2 Poor expressive-receptive
		  language
		3 Poor peer interactions
		4 Fluctuating attention
		5 Weak motivation for task
		  performance
		6 Frequently uncooperative
			A Refine visual perception
			B Increase attending behav-
			  ior
			C Foster independent work
			D Increase vocabulary
			1 Increase conceptual think-
			  ing
			2 Language and general
			  communication skill
			  development
			3 Foster goal directed peer
			  interaction
			4 + 5 Improve attending and
			  motivation for achieve-
			  ment
			6 Decrease negativism

Methods	Results: to be recorded 3 months after admission	Long-term goals	Methods	Long-term results: to be recorded at dis- charge and follow-up evaluation results

To increase assets
a Incorporate visual
  discrimination
  tasks into recrea-
  tional therapy
  and physical
  therapy
b Structured operant
  behavioral milieu
  therapy
c Special education
 	
To decrease pathology
1–2–3 Therapeutic
  education in group;
  individual thera-
  peutic tutoring; in-
  dividual language
  therapy; total milieu
  communications
  skill emphasis
4 Structured milieu
  therapy; individu-
  ally designed behav-
  ioral therapy
5 Group therapy;
  goal-directed educa-
  tional guidance to
  peer interaction
6 Play therapy; milieu
  therapy fostering
  group play
	a–b Improved self-help
	  skills (better eating
	  habits and dressing
	  skills)
	c –1–3–5 See educational
	  report
	4 Decreased negativism,
	  but still present
	6 Improved play skills –
	  minimal motivation
	No spontaneous peer
	  interaction
		1 To solidify short-
		  term gains
		2 To become fully
		  independent in
		  self-help skills
		3 To reach educable
		  range in special
		  education
		4 To tolerate group
		  learning
		5 To participate ac-
		  tively in educa-
		  tional and recrea-
		  tional activities
		6 To derive pleasure
		  from play and from
		  interaction with
		  other children
			1 Same methods as
			  for short-term goals
			2–5 Lessen supervi-
			  sion on self-help
			  activities
			Community outings
			  to train in proper
			  eating habits in
			  restaurants
			To use public toilet
			  facilities
			To behave appro-
			  priately in recrea-
			  tional settings
			3–4–5 Lengthen class-
			  room time
			Advance educational
			  material
			Foster independent
			  learning
			Decrease tutoring
			6 Foster peer interac-
			  tion; provide chal-
			  lenging games and
			  toys tailored to
			  child's mental age
				To be recorded in the
				  first year after dis-
				  charge at
				  3 months
				  6 months
				  9 months
				  12 months
				To be recorded twice
				  a year for the sec-
				  ond and third year
				  after discharge
				To be recorded once a
				  year in year 4 and
				  year 5 after dis-
				  charge

A + 1 Use visual
  perception for
  initiating abstract
  concept formation
D + 2 Exercises in
  vocabulary and
  syntax
B + 4 + 5 Individ-
  ual/small group
  tutoring
C Reward indepen-
  dent work-operant
  techniques
3 Group activities –
  taking turns, give
  and take exercises
6 Behavior therapy
  in therapeutic
  classroom
	Improved attending
	  behavior and moti-
	  vation
	Increased vocabulary
	Decreased negativism
	Small change in com-
	  munication pattern
	Minimal change in peer
	  interaction
	Tolerates group activi-
	  ties but does not yet
	  initiate any
		Mainstreaming
		Independent class-
		  room work
		Normalized com-
		  munication
		Collaborative task
		  oriented attitude
		Age-appropriate
		  peer relations
			Same as for short-
			  term goals
			Adapted from time
			  to time to matu-
			  rational changes	

Table IV (continued)

Admission data	Assets	Pathology	Short-term goals
Social family composition Father 40 years old Mother 38 years old Brother 8 years old	1 Caring and concerned parents 2 They appear motivated to learn new ways of parenting together	1 Communication between couple poor and inadequate to meet needs of family 2 Limited parenting skills as a couple and poor parenting skills by father 3 Mother appears to be insecure, demonstrates poor self-esteem; father frustrated and over-burdened by finances 4 The sibling, Mike, appears at high risk	1 Provide education for behavioral management parenting skills; parent/child interaction sessions 2 Arrange for Mike to come in for a family art session 3 Arrange with the family for a videotape recording of parent-child interactions; review videotape with parents
Emotional (psychiatric) 1 Adjustment reaction of childhood with autistic traits 2 Mental retardation, mild, associated with prematurity and Rh incompatibility 3 Questionable aphasia versus psychotic speech disorder	A Occasionally intends to please B Willing to follow orders for brief periods of time	1 Delayed language with frequent jargon speech 2 Low frustration tolerance 3 Temper tantrums with screaming and kicking 4 Negativism 5 Stereotype movements and posturing 6 Hallucinations? 7 Anxiety and lack of trust in adults 8 Withdrawal from interaction with adults and children	1 Language to be improved towards more communicative speech from the babbling and jargon speech A + 7 decrease anxiety and negativism B + 2 increase frustration tolerance 3 + 4 + 5 + 6 Decrease psychotic symptoms 8 Foster interaction with adults and peers
Medical (pediatric) *Neurological*	Pediatric: in good physical health Neurological: EEG: no clinical seizures diffusely abnormal no focal lesion	No physical problems No anticonvulsive medication	Maintain health status

Methods	Results: to be recorded 3 months after admission	Long-term goals	Methods	Long-term results: to be recorded at discharge and follow-up evaluation results
Couple sessions Family sessions Classroom observations Parent training sessions Therapeutic visits Agency contacts	Excellent collaboration of parents, improved marital relations They learned positive interaction and limit setting Brother referred to individual therapy Parents motivated to continue	Continue same goals to fuller development of the family unit including the patient Normalize family-life situation	Supportive counseling Parent-child interaction training Therapeutic home visits	To be recorded in the first year after discharge at 3 months 6 months 9 months 12 months To be recorded twice a year for the second and third year after discharge To be recorded once a year in year 4 and year 5 after discharge
1 Speech therapy; Therapeutic education A + 7 Milieu therapy; predictable environmental activities in the milieu; clear limit-setting; parent-child interaction training B + 2 Psychotropic medication 3 Psychotherapy 4 Art therapy 5 + 6 + 8 Socializing to be fostered with peers in recreational activities and classroom	1 Speech improvement observed in more frequent occurrence of more communicative speech Jargon (autistic type) speech persists specifically at unstructured times 3-5-6 Psychotic symptoms substantially decreased 2-4 Negativism and low frustration tolerance still evident 7-8 Improved parent-child and staff interaction Minimal peer interaction	1 Fully alleviate psychosis 2 Normalize speech 3 Provide pleasurable age-appropriate play experiences 4 Normalize interpersonal interactions 5 Foster intellectual growth by aiming at full use of potentials 6 Foster emotional maturity	1 Psychotropic medication (possibly in decreasing amounts) 2 Therapeutic education and language therapy 3 Psychotherapy 4-5-6 Milieu therapy to be shifted to home, reintegration into the community and school system	
Control well child care	Has been in good health with exception of ear infection	Well child care	Behind on immunizations: DPT/ODU (B) ordered	

Diagnostic Tools

Each specialist in the diagnostic team will use a set of diagnostic tools, such as evaluation forms, checklists, and psychological and educational standardized tests.

At the end of the diagnostic process the evaluation of each specialist should be discussed by the team and included into a summary tabulation presenting the patient's assets and pathology in five essential spheres: psychological, educational, social, emotional, medical. This tabulation should also include the description of the short-term and the long-term goals, with suggested methods to reach them. Space for recording the results at subsequent dates should be provided.

This format [41] for an ongoing tabulation (the Diagnostic Data and Treatment Chart) of the patient's and the family's progress has been designed by this writer for the John Merck Program in 1975, and since then its use has been introduced by several other programs and agencies.

The case sample recorded on the Diagnostic Data and Treatment Chart (table IV) demonstrates the logical connections between diagnostic assessment, treatment prescriptions and regular reviews (reassessment of the results throughout a patient's total treatment time from admission to discharge and even through regularly scheduled follow-up evaluations).

From among the diagnostic evaluation methods listed in table IV, only the outline of the psychiatric evaluation is discussed here, since the methods of other specialists are covered by the collaborators of this textbook.

The psychiatric evaluation will include the following details: (a) observation of spontaneous behavior and affect; (b) evaluation of the interaction with the examiner and others, attitude, attention span, associations, orientation, memory, thought processes, hallucinations, mood changes, actions and energy level; interaction through nonverbal media: toys, puppets and graphic expression (style and content); (c) stress tolerance evaluation: examiner's silence, pointing out aberrant behavior, exploring painful past experiences and losses, game play – winning/losing, toy play – denial or retrieval of a specific toy.

The use of a checklist for the tabulation of the behavior and of the psychiatric symptoms recorded during the diagnostic evaluation provides the clinician with a baseline psychiatric profile. Priorities can be established from this checklist for the intermediary goals of the treatment plan. By updating the psychiatric profile and behavioral checklist (recording on it also the changes in medication), the patient's progress can be followed throughout the treatment. A psychiatric profile and behavioral checklist form designed by this author is presented in table V.

Table V. Psychiatric profile and behavioral checklist

Name of patient: _____

Name of physician: _____

Baseline date: _____

Review date: _____

Review date: _____

Discharge date: _____

Codes:

i = Improved

w = Worse

√ = Change in medication (and date)

o = Does not apply

Unchanged = Leave blank

Target behaviors and symptoms	Medi-cation change	Code		Target behaviors and symptoms	Medi-cation change	Code	
	Date						
Intellectual delay (MR level)				Ambivalence			
				Intrusiveness			
Self-help skills				Depressive (D) or manic (M)			
Toilet training				Aggressive outbursts			
Dressing				Temper tantrums			
Eating				Self-injury			
Enuresis or encopresis				Passivity			
Self-stimulation-stereotypy				Erratic behavior			
Speech impairment				Withdrawal			
Spatial orientation distance				Delusions			
Short attention span				Hallucinations			
Hyperactivity				Defense mechanisms ( ) type			
Low frustration tolerance				Medical symptoms			
Sleep disturbance				Neurological symptoms			
Negativism				Other (describe)			
Labile affect				Seizures ( ) type			

Treatment

Retarded children need special education; emotionally disturbed children need psychiatric treatment; doubly handicapped MR/ED children
need both psychiatric treatment and therapeutic education. A therapeutic
milieu can provide several supportive services simultaneously. Parents of
MR/ED children need counseling and professional advice.

Goals of the Psychiatric Treatment

(1) Alleviation of symptoms painful or uncomfortable to the patient.
(2) Improvement or disappearance of socially unacceptable behavior patterns. (3) Accumulation of positive affective experiences – love, gratification, acceptance. (4) Realization of the intellectual potential. (5) Accumulation of knowledge, consistent with the level of the retardation.

Evidently, even with our best therapeutic efforts, we cannot promise 'a
genius'. Nonetheless, as the result of our efforts the mentally retarded person will not be emotionally disturbed but happier, healthier, better adjusted
and using his/her intelligence up to the highest potential.

There is evidence that after the alleviation of the psychiatric disorder
the measured intelligence (MA or IQ) is actually increased. In some cases a
quite dramatic accelerated increase of IQ occurs and continues even beyond
the completion of the psychiatric treatment, as evidenced in the psychological report of the following case:

Case 1. [2] Milly (born 3/28/71), a 4-year-old Caucasian girl, was admitted to the John
Merck Program and tested on May 2, 1975. Diagnosis: mental retardation, moderate;
over-anxious reaction of childhood.

Her reaction to the first testing situation was one of diffuse distress, manifested in
fleeing from any attempts at interaction, crying, and running in circles. By observing the
skills of running around without stumbling or holding onto furniture, it could be established that her motor skills were at about the 18-month mental age level at a chronological
age of 4 years, 2 months. This gave her an estimated IQ of 36. Her main psychological
traits during this first observation were high level anxiety, short attention span and negativism. This extensive emotional disturbance interferred with Milly's social and intellectual performance leading to failure in responding to any test item.

On June 25, 1975, Milly was reassessed. Under standardized conditions (Bailey), a
mental age of 1 year, 8 months (IQ = 40) was obtained at a chronological age of 4 years, 3

[2] The names of all the cases quoted in this chapter are changed in order to protect the
anonymity of the patients.

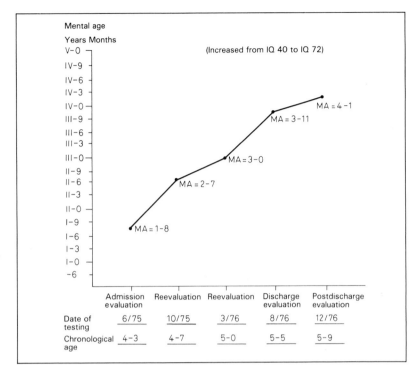

Fig. 1. Accelerated rate of increase in mental age due to decrease in emotional disturbance. Mental growth charted on repeated psychological testing (Milly).

months. During this administration, Milly displayed extreme passivity and lack of motivation which prevented her from passing many of the items.

During the ensuing months it was determined through classroom observation and consultation with Milly's teacher that Milly could indeed accomplish many of the items previously failed. It was decided that by raising Milly's level of interaction through praise and encouragement for performance, she would have a chance to reach her full potential.

On October 27, 1975, Milly was again tested under standardized conditions, and achieved a mental age of 2 years, 7 months (IQ = 56), showing a gain of 11 months mental age in 4 chronological months. Further, a marked decrease in emotional withdrawal was noted. As a result of this test, more refined recommendations were made to improve areas of conceptual skills, such as size relations, counting and performing tasks requiring more abstract thinking.

On February 18, 1976, Milly was retested, revealing a mental age of 3 years, 8 months (IQ = 72), showing a gain of 13 months mental age in chronological 4 months. During this standardized test administration, Milly succeeded on many items previously failed. Recommendations were made in the area of language skills, to prepare her for public school special education classes.

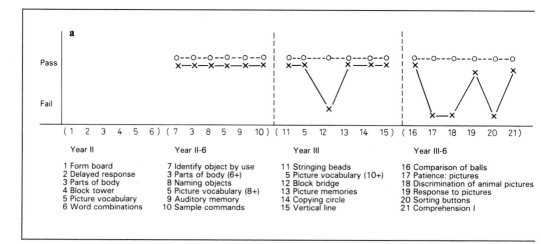

Fig. 2. Qualitative and quantitative changes on the intelligence profile from admission to discharge evaluation. Test-retest results. Sandy: Stanford-Binet (Form L-M) parts I (a) and II (b).

	Admission, X – 7–21–76	Discharge, 0 – 5–9–79
CA	6–0 years	6–10 years
MA	3–6 years	4–2 years
IQ	49	55
Basal age	2–6 years	3–6 years
Ceiling age	5–0 years	6–0 years

In summary, Milly has shown a total gain of 32 IQ points on standardized testing corresponding to an increase of 24 months in mental age. Her test performance changed from moderate trainable to high educable range of retardation (fig. 1).

The improvement reveals that Milly reached her intellectual potential of close to normal when her psychiatric disorder, causing the severe deficits in behavioral adaptation, was alleviated. She received intensive multi-modality treatment as an inpatient.

In another case, the substantial quantitative and qualitative changes in intelligence performance following a 10-month-long inpatient treatment at the John Merck Program are revealed in the psychological profiles recorded at admission and at the time of the child's discharge when the psychiatric disorder was alleviated (fig. 2).

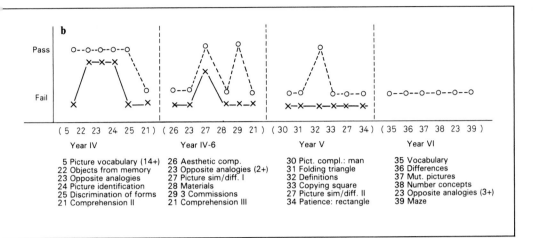

(5   22   23   24   25   21)   (26   23   27   28   29   21)   (30   31   32   33   27   34)   (35   36   37   38   23   39)

Year IV   Year IV-6   Year V   Year VI

5 Picture vocabulary (14+)	26 Aesthetic comp.	30 Pict. compl.: man	35 Vocabulary
22 Objects from memory	23 Opposite analogies (2+)	31 Folding triangle	36 Differences
23 Opposite analogies	27 Picture sim/diff. I	32 Definitions	37 Mut. pictures
24 Picture identification	28 Materials	33 Copying square	38 Number concepts
25 Discrimination of forms	29 3 Commissions	27 Picture sim/diff. II	23 Opposite analogies (3+)
21 Comprehension II	21 Comprehension III	34 Patience: rectangle	39 Maze

Treatment Methods

Factors that cause retardation will often produce associated disorders, such as motor incoordination, perceptual handicap, and emotional instability. All of these have to be treated in their complexities, however individualized, after careful diagnosis and evaluation of each patient.

Mentally retarded persons suffering from multiple handicaps with overlapping symptomatology, require maximum consistency in the environment, in the staff composition, and staff attitude and in all program details, within a carefully designed eclectic treatment program, often including very intricate drug management.

In modern psychiatric practice, based on the interdisciplinary team concept, synthesis of the diagnostic findings and the prescription and monitoring of the multimodality treatment is the primary contribution of the psychiatrist.

The treatment of retarded persons with psychiatric disorders may include one or more of the following methods:

(a)   Etiological treatment of the underlying organic causes
(b)   Medication
(c)   Psychotherapy: individual therapy; group therapy (play therapy); counseling
(d)   Psychiatric milieu and ancillary therapies (psychiatric nursing; art therapy; rhythm and music therapy; recreational and occupational therapy; job training and counseling; psychological support related to practical living experiences)

(e) Behavior therapy
(f) Remedial and/or therapeutic education
(g) Parent and family counseling, or therapy
(h) Social engineering (upgrading and shaping of the home environment; finding community resources of support in housing, in recreation and in the job environment)

Etiological Treatment of Underlying Organic Causes

The etiological treatment of underlying organic causes includes: special diets for metabolic disorders (like in PKU or galactosemia); thyroid hormone substitution in cretinism; anticonvulsive medication, corrective surgery for cardiac anomalies needed by some Down's Syndrome children and orthopedic measures in cerebral palsy; dietary supplements in avitaminosis or malnutrition; medical treatment of high blood pressure, or arteriosclerosis, causing organic brain syndromes and treatment of alcoholism or other substance abuse leading to psychiatric disorders. Of course, the possibility of brain tumor (primary or metastatic) should not be overlooked, especially in frontal lobe and temporal lobe tumors, often manifested in their early stages by psychiatric symptoms. The changes in personality of an adult retardate may be due to a meningeoma causing lack of initiative and aphasia (convexity of the frontal lobe), or causing agitated expansive and short-tempered behavior (basal surface of the frontal lobe) – while sudden inexplainable hallucinations and bizarre behavior may be caused by temporal lobe tumors. Many of these tumors, if diagnosed in time, may be treatable by surgery. Therefore, if a retarded person regresses to a lower level of functioning, or develops psychiatric symptoms the first duty of the physician is to rule out through objective and active diagnostic methods any process of organic brain disease, even if the retarded patient does not complain of the usual early symptoms of headache, dizziness, or visual disturbance. The recognition of some of the degenerative diseases responsible for psychiatric symptoms such as Huntington's chorea, Alzheimer's disease or senile dementia, diagnosed in a retarded person, should not lead to therapeutic nihilism. Rather, the physician should aim at efficient planning for long-term support and care, by keeping the level of functioning at its best at each stage of the disease and by combating the depression frequently associated with these incurable diseases.

In the cases of psychiatric disorders associated with familial cultural deprivation, the etiological treatment will focus on changing the family interaction and on engineering the sociocultural environment, as much as possible, for the benefit of the patient. The removal of the patient from the family to a healthier environment may become necessary.

Table VI. Suggestions for drug treatment of emotionally disturbed retarded persons

1 *Do not treat mental retardation*	6 Select by trial the best-tolerated drug on the lowest possible level
2 Treat the illness of a retarded person	7 Monitor drug levels regularly
3 Establish correct diagnosis	8 Establish drug-free holidays if possible
4 Define target symptoms for relief by drug	9 Stay within safe limits in multiple drug use and avoid chemical incompatibility
5 Treat the person simultaneously by other psychiatric methods	10 Decrease or discontinue drug after a sufficient length of symptom-free state

Use of Psychotropic Medication in Brain-Damaged Psychotic Retarded Persons

Psychotropic medications, in general, do not cure psychiatric illness. By decreasing the acute behavioral symptoms, they help the patient to become accessible to other treatment methods and human interaction. These in turn will provide new and rewarding experiences, which are different from the former psychotic interactions. When normalized interaction patterns have been established, then usually the medication can be decreased and possibly omitted completely. Psychotropic drugs are not indicated for simple mental retardation in the absence of severe subjective distress or behavioral manifestations caused by a psychiatric disorder (table VI).

Medication is needed in cases, when it is otherwise impossible to penetrate the autistic withdrawal and isolation, or the pathological level of anxiety, paired with intense self-destructive impulses. These symptoms would compel the parents, or other caretakers, to apply physical restraints for long stretches of time, making the reaction of the pent-up emotions even more forceful when the restraint is released.

The disruptive behavioral manifestations of the psychotic retarded person should be relieved by antipsychotic medication in order to give the patient a chance to benefit from other therapeutic modalities, which in turn would lead to corrective emotional experiences and to the normalization of their interaction patterns.

It is impossible to provide education, or psychotherapy, or even physical therapy to a psychotic brain-damaged retarded child, with uncontrollable aggression, who at the slightest frustration attacks the environment.

The following case shows that rapid-tranquilization paired with short-term heavy sedation may be necessary to interrupt a pattern of extreme and indiscriminate aggression.

Case 2. Mark, a nonverbal black boy, was admitted to the John Merck Program on 9-2-75 at age 5 years and 3 months.

The presenting problem was uncontrollable aggressive behavior consisting of biting, hitting, pinching, pulling, throwing objects and hitting his head against the wall when frustrated. Family history was negative for epilepsy, mental retardation and mental illness.

Developmental and medical history: pregnancy and delivery uneventful; early milestones delayed, walked at 14 months; speech has never developed; toilet training has been in progress at age two; grand mal seizures started at age 7 months; required frequent hospitalization for uncontrollable seizures in spite of dilantin and phenobarbital maintenance.

At age 2 years, 5 months, when phenobarbital was withdrawn, a status epilepticus developed, leading to a 25-day-long coma followed by a severe decorticated state. He gradually regained his hearing, his sight and motor coordination, but remained nonverbal, giving only grunting and screaching sounds, or screaming loudly. As he became more mobile, it was observed that Mark had become hyperactive and aggressive. Frequently, he was also smearing feces. During this time of early recovery from the coma, a symbiotic relationship started with the mother which developed into a hostile dependent relationship, whereby Mark would abuse the mother to a great extent, hitting, pinching and biting her.

Due to his uncontrollable aggression, day care centers or preschool programs were unable to cope with him. He was readmitted several times to the Children's Hospital because of status epilepticus. He was also hospitalized in a child psychiatric unit. The mother had to be at his bedside most of the time, since staff was unable to cope with him. His aggression and hyperactivity reached such an extent that in one of the hospitals Mark had to be placed in a high crib, with pillows fastened to the side and a mattress on top of the crib, to protect him from injuring himself or others.

Medication at the time of admission to the John Merck Program was: tegretol 200 mg twice a day and valium 2 mg 4 times a day. Grand mal seizures broke through 1–2 times per month.

At admission, the physical and neurological examination and routine lab tests were normal. The EEG revealed theta and delta activity. Slow spike-and-wave, activity was present bitemporally. Photic stimulation produced spike-and-wave forms in the right hemisphere and left temporal region.

Psychiatric evaluation: A nonverbal anxious, hyperactive child, with zero frustration tolerance, short attention span and no awareness of danger, climbing to and jumping from unsafe heights. No eye contact. No stable object relations. Unable to play with toys other than banging them or mouthing them. Uncontrolled aggression to persons and objects. Running aimlessly and biting indiscriminately everybody in this pathway (bit 11 staff members during the first day of hospitalization).

Language: does not follow commands. Reacts to his name only by fleetingly looking at the examiner. No expressive speech. Frequent grunting sounds and high pitched shrill screams were emitted in joy, such as when viewing food.

Psychological evaluation: Bayley Infant Scale, 9/3/75. CA 5 years and 3 months, MA 12.5 months, IQ below 20. Motor development 14.6 months. Vineland Social Maturity Scale: social age 26 months.

The treatment was induced by rapid tranquilization and heavy sedation. This has provided the basis of intensive psychological repatterning.

On the first day of admission a continuous sleep was induced for 5 days (sleeping for about 20–22 h each day), by using a combination of tranquilizers and sedatives (and anti-parkinsonian agents), in addition to anticonvulsive medication. Two nurses, in 12-hour shifts each, were assigned during this phase to provide continuous one-to-one nursing. The physician monitored the drugs by checking the child's physical and neurological status every 4 h. During waking time, the psychological repatterning provided by the nurses consisted of gentle interaction with Mark while feeding and cleansing him, cuddling the child, speaking to him softly, and giving him an occasional kiss on the cheek. Following a gradual decrease of sedatives and tranquilizers after the fifth day, the child's increased alertness was achieved without a returning of the indiscriminate aggression. He developed a temporary symbiotic, but not hostile, attachment to the nurse who provided the patterning. In the next stage gradual change to multiple staff interaction was provided to decrease the symbiosis. Following this sleeping cure the total psychiatric program included: (1) prescription of anticonvulsive medication and Mellaril 50 mg three times a day; (2) behaviorally oriented therapeutic education reinforcing nonaggressive behavior; (3) milieu therapy, and (4) speech stimulation in a total communication framework using sign language. Two years of intensive inpatient treatment, combined with parent-child interaction training sessions, led to decreased aggression in all situations, improved behavior, increased IQ, and emerging verbal language. His attention span remained short and his frustration tolerance remained low. Positive peer interaction was the last to achieve. Complete clinical seizure control was achieved with a combination of dilantin and mysoline, although the EEG remained unchanged.

The psychological repatterning has been the essential factor in this child's intensive multidisciplinary treatment. It has interrupted the previous pathological interactive pattern, through intensive positive interaction, while in a heavily sedated-tranquilized state during the 5 days of the continuous sleep cure. Mark was discharged to a residential educational facility.

Mark's rapid tranquilization was achieved with trifluoperazine and chlorpromazine. For long-range antipsychotic treatment thioridazine H Cl was prescribed as supportive measure to the other treatment modalities. Thioridazine H CL (Mellaril) did not interfere with the established dosage requirements of anticonvulsive medication. As stated before, Mark became completely seizure-free for a period of several years by now as documented in follow-up evaluation. There are no extrapyramidal side effects and electroretinogram remained normal.

The necessity of using major tranquilizers to alleviate life-threatening psychotic states, faces the physician with the problems of severe side effects in some brain-damaged children, such as akathisia and oculargyric crisis with respiratory distress due to muscle spasm, even at very low dosages.

The concomitant use of anticonvulsive and tranquilizing medication is frequently needed and requires special attention in monitoring drug interactions. *Gadow and Kalachnik* [27] determined in a sample of trainable mentally retarded school-children that 10% were medicated for seizure disorder, 4.9% for behavior disorders and 1.8% for both seizures and behavior disorders. The physician should keep in mind that thorazine can produce, in some cases, dilantin toxicity by decreasing the metabolism of dilantin. There is a substantial body of literature on drug interactions [50, 51, 57].

In describing the psychiatric implications of brain damage in children, *Eisenberg* [21] states that 'in the motor sphere one of the most outstanding characteristics is hyperkinesis'. The children with attention deficit disorders caused by hypoarousal [16] respond best to stimulants (ritalin, dexedrine, pamelor, caffeine). These patients' behavior must not be confused with the restless, aggressive behavior of some agitated children, mostly with thalamus or frontal or temporal lobe lesions, whose behavior is characterized by frequent, but targeted aggressive acts, or with the behavior of overanxious, hyperalert children. Children in the last two categories respond to stimulants by erratic and more aggressive behavior or by increased anxiety states. The patients in these categories respond more favorably to tranquilizers.

Combined drug and milieu treatment is suggested by several authors for the treatment of handicapped brain-injured children [44, 46, 75].

If psychotherapy is assisted by concomitant drug therapy it is advisable to terminate the drug therapy before terminating psychotherapy. The decision to terminate drug maintenance therapy should be based on complete psychiatric reevaluation and should be followed by weekly contact for at least 4–8 weeks.

The physician prescribing tranquilizers to the retarded patient with psychiatric disorders should avoid 'changing a patient with an acute psychiatric illness into a permanent neurological invalid' [7]. Close monitoring for side effects and adhering to the lowest possible dosage is necessary. Furthermore, an attempt should be made to decrease or discontinue the drugs after a sufficient symptom-free state (about 6 months to 1 year). Monitoring drug levels for antidepressants is the best tool to assure therapeutic success [29]. It can also help in detecting noncompliance which could lead to symptoms previously thought to be side effects of imipramine in children [62].

A word of caution is in order about undermedicating with tranquilizers due to fear of making a 'zombie' of the patient. *Prescribing less than a clinically effective therapeutic dosage leads to both evils of treatment: the patient is not symptom-free and is exposed to the danger of developing side effects.* Good clinical observation and close monitoring will avoid the 'zombie' effect, while providing symptom relief through slow increase of the dosages of tranquilizers prescribed for the psychotic retarded patient.

The physicians should not function as an agent for social control of violent behavior, as opposed to being healers of the severely mentally ill [43]. The physician's primary role in management is to relieve any medical condition contributing to the developmental deficit or problems of social adaptation [61].

Regarding the ethics of drug treatment the physician should keep in mind, that well used medication is an important treatment toll in lessening the suffering of the retarded patient with psychiatric disorders.

Psychotherapy

The retarded patient often becomes the passive recipient of the therapeutic action, to which he is subjected by the decisions of others.

The overtly stated goal of helping the patient to get better is frequently influenced by the needs of those who refer the retarded person for psychotherapy. The unexpressed goals of the referring persons are usually based on their wishes to make the work of the caretakers smooth and pleasant and to alleviate the distress of the environment caused by the patient's behavior. The goal itself will influence the choice of the method.

The referral may come from the parents, the school, or an agency interested in behavioral changes, with authority to recommend and/or finance the treatment. In these cases, behavior modification techniques, based on *Skinner's* [73] classical theory of selection by consequences, are the most likely methods of choice.

On the contrary, in self-referred cases, such as adult patients (not committed by a court of law), it is the personal pain and suffering that is in the foreground of the need and the indication for the treatment. In these cases drug treatment, combined with individual or group psychotherapy are the most frequently recommended and performed treatment methods.

Psychotherapy Methods

The therapist must address some basic issues inherent in the double handicap of mental retardation and emotional disturbance:

(1) Retarded persons must adjust to the unchangeable consequences of the retardation, including the adjustment to a certain degree of social discrimination because of their retardation.

(2) MR/ED patients must be motivated to use their existing assets for increasing their level of functioning.

(3) The psychiatrist must adapt the treatment to the patient's level of functioning and mental age, while not losing sight of their chronological age and of some specific age-related problems such as puberty, end of schooling, menopause, or an environmental crisis.

(4) The method of therapy should be adapted in range from nonverbal play therapy to dynamically oriented verbal therapy. *Ekstein* [22] describes succinctly these 'two roads to the unconscious ... the play of the child as his major form of dreaming ... the dream of the adult as his major form of playing with thoughts.' In addition to formal play therapy, MR/ED children will learn to interact with each other in small play groups, guided by staff. They learn to use toys appropriately and to interact without undue anxiety or hostility, as illustrated in figure 3, depicting the successive phases of supervised play:

> First, Chad builds a tower, which is toppled by Judy under his angry protest. Next Judy builds and Chad topples her tower by pushing his ball against it. In the last phase the destructive impulses are replaced by cooperative ball play which they both seem to enjoy. Throughout this session the child care worker refrained from actively interfering, but gave verbal support to the child whose 'building' was destroyed by the other.

Psychosis may be aggravated by the difficulties of assessing reality, due to cognitive deficits, or deficits in the cortical processing of sensory perceptions. These symptoms may hinder the psychotherapeutic process. In such cases, when nonverbal behavior is used during psychotherapy it must be very explicit, and occasionally overdramatized, to compensate for their cognitive deficits and their limitations of understanding verbal messages. The therapist's message must be given clearly, repeatedly and concretely.

The therapist's office, or playroom must be set up with the patient's specific needs and handicaps in mind. Some brain-damaged retarded children may need a stimulating environment, while those with hyperactive symptomatology will benefit more from quiet, low-keyed surroundings. Thus, the number of objects, toys and games visible in the therapist's room have to be adapted to the nature of the pathology.

The length of the sessions must be adjusted to the patient's tolerance, from a brief 15-min to the full 50-min session. Severely disturbed retarded patients have low tolerance for being confined with an individual or a group within a given space such as the therapy office or playroom.

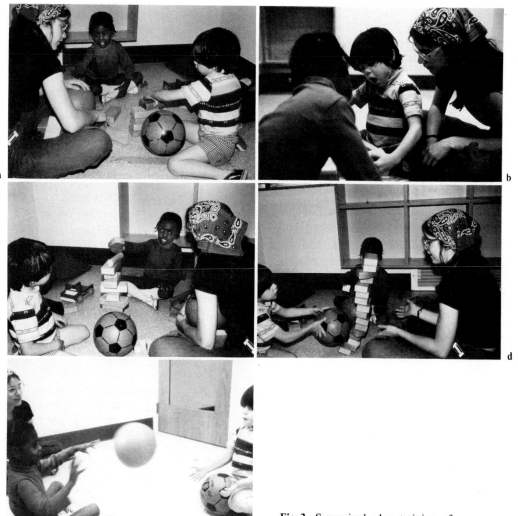

Fig. 3. Supervised play training of MR/ED children.

In psychotherapy it takes special skill to deal with the retarded patient's concreteness of thinking [40], and their greater tendency to develop a symbiotic attachment.

The therapist must help to reality-orient the patient including the understanding of the extent of his handicap. Differentiation between fantasy and reality can be fostered through role playing, interpretation, symbolic use of play materials and actual modeling and demonstration. *Sternlicht* [74] emphasizes the importance of communications through means other than verbal.

When symptoms of depression or aggressive rebellion require therapeutic intervention, the psychiatrist frequently has the task of restoring the patient's self-esteem and to develop a feeling of autonomy, by helping the environment in providing as much freedom of choice for the patient as possible. In the process of extensive physical and intellectual rehabilitation, the emotional needs for play and recreational activities of some brain-damaged retardates may be grossly curtailed. In their struggle to survive and to become physically functional and intellectually competent in school or job setting, they may develop into emotionally starved hard workers carrying the burden of a chronic depression and inability to enjoy age-appropriate play and peer interaction. Some may develop into angry and aggressive teenagers while the more severely depressed would become very withdrawn, or even suicidal.

The following case illustrates the need for psychiatric counseling of the family and of the treatment staff to prevent or alleviate these problems caused by overzealous treatment and rehabilitation.

Case 3. Peter (when seen in consultation by this writer) was a 16-year-old, mildly handicapped and somewhat depressed youngster. Medical history revealed that Peter had a normal early development in childhood. At age 6, he fell off a tree and sustained head injury with fractured skull, epidural hematoma and brain edema, which caused severe brain stem and cerebellar lesions. He recovered after a 2-week-long coma. Residual symptoms were mild right-sided spastic hemiparesis, surgically corrected right abducens paresis, and moderate cerebellar ataxia and speech articulation disorder.

Peter recovered slowly from the decorticated state by regaining his former functions of visual and auditory perception and his speech. During the following 11 years of rehabilitation he reached a level of normal intelligence and good school performance in the public school system. His main handicap was cerebellar ataxia which interferred greatly with his attempts at writing.

Secondary emotional problems developed 4 years after the accident and were treated with psychotherapy for 2 years, on an outpatient basis. Through psychotherapy and social intervention in the environment by his psychiatrist, improvement was achieved at that time.

This youngster has spent about 6 years of his childhood devoted exclusively to the process of his slow, but successful, step-by-step physical rehabilitation. He went through several stages of patterning, followed by orthopedic rehabilitation, each stage requiring hard work and concentrated effort. During all those years, Peter has been essentially a passive recipient of prescribed activities carried out with his mother's help and under professional guidance and supervision.

His formal schooling has required a sustained and equally concentrated effort to manage the competitive work in the public school, in spite of his handicap in writing. His writing was very slow, ataxic and hard to read. He missed out on written tests – not by lack of knowledge, but due to lack of time for writing down the answers.

Peter had no time and no energy for play and for socializing. This left him emotionally starved, missing out on some of the most important aspects in a child's life: 'play' and recreation.

At age 16, new problems of adjustment surfaced. Peter was torn between omnipotent fantasies and defective self-image reflecting the conflict between the wish for autonomy and his great dependency needs. This youngster's life-style and his defenses against despair and unbearable loneliness are centered around hard work while he is aiming toward high achievement.

It is yet to be determined how much emotional independence can be tolerated by Peter, inspite of his present rebellious attitude against parental authority. The goal of his emotional rehabilitation is, at this stage, to help avoid the danger of developing into a self-supporting, lonely robot, since there is a danger of falling into such a life-style by a premature and 'angry' separation.

The therapist has to help the patient learn to tolerate frustration. Playing games of increasing levels of difficulty, introducing both physically and intellectually more demanding tasks are useful to increase the patient's ego strength and frustration tolerance.

The psychotherapy techniques in working with retarded patients should include the management of transference and countertransference. Through the resolution of transference the patient would learn to adapt to his handicap and relate to the environment on a more mature level by using the models developed and understood in transference. The countertransference of the psychiatrist struggling with rescue wishes may lead to overprotective tolerance of aberrant behavior. On the other hand, the psychiatrist may become too active and expect fast behavioral changes, thus overidentifying with the social demands and feeling frustrated for not achieving such changes in short time. In these cases the psychiatrist may lose sight of the primary intrapsychic conflict and give up the patient, to exchange the psychotherapeutic methods for behavioral techniques.

Group psychotherapy may be the choice in selected cases. Normalization and a feeling of 'not being different' may be achieved by mixing retarded and nonretarded disturbed patients and thereby helping them to relate to each other. In the group they learn skills in adapting to the demands of the environment, in spite of their anxieties and often in spite of their anger at the 'nonretarded environment'.

When family therapy is provided by the psychiatrist alone, or in collaboration with the social worker, the therapist must be alert to the surfacing of an unexpected personal pathology of the family members. Some parents, while beginning to have insight into their nontherapeutic handling of the child (either by overprotecting or by rejecting it), may develop feelings of increased guilt. These feelings must be resolved in therapy for a healthier family interaction with the patient. Clinicians frequently underestimate the degree by which the consequences of mental retardation are aggravated by emotional problems. Inadeqate ego control and regressive defensive mechanisms could contribute to the cause of mental retardation itself.

There are no large statistical studies dealing with the evaluation of results of psychotherapy with retardates and there is, according to *Gunzburg* [34], an almost complete lack of follow-up studies. *Luborsky* [48] complains about the lack of measuring instruments in the research of psychotherapy. *Murstein* [55] questions the validity of testing and retesting with the same battery, which, of course, will be inevitable in the cases of brain-damaged psychotic retarded patients who require frequent reevaluations. However, one may consider the patient's ability to 'learn' from the previous testing, as being in itself an indicator of the potential of trainability or educability.

Individual psychotherapy has not been too successful mostly because of the small number of therapeutic sessions delivered and over a short time only [2].

The psychosexual development of retarded children may be beset with problems inherent in the generally delayed development and complicated by parental misconceptions. Therefore parental counseling and counseling of retarded youngsters in this important area is part of the child psychiatric intervention. Much aberrant behavior related to the psychosexual development can be prevented by sexual education of the retarded children (and of their parents).

Psychosexual Development and Sexual Education of Retarded
Children and Counseling of Their Families

The prevention of the complication most feared by parents, namely 'sexual acting out', has to start very early in life by sexual education tailored to the retarded youngster's level of understanding.

Information about puberty and menstruation should be factual (with as few anatomical pictures as possible, since these are usually more frightening than informative). Hygiene of menstruation is an essential topic as well as reassurance that the appearance of blood during the cycle does not mean injury or illness.

One should not start sex education by stories about the horrors of venereal disease or of unwanted pregnancy. Nobody will be deterred by the intellectual knowledge of these dangers from engaging in satisfying one of the most powerful physiological needs which predictably leads to great pleasure.

Of course it is advisable to provide information about VD. This should be done in a matter of fact way, by giving a list of the signs which help detect VD and providing reassurance that these diseases can be treated successfully. This should encourage the retarded person to seek treatment in case of disease.

Pregnancy as a possible consequence of intercourse should also be openly discussed and the feasibility of contraception presented to young women of childbearing age.

Dealing with emergence of masturbation is often considered a 'tabu' subject by parents and teachers alike. When the child discovers the pleasure of masturbation the parents have to teach him/her one rule: 'not here and not now', regarding indiscriminate masturbation in public. This social rule is not different from the rule of toilet training. It is evident that physiologically the bladder and the rectum will empty when they are full. However, the parents teach their children that 'not anywhere but at the toilet' and 'not immediately' at the first urge, but after they reach the bathroom. As it is not expected to refrain forever from voiding and defecating, similarly it should not be expected to suppress the pleasure of masturbation but to learn the need for privacy and the rule of 'not here and not now'.

Another example of social restriction related to a physiological function is the training of proper eating habits: not with your fingers, but with a spoon; do not lean into the soup; use a cup for drinking; do not grab the food from your sister's plate; etc.

Retarded children may take a longer time to learn all the social norms of eating, toilet training and sexual behavior. Retarded children may also develop emotional disturbance related to any of these psychosexual phases of maturation (just like the nonretarded children) during their developing years. The pediatrician or the child psychiatrist may help prevent such emotional disorders through counseling and advice to parents on these subjects.

Successful sexual education starts with coeducational upbringing and by fostering joint recreational activities of girls and boys from early ages on, just like in the nonretarded youngster's upbringing. A retarded woman who grew up overprotected and 'segregated' from male contact is the most likely candidate for sexual promiscuity. The stories of these girls are rather monotonous and alike from case to case: The physiologically mature girl (woman), in the mild or moderate level of retardation, will commute unescorted to school or job. One day a man addresses her 'you are nice' ... she is pleased to hear compliments and is willing to follow him. They have intercourse. During those few minutes she experiences the feeling of being intensely desired, loved, and needed by the partner. A most beautiful psychological experience, which may or may not be paired, at that stage, by the sexual pleasure of orgasm on the woman's part. Then it is all over, until the next man offers the same psychological and sexual pleasure. The experience will be repeated with a predictably pleasant outcome unless she meets a sadist or rapist.

The retarded woman will be likely to seek out male partners in order to feel 'wanted, needed, loved,' even if she must pay for it with the only currency she has – her body.

Coeducational upbringing should provide the retarded woman with opportunities of social contact with men and the psychological experience of the feeling of being liked, being desirable, and ultimately to understand that love is the most beautiful human feeling, which may culminate in sexual interaction. But they must realize that they can be liked without immediately paying with their body for the experience of being desired.

The questions of marriage and the childbearing abilities of retarded women have to be evaluated individually and dealt with in marriage counseling.

Genetic counseling should also be provided as part of the preventive measures to protect the parents from having a defective offspring and to protect the child from being raised in an inadequate family climate. Of course, if there is a healthy spouse or extended family, the retarded mother can get much help in childrearing. Social agencies should also be involved early, if the retarded parent's child is at risk of cultural deprivation, or of developing a psychiatric disorder related to the environmental factors of inadequate parenting.

Psychiatric Milieu

The psychiatric milieu is designed to provide optimal conditions for accurate diagnosis and innovative treatment. In inpatient psychiatric units a stable and predictable environment (the milieu) is created where the staff attitude towards each individual patient is well planned. Some patients may need a firm attitude and limit-setting; some of the unacceptable behaviors of others used for attention gaining may need to be disregarded, while still others may require a substantial amount of individual attention and support from the staff.

In rehabilitation facilities the retarded patient should learn to use group support and gain strength from identifying with well-adapted retarded persons within the therapeutic milieu, by getting to know retardates who are functional and happy. Ultimately, they should attain (within the limitations of the retardation) the highest possible subjective, emotional satisfaction and develop the ability to form enjoyable interpersonal relations.

The prescription of specific staff attitudes toward each patient is based on the diagnostic evaluation and is an important aspect of the treatment in inpatient settings. The individualized treatment prescription will indicate the needed therapeutic attitude towards a given MR/ED patient and his/her family, in order to provide a predictable and consistent environment where all staff members who come in contact with the patient are aware of the required therapeutic attitude for optimal impact.

The following guidelines were developed for the John Merck Program by this writer to clarify the meaning of staff attitude prescriptions for patients with different needs of psychiatric milieu therapy.

Definitions of Staff Attitude Prescriptions
Special Staff Attitudes towards the Child. One or more to be prescribed in order of priority.

(a) Giving support and attention; providing gratification: A particular child is to receive a maximum amount of affection and is provided with pleasurable experiences – smiling at him, praising him, sitting at his side, etc.

(b) Setting limits on child's negative behavior: Being firm with a child without treating him harshly or cruelly. The staff member's attitude is matter-of-fact and business-like.

(c) Reducing excessive stimulation: To act as a calming influence on an over-excited and over-stimulated child. The staff may have to shield the child from too much external stimulation, including noise, and this may involve moving the child quietly away from such sources of stimulation.

(d) Providing a maximum amount of structured activities: Keeping the child on various tasks, thus preventing disorganization and boredom of the child. The staff plans activities and helps the child through those activities.

(e) Encouraging independence: The staff is 'standing back' from the child and expecting the latter to initiate and carry out whatever tasks he is capable of. It implies that the child is capable of more than he had demonstrated in his behavior.

Special Staff Attitudes towards Parents. One or more to be selected in order of priority.

(a) Supportive: This is an attitude of generally enhancing the parent's positive feelings about himself/herself as a 'good enough parent'. It is particularly appropriate in relation to parents who are depressed about their past failures as parents and who feel inadequate as caregivers.

(b) Firm limit setting: The staff deals in a kind but firm manner with a parent's excessive demands on the staff. This attitude has top priority when a parent maliciously misquotes statements of one staff member to another, becomes overly ingratiating, or attempts to interact with the child in a manner contrary to the treatment plans.

(c) Concrete, educational approach: This means dealing with the parent primarily by providing concrete information. It presupposes that the parent needs certain facts about the child and his management, and that the parent can make good use of these facts.

(d) Encouraging parent-child bonding: The staff facilitates the improvement of the parent-child relationship. It means giving the parent support in specific areas of relating to the child. This can be done by emphasizing the positive aspects of the child when speaking to the parent, or by demonstrating to the parent the positive staff interaction with the child.

(e) Encouraging parent-child separation: The staff supports the parent's emotional detachment from the child. It can be done by emphasizing the child's needs for autonomy and independence, and by concrete demonstration of allowing the child such independence.

The attitude therapy as part of the intervention in the psychiatric milieu is carried out essentially by nursing personnel. Therefore, nurses, aides and child care workers have to be trained in this technique.

Ongoing day-to-day communication reaching the whole staff about any changes in a given patient's attitude therapy can be achieved by a brief, concise morning report given by the head nurse each day for the total staff.

Special Contributions of the Nursing Services to the Psychiatric Treatment of Retarded Patients

The nurse will gather information by use of a questionnaire, filled out in advance by the parents, and by personal interview of the parents or other caregivers. The use of this information is intended to help make the patient's adjustment to the treatment program easier. It would also include items like favorite foods and disliked foods, allergies, and any special routines that mother follows with her children in eating, dressing, and toilet training techniques.

On the day of admission the staff nurse will assist the physician in the physical examination. Following the examination, the nurse will take the patient on a tour of the facility and will frequently 'special' the patient for the rest of the day. This one-to-one relationship helps in the psychological preparation of the patient for medical tests (blood work-up, EEG, X-rays), while the nurse carefully notes any symptoms and the reactions of the patient to the environment.

The Role of Coordinator

The coordinator's job is not a separately budgeted staff position but it is a special assignment of a member of the nursing staff (the position being that of an aide, a child care worker, or a nurse) in addition to the other daily duties of that particular staff member.

Each patient comes to the psychiatric program with individual needs and problems and each coordinator must establish a relationship with the patient to meet these needs. The coordinator is an advocate for the patient and a contact person with the program staff and the family. The coordinators participate in the treatment review conferences by presenting to the team their observations of the patient's behavior in the milieu and are responsible for informing the rest of the staff of any specific programs or changes prescribed at the treatment review team meetings. The parents or other relatives are informed by the coordinator of the concrete steps in the patient's development and of the type and timing of scheduled tests, group outings to the community, etc. In return, the coordinator provides the team and other staff members with information of any questions or problems shared by the family. Coordinators may function as models in therapeutic play sessions for parents and siblings.

There are children whose parents are not involved with them. In these situations a one-to-one 'mothering' relationship is established between the coordinator and the child. The objective is to help the child's ego development by fostering positive interpersonal relationships with other children and adults, as shown in the following case.

Case 4. David was admitted to the John Merck Program on March 3, 1975 at age 5 years, 8 months.

Diagnosis: mental retardation (severe), unspecified childhood psychosis with autistic features, IQ 32.

David's father left the family shortly after his birth. The mother, who was employed before her marriage, went on welfare after the divorce and moved in at first with her inlaws in this country, but could not stay long because of David's disturbed behavior – next she returned to Europe to her widowed mother, but David's disruptive behavior challenged the grandmother's tolerance to its limits. Thus, mother and child have returned once again to the US. By age 3½ David was still nonverbal and not toilet trained; he was severely withdrawn and anxiously restless. David was self-abusive and aggressive. He was endangering himself by pushing objects into electrical outlets, pulling pots off the hot stove, running into the street if not constantly 'held by the hand', by mother. The mother was exhausted and depressed by the child's autistic, hostile-dependent behavior. She attempted to care for him, but was unable to establish a close emotional relationship with him. David was admitted as an emergency, because the mother stated that she 'doesn't feel she can be responsible anymore, she may harm the child if he remains with her'. This child had very negative experiences in human contact.

The coordinator had to take into account the factors which hindered David's emotional development, and she had to counteract them.

After David entered the Merck program, weekly visits were set up with the mother and the interaction between mother and son were guided by the coordinator. What happened at the end of visits, when the mother left, was a pathetic reflection of David's behavior. He would stand for a long time at the glass door at the end of the corridor (after she has left) and wave after her. To overcome this separation trauma, the coordinator initiated a game of bye-bye with inanimate objects. Dolls were told bye-bye and taken to an adjacent room, then brought back and greeted with 'hello' repeatedly. The next phase was role playing to teach David that he can also be the leaving party. The procedure was the following: the coordinator stood on the inside of the glass door waving to David who went out for a few minutes with another staff member and then came back. This provided David with the experience that it is not always he who is left behind, but that somebody else can remain there and wave to him when he leaves. This helped David 'feel', rather than understand, that those who leave will come back. This game has evolved further with appropriate staff interaction upon their departure, by David waving bye-bye to them. David learned to play a game of hide and seek with staff members and other children, while he employed the 'waving goodbye' gesture.

The visiting sessions with the mother ended when the mother left the country with no forwarding address. Legal, guardianship was established. In the meantime, David had to cope with the mother's loss. He understood verbal speech (although he did not speak), therefore, his mother's leaving had to be communicated to him. It was the coordinator's responsibility to tell David of his mother's leaving, and to support his responses to this loss. To substitute for the loss of his mother, the coordinator established a one-to-one relationship with David through several activities, including play sessions, taking him outside for walks, and eating meals with him. With this approach, an attachment was formed. David demanded infantile gratifications and exploded with rage and aggression when his needs were frustrated. His relationship with the coordinator was expressed in his attempts to satisfy his needs. When he became anxious he would seek her out, either to be held, or just to remain close to her, until he calmed down. Further evidence of the early stages of his attachment was David's difficulty of separating from her. With time through this one-to-one relationship substantial changes were achieved in David's behavior, leading to better frustration tolerance, by establishing the basic trust he had never experienced before.

During his inpatient treatment David received therapeutic education, speech therapy, art therapy, in addition to play therapy with the coordinator, supervised by a staff child psychiatrist.

When he was discharged to a group home and school in the community David was no longer self-abusive or aggressive, although he still remained rather withdrawn. He used sign language to communicate and verbal language was emerging. Follow-up visits revealed further progress.

Art Therapy and Music Therapy

Both these ancillary treatment methods can be suitably adapted to the needs of the MR/ED patient of any age.

The diagnostic evaluation through the graphic art media is helpful in understanding the patient's unconscious wishes, fantasies and their self-image. The drawing of the human figure can be used for rating the mental age [31] and for interpreting unconscious conflicts. Distortions of the body image concept are also reflected in the human figure drawings of MR/ED patients [37, 38]. The spontaneous expression through the art media (drawing, painting, clay-work, etc.) may reveal psychopathology even before clinical symptoms necessitate therapeutic intervention. Therefore periodical art-diagnostic evaluation within the school setting, of retardates at risk for emotional disturbance, may become a valuable tool in early case-finding efforts leading to preventive measures. *Thompson* [79], however, questions the reliability of scoring drawing tests.

Art media can be used in the course of psychotherapy with retarded children, specifically in helping them to establish an acceptable body image, including the acceptance of a visible physical handicap, such as hemiplegia, spasticity, hydrocephalus, etc. Expression of feelings, in a nonverbal way, may help retarded patients at any age to abreact some of the conflicts which are inaccessible to the consciousness, or for which they may not possess the proper vocabulary. Art therapy enables the nonverbal child to express himself in a concrete form. It facilitates the verbal patient's ability to articulate his feelings [39]. Children and adolescents can often express themselves and relate only through the shared artistic experience [28].

The active creative work, especially if it is an enjoyable experience, will help reestablish the patient's self-esteem. Art therapy should be used as a tool in the total rehabilitation of MR/ED patients.

Rhythm and music therapy are quite useful methods in structuring group interaction of MR/ED patients. They also help in body awareness, and may transform the customary clumsiness of many retardates into more graceful motor patterns [42]. Listening skills improve and even the attention of the hyperactive retarded child can be channelled into a more sustained pattern of activity through the use of music and rhythm therapy. Music and rhythm may be the only social contact initiated by an autistic retarded child, who may be willing to change the rhythm of his spontaneous twirling and to adapt it to the speed of the music engineered by the therapist. An anxious or negativistic child may accept 'hand holding' during a group dance. Music as an art media is a most versatile tool in the hands of a trained therapist in the treatment of MR/ED patients.

Behavior Therapy

In the cases of retarded person with psychiatric disorders the psychiatric treatment methods may have to be combined with other methods of rehabilitation in an effort to treat the total patient.

Behavioral therapy is the most frequently used intervention in the school system to cope with the emotional problems of mentally retarded children. The behavior modification techniques can help in establishing (or reestablishing after temporary regression) the basic self-help skills, such as toilet training or appropriate eating habits. Behavioral therapy can eliminate the symptoms of emotional disturbance by consistently rewarding the desired behavior. It can also help in lengthening the attention span in classroom situations.

Clinical psychologists by their special training are key staff members of the psychiatric team by providing specialized treatment prescriptions for behavioral therapy; they will train the staff in these methods and supervise the patient's progress in the behavioral program.

Areas of behavior for which behavioral programs are widely used include procedures involved in reducing self-stimulatory behavior and aggressive behavior, such as tantrumming at mealtime, book destruction, screaming, and inappropriate touching of people. For clinical samples, see *Shapiro* [this book].

Other programs can help increase a child's expressive language, improve the eye contact and attention span of a withdrawn child, or improve self-management in classroom behavior. *Marks* [49] reported behavioral methods useful in reducing a variety of sexual deviations (paraphilias).

The need for longitudinal behavioral observation in a diagnostic classroom has been proven in the following case. The clinical decision to recommend a change to inpatient treatment from partial hospitalization was based on behavioral observations.

Case 5. Barbara, a 10-year-old Caucasian girl, was admitted to the John Merck Program on March 14, 1975. Diagnosis: profound mental retardation (IQ was under 10) and early infantile autism. She was a severely withdrawn, negativistic, extremely anxious, nonverbal and self-abusive child. She had a history of tantrums, consisting of head banging, wrist biting, and screaming.

Barbara was originally admitted as a partial care patient, who attended the program from 8:30 a.m. to 4:30 p.m., Monday through Friday.

Figure 4, a behavioral chart, is a record of the frequency of Barbara's temper tantrums in the first 3 weeks in the day-patient program. It shows the increase in pathology following each weekend at home. These observations led to the decision to have her admitted as an inpatient. In the structured inpatient milieu Barbara's tantrums have rapidly decreased from 14.3 per day to less than 1.6 per day. By the 14th week of treatment they have essentially disappeared.

Barbara's behavioral program has been assisted by psychotropic medication. She received Mellaril 50 mg twice a day.

Barbara made steady progress. However, on the 12th week of treatment, suddenly, her anxiety increased and as a consequence the number of temper tantrums raised sharply. It was assumed that this relapse was caused by increased environmental stress due to the admission of two very aggressive and disruptive children to the same ward. Barbara's medication was adjusted at this point by increasing the dosage from 50 mg of Mellaril twice a day to 50 mg of Mellaril three times a day. This brought about a very dramatic change, by decreasing her anxiety and increasing her stress tolerance. As a result the number of temper tantrums decreased. Figure 5 is a record of this phase of Barbara's treatment, which proves that in order to cope with increased environmental stress this child required a slight increase in the dosage of medication.

Behavioral programs are the most promising methods of intervention in the following grossly inappropriate behaviors which occur primarily in institutionalized MR/ED adults (the so-called 'back ward' syndromes): smearing excrements, disrobing, ruminating, excessive public masturbation, and continuous indiscriminate object destruction. Usually several patients indulge in the same aberrant behavior on a given ward. In some hospitals one could consider these symptoms as endemic.

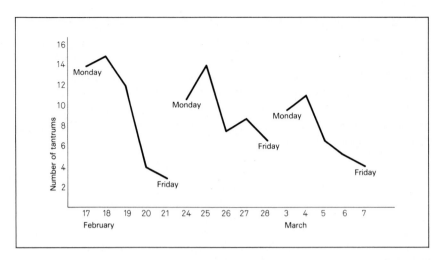

Fig. 4. Behavioral observation chart. Record of first 3 weeks in a day-patient program, outlining the regression following the weekends at home. These observations led to the decision to have her admitted as an inpatient.

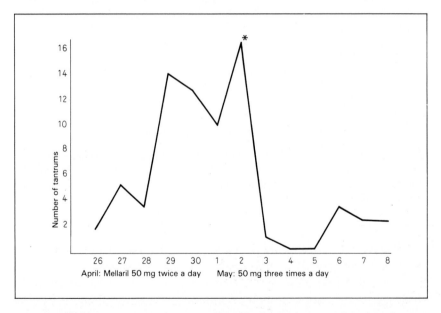

Fig. 5. Behavioral observation chart. Record of Barbara's 11th, 12th and 13th weeks in the program. Note (*) decrease in tantrums following slight adjustment in Mellaril from 50 mg twice a day to 50 mg Mellaril three times a day.

Behavior modification in these cases will be more successful if at the start of the new treatment the patients are transferred to a different ward where the staff-patient interaction is not yet entangled into a vicious circle of acting out and punishment or to a ward where 'total staff apathy' has not yet set in.

The psychologist should motivate the staff and train them in behavioral techniques, ultimately helping not only the patients, but increasing staff morale by providing them with a successful tool of handling these very distressing symptoms of emotional disturbance in a population of institutionalized retardates.

Other Treatment Methods

The treatment of MR/ED persons may necessitate other ancillary treatment methods such as physical therapy, language therapy (including sign language and traditional speech therapy), and dental intervention. Special education with both academic and therapeutic tutoring are integral parts of the total multimodality treatment of school age children.

Further details on these treatment methods are not given in this chapter since they are covered in other parts of this textbook.

Family Involvement and the Role of the Social Worker

Brain-damaged, MR/ED children exert a profound influence on their family. *Goldenberg and Levine* [30b] have proven the mutual influence exerted on each other by the mentally subnormal patient and his family. The family may literally assign one or more members to fulfill the role of the damaged child's entire care. This person will deny his own needs during the 'heroic stage' of total devotion to the process of rehabilitation [82]. In time, martyred family members become increasingly irritable and angry.

The family's attitude toward the brain-damaged, MR/ED child will greatly influence the child's expectations of himself and of his environment. If the caretakers tend to be irritable, depressed, or anxious, the likelihood is great that the child will be increasingly angry, guilty, anxious and ambivalent.

Retarded persons suffering from a psychiatric disorder, frequently require institutional care; many of them are on waiting lists, for years. Caring for these patients in their home can lead to a family disaster, caused by the parent's exhaustion. Nervous breakdown of parents and siblings is not uncommon under the strain of the constant demands on the family's time, energy and emotional resources. The families do not have the skills to deal with the vulnerable MR/ED child. Therefore, they require support, guidance and sometimes more intensive therapeutic intervention.

The family of any doubly-handicapped child will have more than its share of bad days with their child. With a reserve of positive experiences behind them, they will have greater strength to cope with problems when they do arise. A better ability on the parents' part to handle the child would, of course, ease the tension in the family and, in turn, a lessening of tension would make it easier for the child to cope within the structure of the system.

The social workers focus on the family system and its individual members as they effect, and are effected by, the one who has become the patient. The assets and the pathology in the precarious balance of the family system provide the parameters of intervention.

For adult retardates social services fulfill an essential role in the preparations for discharge from large institutes. The social worker provides guidance and support to the families of retardates who after long years of institutional care return to the family home. Supervision and if necessary supportive therapy is the social worker's contribution to the adjustment of retarded adults who are on their way to gradually achieving higher levels of independence in community living.

Discharge Planning and Follow-Up Evaluations

The success of discharge planning, especially after long-term institutionalization, depends on the availability of appropriate facilities in the community [7]. In the conclusion of the mental health service systems report, *Borus* et al. [13] emphasize the need for financial support for Neighborhood Health Centers, for the coordination of primary health care and mental health care, and for professional education. *Goldberg* et al. [30] found that patients with a psychiatric diagnosis used general health care facilities for almost twice as many visits per patient, than those without psychiatric diagnosis. We assume that discharged MR/ED patients would utilize to a great extent neighborhood services (where available). *Heiman and Shanfield* [35] found that patients under 20 and over 65 years stay longer in hospitals for each diagnosis, possibly due to problems of disposition, since both groups are often unable to live alone or to return to their previous homes. This would certainly apply to the difficulties encountered in discharging MR/ED patients, even after the alleviation of their psychiatric disorder. The single most important obstacle to deinstitutionalization is the great resistance of most communities to accepting mentally or emotionally handicapped persons. The readjustment of black high-risk adolescents in the community is discussed by *Wyatt* et al. [83]. The well known outcry 'Group homes – anywhere but here' [33] can be heard throughout the nation as a vivid documentation of existing discrimination. The problems of deinstitutionalization are dealt with by *Braun* et al. [14].

It is advisable to start working on the discharge plans from the moment of the admission. The willingness of the psychiatric staff to serve as consultants, on an informal basis, to the agencies and schools which accept former patients, is an effort which brings about the collaboration of agencies and more ready acceptance of discharged MR/ED patients in the community.

In the case of children who require long-term hospital treatment or institutional care, the casework with their families increases the patient's chances of smooth readaptation into the family.

The following case shows the complicated process of reintegration into the family of a MR/ED child following the completion of his inpatient treatment.

Case 6. Barry was an 8-year-old child who spent 5 months in the residential program of the John Merck Program. Diagnosis: mild mental retardation. Behavior disorders related to temporal lobe pathology. Unspecified psychosis with depressive features and severe aggression. Because of Barry's psychosis, past EMR (educable mentally retarded) classroom placement in the community had not met his needs and by the time of admission his behavior had totally disrupted the family system. Parents in this lower-middle class family are middle-aged, with an older son aged 20 and daughter aged 23 who also live in the home. There were multiple family problems and stresses including a symbiotic relationship between the neurotic mother and Barry, dysfunctional marital relationship and an inappropriate parental-child role assumed by the sister. The father was detached and the brother had withdrawn emotionally.

During Barry's adjustment in the program, the social worker met with the family weekly. After assessing their needs, caseworker aimed at the following goals: (1) help the parents (especially the symbiotic mother) deal with the loss of Barry's presence in the home, and to cope with the reality of Barry's retardation and emotional problems; (2) to realign mother and father in their appropriate roles as parents, while easing the sister out of her role as parental substitute; (3) to give support and build ego strength in this very anxious mother; (4) to help the family to understand, set and maintain appropriate and consistent limits with Barry; and ultimately (5) to smoothly reintegrate Barry into a more functional family system. The details in which this last goal was achieved are presented here.

As positive changes began to develop in terms of Barry's behavior on the unit, the family for the first time began to see hope for the future. It was important to keep the family's hopes realistic, within the boundaries of the child's potential; but it was equally important to build on that hope when it first appeared so that they could accumulate a reserve of positive experiences in their interaction with the child.

Barry's reintegration into the family required the following process: when the child had made sufficient progress in developing cooperative, socially acceptable behavior on the unit, trial home visits were carefully planned to assure that the methods used by the family in handling Barry's daily routines would elicit a positive response from Barry. Family cooperation was required in setting priorities in dealing with the problems they had at home with Barry. The family had to learn effective methods to deal with specific problems.

Initially, Barry's family agreed upon the three most controversial and disruptive issues: (1) Barry's obsessive opening of the refrigerator door; (2) bath routine; (3) bedtime routine. They agreed to target one problem at a time. Before each home visit, the family participated in planning sessions, where the social worker wrote out the program plan for them in a personal step-by-step format. While targeting one problem, they circumvented the others, to avoid possible negative experiences until the current target problem was successfully controlled.

For example, while dealing with Barry's refrigerator obsession, the home visits were limited to daytime visits, thus eliminating the family's having to bath or put Barry to bed. Predictably, Barry tested the new limits. However, the family was consistent in handling the target behavior and setting appropriate limits, using popsicles as primary reinforcers and praise as a secondary social reward for complying. By the end of the second home visit, the target behavior was successfully controlled. The social worker suggested the bedtime routine rather than the bath routine as target behavior for the first overnight visit and asked mother not to bath Barry at home. If negative behavior had occurred at bathtime it could have escalated and carried over to the bedtime routine, thereby destroying the possibility for a positive experience there. By this time Barry got used to sleeping in a single bedroom on the ward. By consistently following at home the program plan (which they themselves helped formulate), the family put an end to the nightly trauma of the past 8 years. In one night they were successful in getting Barry to sleep in his own bed in his own bedroom, rather than allowing him to replace father in the parent's bed.

During the next overnight home visit, the bath routine was targeted, the family was equally successful. Barry no longer manipulates his mother into arguing with him at bathtime, which in the past would bring father storming in from the livingroom.

Throughout the reintegration process, the family continued to meet with the social worker. She gave them adequate support, praise, guidance and interpretation. The mother was very cooperative in writing follow-up comments on the home visits which provided an added therapeutic tool and helped her become more thoughtful about her actions and her observations. In this case both Barry and the other family members were strengthened by these positive experiences. Family tension has diminished substantially and the entire family system, in turn, has become more functional.

By recording the changes and improvement in the patient's symptomatology and the changes and improvement in the family dynamics, it becomes evident that they are strongly interrelated. Like two sides of a coin – on the one hand the improvement of the patient helps lessen the family stress and pathology, and on the other hand the lessening of the family pathology (through social case work or therapy) has a profound impact on the level of improvement achieved by the patient. This relationship is especially noticeable in the level of maintaining the therapeutic gains after the discharge of the patient from the treatment program.

The findings recorded in table VII are the result of the assessment of the respective levels of improvement in the first 26 discharged patients from the John Merck Program and their families. The ratings made by 2 independent raters were based on the data in the patient's medical records. Table VII shows the relationship between the level of improvement achieved in the family and the improvement of the child, as measured at the time of discharge from the program and at the time of follow-up evaluations one year after discharge. Significant level of improvement in the family attitude and behavior was parallelled by significant improvement of their children. In cases where the family interaction (and pathology) did not improve during the child's hospitalization, the children themselves showed much less improvement and some of them have regressed after discharge as recorded during their follow-up evaluations.

Prevention

The physician's role in prevention includes, among others, genetic screening for Down's syndrome [1], and advising about the possibility of intrauterine surgery, a topic which lately raised ethical questions [6]. In the case of young MR/ED children, prevention of child abuse should be foremost on the physician's mind, since these children as a group are more vulnerable to mental, physical and sexual abuse [26, 64, 80, 81].

In adult cases, instruments like 'The Schedule of Recent Experience' [52] may be useful in evaluating the potential environmental stress for instituting preventive support. *Ripley and Dorpat* [68] in their historical review of life change and suicidal behavior quote the following life situation among the factors assessed: 'being thrust into independence, but lacking the

Table VII. Correlation of the levels of improvement in 26 patients and their families: all 26 were emotionally disturbed retarded children (ages 3–12) treated at the John Merck Program

	Number of subjects in each category							
	families (n = 26) discharge evaluation	patients (n = 26)			follow-up evaluation			
		discharge evaluation						
		significant improvement	moderate improvement	slight improvement	continued improvement	plateau	regression	not yet returned for follow-up
Significant improvement	7	7			7			
Moderate improvement	2	1[1]		1	1	1		
Slight improvement	9	1[2]	3	5	2[3]	2	2	3
Not improved	8	1	1	6	1	1	4	2
Total	26	10	4	12	11	4	6	5

[1] Child removed from family to institutional care.
[2] Child removed from family to institutional care.
[3] One of these is the same child mentioned in footnote 2.

skills to cope with new responsibility'. This is a frequently encountered situation in deinstitutionalized retarded persons. Concomitant variations between stressing events and the evolution of pathology in a group of youngsters has been demonstrated by *Amiel-Lebirge and Pichot* [4]. On the other hand, *Caplan's* [15] findings have demonstrated that adequate support may prevent mental and physical illness in persons exposed to high stress. *Masuda and Holmes* [52] show the clinical significance of life events. These findings point to the need for early detection and possible prevention of depression in retarded children, since childhood depression is in most cases reactive to life's stresses [32, 60]. Childhood depression is usually manifested in atypical symptoms [10], and recognition of its early stages is difficult. Rating scales for depression in children are still in experimental stages [47]. Preventive support during the retarded children's stressful life situations should be provided before depression occurs.

Recognizing the specific constellations predisposing to the breakdown of already deficient adaptive mechanisms of retarded persons is the first step in prevention.

The child who cannot keep up with the academic demands of the school may become depressed and give up all efforts. In other cases he may realize that he can fight better than the other kids in his class and, therefore, he will 'excel' in bullying them or in destroying school property.

The teenager and adult retarded person may resort to pathological reaction formation under the stress of discrimination when they realize that their nonretarded peers exclude them from their 'in-groups', or use them for menial tasks. The need to be accepted may motivate a retarded youngster to join a youth gang. Of course, it is usually the retarded youngster who is apprehended first, frequently without actually understanding the context of the illegal action in which he is involved.

Prevention should aim at providing appropriate experience in social interaction, through supervised recreation and sports. This should be extended into community facilities as much as possible mixing retarded and nonretarded persons.

Conclusions

The goal of treatment is to alleviate the patient's personal suffering and the difficulties in adapting to the social environment. There is a considerable need to compromise in setting goals. Individual goals are limited goals.

It is advisable to set intermediary goals repeatedly during the treatment, and to institute control points at set intervals for the re-evaluation and reassessment of progress. It is at those points that action can be taken to change treatment methods.

The multimodality treatment delivered by several specialists and support personnel must be orchestrated by designating unambiguously one person, usually the psychiatrist, to be responsible for coordination and overview. While several specialists deal with their 'part' – the target symptoms – the psychiatrist is concerned with the total treatment of the patient.

Therapeutic alliance must be established with the patient, the family and other caregivers. A prerequisite for securing their cooperation is to provide the family with detailed information derived from the diagnostic assessments. They should be informed of the prognosis, the outlined goals, and the treatment plans as these emerge during the initial evaluation and during the scheduled reassessment checkpoints. Flexibility is required in the use of the traditional psychiatric methods. Prevention of secondary emotional problems, associated with the adjustment to the fact of being mentally retarded in a 'nonretarded' society, can be achieved by early counseling of the family and/or other caregivers.

References

1   Adams, M.M.; Erickson, J.D.; Layde, P.M.; Oakley, G.P.: Down's syndrome. Recent trends in the United States. J. Am. med. Ass. *246:* 758–760 (1981).

2   Albini, J.L.; Dinitz, S.: Psychotherapy with disturbed and defective children. An evaluation of changes in behavior and attitudes. Am. J. ment. Defic. *69:* 560–567 (1965).

3   American Psychiatric Association: Diagnostic and statistical manual of mental disorders; 3rd ed. (American Psychiatric Association, Washington 1980).

4   Amiel-Lebirge, F.; Pichot, P.: Variation concomitante entre evénements stressants de la vie et évolution de la morbidité psychique dans une groupe de jeunes. Annls méd.-psychol. *139:* 1–10 (1981).

5   Balthazar, E.E.; Stevens, H.A.: The emotionally disturbed mentally retarded. A historical and contemporary perspective (Prentice-Hall, Englewood Cliffs 1975).

6   Barclay, W.R.; McCormick, R.A.; Sidbury, J.B.; Michejda, M.; Hodgen, G.D.: The ethics of in utero surgery. J. Am. med. Ass. *246:* 1550–1555 (1981).

7   Baruk, H.: Psychanalyse ou blocage pharmacologique dans la culture des handicapés mentaux. Annls méd.-psychol. *139:* 335–351 (1981).

8   Beier, D.C.: Behavioral disturbances in the mentally retarded; in Stevens, Heber, Mental retardation, pp. 453–487 (University of Chicago Press, Chicago 1964).

9   Bellak, L.: Psychiatric aspects of minimal brain dysfunction, pp. 208 (Grune & Stratton, New York 1979).

10 Belmont, H.S.: Confusing varieties of depression in childhood. Pennsylvania med. *84:* 41–43 (1981).

11 Bernstein, N.R.: Diminished people (Little, Brown, Boston 1970).

12 Bernstein, N.R.: Mental retardation; in Nicholi, The Harvard Guide to Modern Psychiatry, pp. 551–567 (Belknap Press of Harvard University Press, Cambridge, 1978).

13 Borus, J.F.; Burns, B.J.; Jacobson, A.M.; Macht, L.B.; Morrill, R.G.; Wilson, E.M.: Coordinated mental health care in neighborhood health centers, Series DN, No. 3, National Institute of Mental Health, DHHS Publication No. (ADM) 80-996 (Superintendent of Documents, US Government Printing Office, Washington 1980).

14 Braun, P.; Kochansky, G.; Shapiro, R.; Greenberg, S.; Gudeman, J.E.; Johnson, S.; Shore, M.F.: Overview. Deinstitutionalization of psychiatric patients. A critical review of outcome studies. Am. J. Psychiat. *138:* 736–749 (1981).

15 Caplan, G.: Mastery of stress. Psychological aspects. Am. J. Psychiat. *138:* 413–420 (1981).

16 Conners, C.K.: Clinical use of stimulant drugs in children (American Elsevier, New York 1974).

17 Czeizel, A.; Lanyi-Engemayer, A.; Klujber, L.; Metneki, J.; Tusnady, G.: Etiological study of mental retardation in Budapest, Hungary. Am. J. ment. Defic. *85:* 120–128 (1980).

18 Editorial Notes: 'Most in need' program: a talk with its director. Alcohol Drug Abuse Mental Health Agency News, vol. IV, No. 18, 1–2 (October 6, 1978).

19 Editorial Notes: NIMH launches most in need program. Am. Family natn. Action-Overview, vol. I, No. 4, 2 (June–July, 1978).

20 Editorial Notes: A new NIMH program on children seeks to orchestrate the professions. Behav. Today, 2–3 (August 7, 1978).

21 Eisenberg, L.: Psychiatric implications of brain damage in children. Psychiat. Q. *31:* 72–92 (1957).

22 Ekstein, R.: Some thoughts concerning the clinical use of children's dreams. Bull. Menninger Clin. *45:* 115–124 (1981).

23 Federal Register: *42:* 163: 42481, 121a 121 (August 23, 1977).

24 Federal Register: *42:* 163: 42982, 121a 128 (August 23, 1977).

25 Frazier, A.; Lisonbee, L.K.: Adolescent concerns with physique. School Rev. *58:* 397–405 (1950).

26 Frodi, A.M.: Contribution of infant characteristics to child abuse. Am. J. ment. Defic. *85:* 341–349 (1981).

27 Gadow, K.D.; Kalachnik, J.: Prevalance and pattern of drug treatment for behavior and seizure disorders of TMR students. Am. J. ment. Defic. *85:* 588–595 (1981).

28 Gibson, R.W.: The creative arts therapies. An overview. Natn. Ass. Private Psychiat. J. *11:* 4–6 (1979).

29 Glassman, A.H.: Blood-level measurements of tricyclic drugs as a diagnostic tool. Psych. Annls *11:* 14–23 (1981).

30a Goldberg, I.D.; Regier, D.A.; Burns, B.J.: Use of health and mental health outpatient services in four organized health care settings. National Institute of Mental Health, Series DN No. 1, DHHS Publication No. (ADM) 80-859 (Superintendent of Documents, US Government Printing Office, Washington 1980).

30b Goldenberg, I.; Levine, M.: The development and evolution of the Yale psycho-
     educational clinic. Int. Rev. appl. Psychol. *18:* 101–110 (1969).
31   Goodenough, F.L.; Harris, D.R.: in Goodenough-Harris Drawing Test: Ages 3–15,
     Revision and Extension of the Goodenough intelligence Test (Brace Jovanich, Inc.,
     1926–1963).
32   Graham, P.J.: Depressive disorders in children. A re-consideration. Acta paedopsy-
     chiat. *46:* 285–296 (1980–1981).
33   Group Homes: Anywhere but here. Institutions etc. *3/4:* 1–3 (April, 1980).
34   Gunzburg, H.C.: Psychotherapy with the feeble-minded; in Clarke, Clarke, Mental
     deficiency. The changing outlook, pp. 365–392 (Methuen, London 1965).
35   Heiman, E.M.; Shanfield, S.B.: Reflections on length of stay. Psychol. Annals *11:*
     64–67 (1981).
36   Hersh, S.P.; Platt, L.J.: Personal communication. The 'most in need'. NIMH Pro-
     gram Update (December, 1981).
37   Jakab, I.: Le rôle diagnostique du contenu et du style des dessins d'enfants. Annls
     méd.-psychol. *116:* 1–16 (1958).
38   Jakab, I.: Graphic expression of the emotional troubles of retarded children. Confinia
     psychiat. *10:* 16–27 (1967).
39   Jakab, I.; Howard, M.: Art therapy with a 12 year old girl who witnessed suicide.
     Psychother. Psychosomat. *17:* 309–324 (1969).
40   Jakab, I.: Psychotherapy of the mentally retarded child; in Bernstein, Diminished
     people, chap. 11, pp. 223–263 (Little, Brown, Boston 1970).
41   Jakab, I.: The psychiatric treatment of severely brain-injured children in Noshpitz, et al.,
     Basic handbook of child psychiatry, vol. 4, pp. 663–673 (Basic Books, New York 1979).
42   Kannas, G.; Gerber, M.: Body-awareness and learning of self-expression through
     rhythm and movement; in Jakab, Art interpretation and art therapy, psychiatry and
     art, vol. 2, pp. 124–130 (Karger, Basel 1968).
43   Klerman, G.L.: Reimbursement and psychotherapy. What if they want proof? Roche
     report. Front. Psychiat. *11:* 12–13 (1981).
44   Klapman, H.; Baker, F.B.: The task force treatment. Intensified use of the milieu for
     the severely disturbed child. Am. J. occup. Ther. *17:* 239–243 (1963).
45   Klicpera, C.; Heyse, I.L.: Der Einfluss einer leichten zerebralen Dysfunktion auf die
     Ausprägung und die langfristige Entwicklung von Verhaltensstörungen bei Kindern.
     Acta paedopsychiat. *47:* 9–18 (1981).
46   Knight, D.: The role of varied therapies in the rehabilitation of the retarded child.
     Occupational therapy. Am. J. ment. Defic. *61:* 508–515 (1957).
47   Kovacs, M.: Rating scales to assess depression in school-aged children. Acta paedo-
     psychiat. *46:* 305–315 (1980–1981).
48   Luborsky, L.: Research problems in psychotherapy. A three-year follow-up; in
     Strupp, Luborsky, Research in psychotherapy. Proc. Conf., Chapel Hill 1961,
     pp. 308–329 (French Bay, Baltimore 1962).
49   Marks, I.M.: Review of behavioral psychotherapy. II. Sexual disorders. Am. J. Psy-
     chiat. *138:* 750–756 (1981).
50   Martin, E.W.: Techniques of medication (Lippincott, Philadelphia 1969).
51   Martin, E.W.: Hazards of medications (Lippincott, Philadelphia 1971).
52   Masuda, M.L.; Holmes, T.H.: Variations in life events in different groups. Clinical
     significance. Psychiat. Annls *11:* 48–65 (1981).

53   McDonald, M.C.: NIMH project aims at national child policy. Psychiat. News *XIII:* 30–31 (1978).

54   Menolascino, F.J.: Emotional disturbances in mentally retarded children. Am. J. Psychiat. *125:* 168–179 (1969).

55   Murstein, B.I.: Handbook of projective techniques (Basic Books, New York 1965).

56   Nicholi, A.N., Jr.: The adolescent; in Nicholi, The Harvard guide to modern psychiatry, pp. 519–541 (Belknap Press of Harvard University Press, Cambridge 1978).

57   Niedermeyer, E.: Modern problems of pharmacopsychiatric – epilepsy, vol. 4, (Karger, Basel 1970).

58   O'Gorman, G.: Psychosis as a cause of mental defect. J. ment. Sci. *100:* 934–943 (1954).

59   Orvaschel, H.; Sholomskas, D.; Weissman, M.M.: The assessment of psychopathology and behavioral problems in children. A review of scales suitable for epidemiological and clinical research (1967–1979), National Institute of Mental Health, Series AN No. 1, DHHS Publication No. (ADM) 80-1037 (Superintendent of Documents, US Government Printing Office, Washington 1980).

60   Pearce, J.B.: Drug treatment of depression in children. Acta paedopsychiat. *46:* 317–328 (1980–1981).

61   Pearson, P.H.: The physician's role in diagnosis and management of the mentally retarded. Pediat. clins N. Am. *15:* 835–859 (1968).

62   Petti, T.A.; Law, W.: Abrupt cessation of high-dose imipramine treatment in children. J. Am. med. Ass. *246:* 768–769 (1981).

63   Phillips, I.; Williams, N.: Psychopathology and mental retardation. A study of 100 mentally retarded children. I. Psychopathology. Am. J. Psychol. *132:* 1265–1271 (1975).

64   Price, J.M.; Valdiserri, E.V.: Childhood sexual abuse. A recent review of the literature. JAMWA *36:* 232–234 (1981).

65   Proc. 1980 HEW Conf. Needs of Emotionally Disturbed/Developmentally Disturbed Individuals (HEW, Bethesda 1980).

66   Project Challenge: Residential services plan update of resources and needs, p. 33 (State of Connecticut Department of Mental Retardation, 1979).

67   Provence, S.; Marsh, E.J.: Definition of children with emotional, psychotic, and personality problems who are retarded. Appendix 1; in Joint Committee on Retarded Children, section of 'Miles to go' report of the Mental Retardation Planning Project, March, 1966. A Connecticut State Department of Health Publication (1966).

68   Ripley, H.S.; Dorpat, T.L.: Life change and suicidal behavior. Psychiat. Annls *11:* 32–47 (1981).

69   Russell, A.T.; Tanguay, P.E.: Mental illness and mental retardation. Cause or coincidence? Am. J. ment. Defic. *85:* 570–574 (1981).

70   Rutter, M.: Psychiatry, in Wortis, Mental retardation. An annual review, vol. 3, pp. 186–221 (Grune & Stratton, New York 1970).

71   Schaar, K.: National Institute of Mental Health Floats New Child Initiative. Am. psychol. Ass. Monitor *9:* 1, 13 (1978).

72   Schenk, L.; Bear, D.: Multiple personality and related dissociative phenomena in patients with temporal lobe epilepsy. Am. J. Psychiat. *138:* 1311–1316 (1981).

73   Skinner, B.F.: Selection by consequences. Science *213:* 501–504 (1981).

74 Sternlicht, M.: Psychotherapeutic techniques useful with the mentally retarded. A review and critique. Psychiat. Q. *39:* 84 (1965).
75 Stock, D.: An investigation into the interrelations between the self-concept and feeling directed toward other persons and groups. J. consult. Psychol. *13:* 176–180 (1949).
76 Szymanski. L.S.: Individual psychotherapy with retarded persons; in Szymanski, Tanguay, Emotional disorders of mentally retarded persons, chapt. 10, pp- 131–147 (University Park Press, Baltimore 1980).
77 Tarjan, G.: Sex: A tri-polar conflict in mental retardation; in Zyman, Meyers, Tarjan, Sociobehavioral studies in mental retardation. Monogr. AAMD, No. 1, pp. 175–183 (1973).
78 Tawney, J.W.; Knapp, D.S.; O'Reilly, C.D.; Pratt, S.S.: Programmed environments curriculum. A curriculum handbook for teaching basic skills to severely handicapped persons. Bureau of Education for the Handicapped, p. 558 Charles E. Merrill, 1300 Alum Creek Dr., Columbus, OH 43216 (1979).
79 Thompson, A.: How able children fall below normal scores on drawing tests; in Jakab, Psychiatry and art, pp. 194–199 (Karger, Basel 1966).
80 Vesterdal, J.: Psychological mechanisms in child-abusing parents. Paediatrician *8:* 145–151 (1979).
81 Weeks, R.: The sexually exploited child. South. med. J. *69:* 848–852 (1976).
82 Wilkin, D.: Caring for the mentally handicapped child (Croom, Helm, London 1979).
83 Wyatt, G.E.; Reardon, E.F.; Bass, B.A.: The readjustment of black, high risk adolescents to the community. J. Community Psychol. *5:* 72–78 (1977).

13 The Psychopharmacology of Emotionally Disturbed and Mentally Retarded Children and Adolescents

Paul A. Andrulonis

'Anyone who hopes to learn the noble game of chess from books will soon discover that only the opening and closing moves admit of an exhaustive systematic presentation and that the infinite variety of moves which develop after the opening defy any such description. This gap in instruction can only be filled by a diligent study of games fought out by masters ... In what follows, I shall endeavor to collect together for the use of therapists some of the rules for the beginning of the treatment. Among them there are some which may seem to be petty details, as, indeed they are. Their justifications is that they are simply rules of the game which acquire their importance from their relation to the general plan of the game.'

Sigmund Freud

As an early researcher in pharmacology, *Freud* knew that any rules which can be laid down for the treatment of psychiatric patients had definite limitations. After periodic reviews of the literature and years of doing research in psychopharmacology, I am deeply aware that the work of clinicians and researchers has produced much data but few conclusions for the physician treating emotionally disturbed and mentally retarded children with behavior-modifying medications. It is most important that the individual physician treating the individual child be aware of the possibilities for help and the potential for harm of utilizing psychotropic medications. There are indeed no 'magical bullets' in the form of medications which will 'cure' any child. We must be honestly humble and accept that '... the intellectual's role will be to say that the king is naked when he is, and not to go into raptures over his imaginary trappings'. This warning by *Albert Camus* will focus our attention on the conclusion that psychotropic medications have a relatively small place in the general treatment program of an emotionally disturbed and mentally retarded child.

The purpose of this paper is to help the clinician use medications in a limited, but safe and clinically responsible manner. Since in child psychiatry, with the possible exception of the hyperactive and attention-deficit nonretarded child, medications do not provide dramatic help in specific psychiatric syndromes, the emphasis will be on symptom relief followed by diagnostic considerations. Unlike in adult psychiatry, the psychotic child is not always treated with phenothiazines nor the depressed child with antidepressants. Psychotropic medication in children usually decreases symptoms such as hyperactivity, aggression, self-mutilation, excitability, attentional deficit, enuresis, and at times, delusions and hallucinations. Hopefully then, the medication will allow the child more self-control in order that more important modalities such as better parenting, special education, psychotherapy, behavior modification, language therapy, day treatment, and residential care are more effective.

Case Examples

Case 1. George, a 3½–year-old developmentally delayed child, presented with symptoms of hyperactivity and aggression towards others making him unmanageable in a regular preschool program. After enrollment in the Children's School of the Institute of Living, a special therapeutic education program, George was started on low dosages of methylphenidate. He became at times mildly agitated and tearful and at other times lethargic and sleepy. A short trial of diphenhydramine was effective in calming him without causing significant side effects. That medication was then discontinued after his behavior improved in the highly structured special education classroom.

Case 2. Mary, a 5-year-old mentally retarded autistic child, developed serious self-abusive behavior. Thioridazine has been effective in decreasing the self-abusing behavior and making Mary more manageable in the classroom. At the same time, however, Mary seemed less available to learn and so the medication has been maintained at a lower dose level which has allowed Mary to progress developmentally while being in better control.

Case 3. Tom, an 8-year-old mildly retarded child, presented with symptoms of an attention disorder, severe hyperactivity, and impulsivity. Methylphenidate at the level of 0.8 mg per kg has provided a dramatic relief of such symptoms allowing steady developmental progression. When taken off his medication, Tom rapidly regresses over 24–72 h requiring a reinstitution of the methylphenidate.

Case 4. Michael, a 10-year-old moderately retarded child, presents with symptoms of Gilles de la Tourette's syndrome. A trial of low dose haloperidol decreased his capacity to learn but ameliorated the symptoms of Tourette's syndrome. A switch to clonidine provided continued symptomatic relief without decreasing the child's capacity to learn.

Case 5. John, a mildly retarded schizophrenic child, demonstrated severe pan anxiety, hallucinations, delusions, hyperactivity, impulsivity, aggression and a thinking disorder. 1 mg of haloperidol t.i.d. has alleviated the anxiety, hyperactivity, aggression, impulsivity, and thinking disorder. He remains delusional with infrequent auditory hallucinations but has been able to function more comfortably and at a higher developmental level. John, currently 12 years old, became psychotic at the age of 11.

Case 6. Tim, a 15-year-old moderately retarded autistic adolescent, has been successfully treated with medications over the years. At the age of 8, symptoms of hyperactivity and impulsivity responded to dextroamphetamine. Between the ages of 13 and 15 years, his psychotic symptoms have responded to trifluoperazine.

Case 7. Gloria, a 16-year-old moderately retarded, deaf, rubella-autistic adolescent, developed symptoms of severe aggression, self-mutilating behavior, excitability, and impulsivity beginning with menarche. Perphenazine, 4 mg t.i.d., has been of substantial benefit in decreasing this symptomatology and allowing behavior modification techniques to be effective.

Case 8. Paul, an 18-year-old mildly retarded schizophrenic, had been placed on moderate dosages of fluphenazine and later haloperidol continuously over a 6-year period. After referral to the Institute of Living, Paul was slowly tapered off of his phenothiazine medication because of an absence of true psychotic symptoms. Paul demonstrated symptoms of a withdrawal dyskinesia and continues to show a tardive dyskinesia picture with mild facial tics, restlessness, and finger and toe movements.

Basic Principles

Many of the basic principles in medicating a mentally retarded, emotionally disturbed child are illustrated by the case examples. The first and most important of these is for the physician to do no harm to the child and if in doubt, *not to medicate,* without an expert consultation. As will be described under the various classes of psychotropic medications, the physician must have an up-to-date knowledge of all medication side effects. Cardiac, liver, blood, cognitive, emotional, and neurological side effects are common particularly if high dosages of medication are utilized.

A second principle is that medications are prescribed according to the symptoms a child presents, with careful consideration of but not emphasis on psychiatric diagnosis. As illustrated in case No. 6, a child may require one class of medication at an early stage of development and a totally different class of medication at a later stage. This third principle of recognizing the importance of a child's chronological age in medication choice is often unappreciated by clinicians. Case No. 1 illustrates that preschoolers are most difficult to medicate and that usually an initial trial of diphenhydramine is indicated before utilizing stimulants or penothiazines.

Principle number four is regarding the actual administration of the medication. Generally medications in children should be administered in small dosages with a gradual buildup until symptom relief occurs. Because of the child's and adolescent's high metabolic rate, all medications should be given in divided dosages. Medications should be administered for relatively short periods of time (1–3 months) after symptom relief. The child or adolescent should then be slowly tapered off of the medication in order to see if the medication is still necessary and to look for signs of hidden side effects, such as, dyskinesias. Principle number five is that a child should not be given a medication unless the presenting symptomatology has lasted for a significant period of time and has interfered with the child's adaptation and functioning. This allows clinical justification for the risk of medications and enables one to meaningfully explain to the child, adolescent, and parents the need for medications. Since the emphasis is on symptomatology, functioning, low dosages, and short medication trials, medication holidays or summers off a medication usually are not pertinent.

Principle number six is that whenever possible a medication should be prescribed in a dosage according to milligrams per kilogram of body weight. This will remind the physician not only of the above-mentioned principles but also of the need to adjust the dosage as the child gets bigger.

Principle number seven is that a positive or a negative clinical response to a certain medication does not allow one to make a clinical diagnosis of a child or adolescent. For example, a small but significant percentage of autistic children do respond to stimulants. Also a small but significant number of mentally retarded hyperactive children with attentional deficits respond to phenothiazines but not to stimulants. The clinician must continually be aware that many mentally retarded, emotionally disturbed children have symptomatology reflecting their being multiply handicapped. The child might in addition to being mentally retarded, show signs of autism, schizophrenia, hyperactivity, aggressive conduct disorder, and episodic dyscontrol. This principle further implies that if a child fails to respond to a certain medication, another medication should be tried before the child is considered 'medication-resistent'. For example, some children respond to methylphenidate but not to dextroamphetamine, while others selectively respond only to pemoline. Also many children respond selectively to one phenothiazine but not to another. This does not mean, however, that children also deserve, necessarily, a trial on medication combinations. Only a very small percentage of children require this. It is especially important to note that there is seldom, if ever, justification for a child to be on three psychoactive medications. Such combinations are dangerous, enhance routine side effects, and can produce special harmful side effects.

Finally, principle number eight is that children require an initial and then periodic physical examinations and blood studies pertinent for the particular medication that the child is receiving. This is particularly important in the case of phenothiazines, anticonvulsants, and the rarely used antidepressants or lithium carbonate.

Stimulant Medications

Of all psychoactive agents used in child psychiatry, the best documented are the effects of psychomotor stimulants beginning with the classic study by *Bradley* in 1937 [1]. The efficacy of stimulant medications for nonretarded children aged 6–12 years with nonpsychotic hyperkinetic or hyperkinetic-aggressive behavior is established [2–10]. Such research found that stimulants decrease symptoms of hyperactivity, short attention span, impulsivity, and low frustration tolerance. It is doubtful, however, that stimulants should be utilized if a child has only a learning disability. Of course, mental retardation per se does not merit stimulant or other types of medications unless certain definitive symptomatology such as hyperactivity coexists with the cognitive handicap. *Lipman* et al. [11] report that some 33 publications in the literature are not encouraging regarding the efficacy of stimulants for mentally retarded children. These same authors, while maintaining that stimulant medications have had little impact on the pharmacotherapy of mentally retarded children, nevertheless, state that adequately designed studies to test the behavioral and cognitive effects of the stimulants in this group are urgently needed. Since as previously mentioned, researchers have found that stimulant medications are not helpful in non-hyperactive children with pure learning disorders [12, 13], it makes no clinical sense to use these or any other type of medications on mentally retarded children without the described target symptoms which may respond to medications.

Methylphenidate, dextroamphetamine, and pemoline are all equally effective for hyperactive children, although a small number may respond to one medication and not to one of the others. Dextroamphetamine is often considered the drug of first choice for hyperactive children because of its relatively inexpensive cost. Another disadvantage of methylphenidate is that it should not be administered with meals but rather at least ½ h before eating. While dextroamphetamine and methylphenidate have half-lives of 6 or 4 h, pemoline can be given in a single morning dose. While methylphenidate and Dexedrine require approximately a 2-week trial, pemoline does not reach its maximum effectiveness until 6 weeks. The dose range for dextroamphetamine is approximately 2.5–30 mg/day, for methylphenidate 5–60 mg/day, and for pemoline 18.75–112.5 mg/day. Methylphenidate seems most effective at approximately 0.3 mg/kg to enhance attention and at 0.8 mg/kg to reduce hyperactivity.

The most frequent side effects of stimulant medications are anorexia, irritability, and insomnia. Other side effects include sadness, nausea, headache, abdominal cramps, thirst, and tremor. Methylphenidate may cause a mild elevation of resting pulse and diastolic blood pressure. Although, initially, methylphenidate and dextroamphetamine were reported to decrease height and weight of hyperactive children [14, 15], more recently *Oettinger* [verbal report] has found that the long-term use of methylphenidate in nonretarded MBD children did not effect ultimate height nor the expected growth rate. This researcher concludes that children with MBD are physiologically immature as shown by bone age determinations and continue to grow for a longer period of time than other children. Similar studies need to be done on retarded children. Rare side effects of stimulants include delirium, facial tics, Tourette's syndrome, dyskinesia, and hallucinosis. Nonretarded hyperactive adolescents also respond positively to stimulant medications [16] and usually report no euphoria and little tolerance. Stimulants therefore appear to have a role in treating mentally retarded adolescents with hyperactivity and attentional problems.

The clinician must be aware that mentally retarded autistic, schizophrenic, or borderline psychotic children may become more disturbed on stimulant medications regardless of their age.

Major Tranquilizers

Phenothiazines, particularly thioridazine and chlorpromazine, are the most frequently prescribed medications for the mentally retarded. Various surveys of institutions consistently find that over 50% of mentally retarded residents are on such medications. Tragically, many of these mentally retarded children do not require such medication and are on maximal dosages for extended periods of time. Many institutionalized retardates are also inappropriately on two or more major tranquilizers.

In contrast, sound medical practice dictates that such major tranquilizers be reserved for mentally retarded children and adolescents with severe, otherwise unmanageable, behavior disorders characterized by extreme agitation, hyperactivity, impulsivity, aggression, or psychosis. Even when useful for such serious behavioral dificulties, the major tranquilizers often decrease cognitive-learning performance. While classroom behavior might improve, actual educational achievement often suffers when a retarded child is on such a medication.

Major tranquilizers which have been used with some but limited success in mentally retarded schizophrenic, autistic, hyperactive, aggressive, or acutely psychotic mental retardates include chlorpromazine, thioridazine, promazine, perphenazine, trifluoperazine, and haloperidol. Haloperidol and clonidine [17] have a role in low dosages regarding the treatment of Gilles de la Tourette's syndrome.

The physician should start at the lowest recommended dosage of a major tranquilizer with gradual increases over 1–3 weeks until a clinical response. A minimum of 3 weeks are needed to establish efficacy and dosage before switching to another medication. As stated under 'Basic Principles', children should be tapered off of such medication every 3–6 months to assess whether or not the medication is still needed and to avoid side effects.

Common side effects of major tranquilizers in children include drowsiness, weight gain, increased appetite, dry mouth, photosensitivity (especially chlorpromazine), enuresis (especially thioridazine), and neurological symptoms of drooling, rigidity, tremor, akathisia, dystonia, and akinesia. Thioridazine with its extreme anticholinergic properties is beginning to decline as a most popular medication. It remains, however, together with chlorpromazine as the most firmly established efficacious phenothiazine for mentally retarded children. Chlorpromazine, in particular, decreases the seizure threshold in epileptic mentally retarded children. Although abnormalities in laboratory studies are rare in children on phenothiazines, weekly alkaline phosphatase, SGPT, SGOT, and CBC, and urinalysis should be done for one month, monthly for three additional periods, and then at least yearly.

Tardive and withdrawal dyskinesias occur in children and adolescents treated with major tranquilizers [18–20]. In retarded or nonretarded children and adolescents the dyskinesia manifests itself by buccolingual-masticatory movements, facial tics and grimaces, choreoathetoid, ballistic, and myoclonic movements of the extremities and trunk, torticollis, abnormal posturing, generalized motor restlessness, and ataxia. Such tardive dyskinesia can be seen with low dose, short-term treatment, as well as in high dose, longer-term therapy. A more benign withdrawal dyskinesia might be avoided by gradually rather than abruptly reducing medication dosages. Such dyskinesias usually remit within 8 or 12 weeks. Once the dyskinesia persists for 6 months or longer they should be labeled tardive dyskinesia. Acute dyskinesias have been reported in patients on methylphenidate, dextroamphetamine, antihistamines, ethosuximide, carbamazepine, and phenytoin.

An anticholinergic psychosis [21] can result from utilizing high dosages of major tranquilizers or combining phenothiazines, antiparkinsonian drugs, and tricyclic antidepressants. The signs of this syndrome include dilated and poorly reactive pupils, confusion, disorientation, flushed face, visual hallucinations, tachycardia, restlessness, hyperactivity, agitation, ataxia, and decreased motor coordination. Generally, physostigmine is the treatment for an anticholinergic psychosis. A potentially lethal consequence of treatment with high-potency neuroleptics such as haloperidol, thiothixene, or piperazine phenothiazines in therapeutic dosages is the neuroleptic malignant syndrome. This syndrome is characterized by muscular rigidity, hyperthermia, altered consciousness, and autonomic dysfunction [22]. Depot fluphenazine injections are a common causative agent. Treatment consists of early recognition, immediate discontinuation of psychotropic medications, and the prompt institution of intensive, supportive medical and nursing care.

Therefore, because of the potential serious side effects of major tranquilizers, such medication should be reserved for either psychotic or severely aggressive and hyperactive mentally retarded children and adolescents who are a potential danger to themselves or others or who are severely impaired in their functioning.

Antidepressants and Lithium Carbonate

The concept of depression as a major syndrome in children and adolescents is a relatively new one. The subject of depression in the mentally retarded is not only seldom written about but also infrequently appreciated. Even DSM-III does not recognize a specific depressive syndrome in children. Clinicians and writers continue to talk about nonspecific 'depressive equivalents' in children and adolescents. There have not been any well-controlled and -designed studies on significant numbers of children treated specifically for depression by antidepressants in this country. In fact, tricyclic antidepressants and MAO inhibitors are not approved as treatment for depression in children. Only imipramine has approval by both the Physicians' Desk Reference (PDR) and the Federal Drug Administration (FDA) for its use in enuresis for children of 6 years or older. Imipramine has also been reported as useful for children with school phobia, hyperkinesis, impulsivity, or aggression [23–26]. Amitriptyline has also been reported as sometimes effective in hyperkinetic, depressed, or aggressive children [27–29]. Imipramine has not been found effective for retarded autistic or schizophrenic children [30] while nortriptyline may have a very limited role for retarded autistic children [31]. Tricyclic antidepressants may be useful for seriously depressed nonretarded adolescents, but there is no clinical or research evidence that they are possibly effective for depressed retardates. There is no role at this time for the use of the monoamine oxidase inhibitors in the treatment of emotionally disturbed retardates.

The dosage utilized for imipramine is in the range of 1–2.5 mg/kg/day. Imipramine is definitively effective in treating enuresis in this dosage range. The FDA has not approved the clinical use of imipramine at a dosage higher than 2.5 mg/kg/day. Investigational protocols for imipramine cannot exceed 5 mg/kg/day with recommended EKG monitoring when these dose limits are approached. The half-life of imipramine is 15 h in children, while amitriptyline and nortriptyline half-lives are 24 h in children.

The most frequent side effects with tricyclic antidepressants are: anorexia, drowsiness, insomnia, dry mouth, constipation, and irritability. There is no question regarding the cardiotoxic potential of the tricyclics [32]. Several overdose deaths have occurred in children on imipramine [33, 34]. Most of the severe toxic effects and deaths occurred at doses above 10 mg/kg/day of imipramine in children. There is a report [34] of a sudden death in a child on a single daily dose of 14.7 mg/kg of imipramine, and a lethal dose in an adult reported at 8 mg/kg/day [35]. Imipramine and amitriptyline also have epileptogenic properties in susceptible individuals and adolescents.

Although not studied in retarded children, imipramine seems to lose its effectiveness in the treatment of hyperkinesis with the child's behavior often deteriorating after 2 or 3 months of treatment [5, 36].

Lithium carbonate is not established as effective for any specific symptoms or syndromes in mentally retarded children and adolescents. Lithium has been used with equivocal results in nonretarded children with 'manic-depressive-like' conditions [36]. Lithium may be effective in some retarded psychotic children and adolescents through its reduction of hyperactivity, psychotic speech, stereotype behavior, and aggression [37, 38]. The assessment of the efficacy of lithium in retarded children and adolescents depends on further exploration. It may prove of value in certain behavioral profiles of treatment-resistant severe disturbances characterized by hyperactivity, aggressiveness, explosiveness, and mood swings.

Side effects of lithium in children and adolescents include irritability, lethargy, motor retardation or excitement, ataxia, and drooling. Lithium can also cause diabetes insipidus manifested by polydipsia and polyuria, seizures, hypothyroidism, and renal dysfunction. Although the serum lithium level may need to be approximately 1.0 mEq/l during treatment of an acute disturbance, a maintenance lithium level of 0.4–0.6 mEq/l causes fewer side effects while maintaining efficacy. Dosage should be reduced if moderate tremors, nausea, vomiting, diarrhea, and muscle stiffness exists. Severe toxic signs requiring discontinuation include muscle weakness, hypertonia, rigidity, confusion, or seizures. Serum creatinine, urinalysis, blood electrolytes, T_3 and a CBC need to be done prior to lithium treatment with the T_3, serum creatinine, urinalysis, and serum lithium levels being done periodically afterwards.

Sedatives, Antianxiety Agents, and Anticonvulsants

Diphenhydramine is an antihistamine in the class of ethanolamines and exerts a depressant effect on the central nervous system. This medication might be tried prior to stimulants for mentally retarded hyperactive preschool children. It also may have a role in older hyperactive aggressive, or even schizophrenic retarded children in dosages of 2–25 mg/kg/day and up to 600 mg daily in divided dosages. An average dose is usually 100 mg daily or 6 mg/kg/day. Many retarded children, however, suffer from excessive sedation on this medication and usually older children and adolescents soon develop tolerance to it. Other side effects include headache, restlessness, dryness of the mouth, and constipation. Very rarely facial tics or dyskinesia are reported. Diphenhydramine elixir is not recommended for children with behavior disorders because such children often become irritable and hyperactive to its 14% alcohol content.

Chloral hydrate, flurazepam, and the new compound temazepam in low dosages are useful hypnotics if used for short periods of time. Chloridazepoxide and diazepam have a very limited role in treating mentally retarded children but might be considered in low dosages to treat situational anxiety. Often, however, mentally retarded children, epileptics, borderline psychotic, or schizophrenic children develop a 'paradoxical reaction' to such agents with a loss of control, a worsening or precipitation of a psychosis, and an increase in hyperactivity and aggressiveness [39]. Although its effectiveness remains undocumented, diphenhydramine is probably the drug of choice in the management of transient anxiety states in mentally retarded children and adolescents.

Anticonvulsants including barbiturates and diphenylhydantoin should be used only as anticonvulsant medications in children. Barbiturates often cause an increase of disorganization and hyperactivity in emotionally disturbed mentally retarded children. Carbamazepine is the only anticonvulsant which seems to have potential in treating severely disturbed mentally retarded children and adolescents particularly if they are also epileptics. More research needs to be done on this interesting compound which may have antipsychotic, antidepressant, and anticonvulsant properties.

Concluding Remarks

The psychopharmacology of emotionally disturbed, mentally retarded children and adolescents largely remains on an 'empirical basis'. Certainly, psychotropic medications should not be used in the treatment of mild disturbances of mentally retarded children and adolescents. When, because of the severity and duration of symptoms, psychotropic medications are needed, the physician must utilize them only as an adjunct to a total treatment modality for such children. Medications should never be the sole treatment. Hopefully, the medications can help some children become more amendable to special education, rehabilitation, behavior modification, psychotherapy, and social adaptation in a family, halfway house, or an institution. The hazards of drug treatment should always be weighed against the dangers of the nonmedicated child. Physicians should utilize low dosages, divided dosages, and short trials whenever possible. The clinician should be aware, for example, that symptom relief by medications may decrease the retarded child's ability to learn.

In mentally retarded children the superiority of one psychotropic medication over another is infrequently documented. Many physicians base medication decisions on their own unique past clinical experiences. Therefore, well-designed and adequately analyzed studies must be done before any generalizations can be made about psychotropic medication effects on the behavior, mood, or thought processes in the mentally retarded [11].

From a review of the literature one becomes painfully aware that psychopharmacologic research for the mentally retarded has been grossly neglected. In textbooks of pediatric psychopharmacology it is usually not even mentioned. Mentally retarded children and adolescents should be helped by medications and not harmed by them which is perhaps the more frequent result. The most tragic example of this is the fact that the majority of mentally retarded children and adolescents in institutions are maintained on neuroleptic medications for extended periods of time and for no good clinical reason. Such individuals are medicated simply to be controlled rather than to be helped. Such retardates then become victims rather than patients.

Table I. Clinically useful psychotropic agents in the treatment of mentally retarded, emotionally disturbed children and adolescents

Medication	Indications	Daily dosage range[1]	Special remarks
1 Dextroamphetamine sulfate Dexedrine, eskatrol	A distractability, attention deficit B hyperactivity C impulsivity, aggression	A ages 3–6 years: 2.5–15 mg/day B ages 6–12 years: 5–40 mg/day C 1.5 mg/kg/day is the maximum dose	A not recommended for children less than 3 years of age B may induce or worsen a psychotic process C main side effects: irritability, insomnia, anorexia
2 Methylphenidate HCL (Ritalin)	same as dextroamphetamine	A ages 6–12 years: 10–60 mg/day B dose range: 0.1–3.0 mg/kg/day	A not recommended for children less than 6 years of age B medication must be given ½ h before or between meals
3 Pemoline (Cylert)	same as dextroamphetamine	A ages 6–12 years: 18.75–112.5 mg/day B mean dose: 0.5–2.7 mg/kg/day	A not recommended for children less than 6 years of age B in contrast to other stimulants, it may be administered in one daily dose
4 Imipramine (Tofranil)	A adolescent depression B hyperactivity refractory to other medications C enuresis	A ages 6 years and older: 25–100 mg/day B dose range: 0.5–5 mg/kg/day	A not recommended for children less than 6 years of age B approved only for enuresis in children by the PDR and FDA C FDA maximum daily dose: 2.5 mg/kg/day for routine clinical use and 5 mg/kg/day for improved investigational use D major cardiac side effects and deaths

Drug	Indications	Dosages	Comments
5 Diphenhydramine (Benadryl)	A hyperactivity, aggression, and distractibility in preschoolers B psychosis or hyperactivity in school age children C situational anxiety D insomnia	A ages 3–6 years: 25–150 mg/day B ages 6–12 years: 50–600 mg/day C dose range: 2–10 mg/kg/day	A often loses its clinical effectiveness after a short period of time B usually not useful for adolescents C excessive sedation is a common side effect
6 Chlorpromazine (Thorazine)	A psychosis B severe hyperactivity, aggression	A ages 3–6 years: 5–100 mg/day or 0.5–3 mg/kg/day B ages 6–12 years: 25–100 mg/day or 1–9 mg/kg/day C ages 12 years and older: 75–500 mg/day	A lowers the seizure threshold B sedating C permanent dyskinesias can be a side effect
7 Thioridazine (Mellaril)	same as chlorpromazine	A ages 2–12 years: 0.5–3.0 mg/kg/day B ages 12 years and older: 3–6 mg/kg/day to a maximum of 600 mg/day	A anticholinergic side effects are a common problem B enuresis is a side effect same as chlorpromazine C
8 Trifluoperazine (Stelazine)	same as chlorpromazine	A ages 6–12 years: 0.05–0.5 mg/kg/day B ages 12 years and older: 5–20 mg/day	same as chlorpromazine but less sedating
9 Haloperidol (Haldol)	A same as chlorpromazine B Gilles de la Tourette's syndrome	A ages 6–12 years: 0.025–0.5 mg/kg/day B high dosages for the short-term treatment of acute psychoses	A lower dosages often useful for Tourette's syndrome B useful for acute psychoses C same as chlorpromazine but less sedating and more likely to cause dyskinesia

Table I (continued)

Medication	Indications	Daily dosage range[1]	Special remarks
10 Thiothixene (Navane)	same as chlorpromazine	A ages 12 years and older: 0.05–0.3 mg/kg/day B dose range: 3–20 mg/day	A FDA approval for patients over 12 years of age only B same as chlorpromazine
11 Lithium carbonate (Lithane, Eskalith, Lithonate)	A mania or severe cyclic mood and behavioral changes B severe aggression or self-mutilation not responsive to other medications	A ages 12 years and older: 0.25–1.5 mEq/l B blood levels can be maintained at lower levels for maintenance than for acute treatment	A not recommended for children less than 16 years of age except for treatment-resistent children B major kidney complications C neurological side effects are not uncommon in retardates
12 Clonidine HCL (Catapres)	A Gilles de la Tourette's syndrome B utilized only if Tourette's is non-responsive to haloperidol or phenothiazines	A ages 8 years and older: 1–2 µg/kg/day or 0.05–0.30 mg/day	A less sedating than haloperidol B dry mouth and increased salivation common side effects C prior cardiac assessment necessary before treatment

[1] Medications in children and adolescents should generally be given in divided dosages.

The hope of this paper is that general good clinical principles will be maintained in order that emotionally disturbed and mentally retarded children and adolescents can receive limited but definitive help from medications when indicated. Refer to table I for a general summary of clinically useful psychotropic agents.

References

1   Bradley, C.: The behavior of children receiving benzedrine Am. J. Psychiat. *94:* 577 (1937).
2   Conners, C.K.: Psychological effects of stimulant drugs in children with minimal brain dysfunction. Pediatrics *49:* 702 (1972).
3   Denoff, E.; Davids, A.; Hawkins, R.: Effects of dextroamphetamine on hyperkinetic children. J. learn. Disabil. *4:* 491 (1971).
4   Wender, P.: Minimal brain dysfunction in children, pp. 87–108 (Wiley, New York, 1971).
5   Katz, S.; Saraf, K.; Gittelman-Klein, R.; Klein, D.: Clinical pharmacological management of hyperkinetic children. Int. J. ment. Health *4:* 157 (1975).
6   Millichap, J.G.: Drugs in the management of minimal brain dysfunction; in Klein, Gittelman-Klein, Progress in psychiatric drug treatment, pp. 675–688 (Brunner/Mazler, New York 1975).
7   Millichap, J.G.; Johnson, F.: Methylphenidate in hyperkinetic behavior: relation of response to degree of activity and brain damage; in Conners, Clinical use of stimulant drugs in children, pp. 130–139 (Excerpta Medica, The Hague 1974).
8   Winsberg, B.G.; Press, M.; Bialer, I.; Kupretz, S.: Dextroamphetamine and methylphenidate in the treatment of hyperactive/aggressive children. Pediatrics *53:* 236 (1974).
9   Conners, C.K.; Eisenberg, L.: The effects of methylphenidate on symptomatology and learning in disturbed children. Am. J. Psychiat. *120:* 458 (1963).
10 Gittelman-Klein, R.: Review of clinical psychopharmacological treatment of hyperkinesis; in Klein, Gittelman-Klein, Progress in psychiatric drug treatment, pp. 661–674 (Brunner/Mazel, New York 1975).
11 Lipman, R.S.; DiMascio, A.; Reatig, N.; Kirson, T.: Psychotropic drugs and mentally retarded children. Psychopharmacology (Raven Press, New York 1978).
12 Gittelman-Klein, R.; Klein, D.F.: Methylphenidate effects in learning disabilities. Archs gen. Psychiat. *33:* 655–664 (1976).
13 Gittelman R.: Indications for the use of stimulant treatment in learning disorders. J. Am. Acad. Child Psychiat. *19:* 623–636 (1980).
14 Safer, D.; Allen, R.; Barr, E.: Depression of growth in hyperactive children on stimulant drugs. New Engl. J. Med. *287:* 217 (1972).
15 Safer, D.; Allen, R.: Factors influencing the suppressant effects of two stimulant drugs on the growth of hyperactive children. Pediatrics *51:* 660 (1973).
16 Lerer, R.; Lerer, M.: Response of adolescents with minimal brain dysfunction to methylphenidate. J. learn. disabil. *5:* 223–228 (1977).

17   Cohen, D.; Detlor, J.; Young, J.G.; Shaywitz, B.: Clonidine ameliorates Gilles de la Tourette syndrome. Archs gen Psychiat. *37:* 1350–1357 (1980).

18   McAndrew, J.B.; Case, Q.; Treffert, D.: Effects of prolonged phenothiazine intake on psychotic and other hospitalized children. J. Autism Childh. Schiz. *2:* 75 (1972).

19   Polizos, P.; Engelhardt, D.; Hoffman, F.: Neurological consequences of psychotropic drug withdrawal in schizophrenic children. J. Autism Childh. Schiz. *3:* 247 (1973).

20   Gualtieri, C.T.; Barnhill, J.; McGimsey, J.; Schell, D.: Tardive dyskinesia and other movement disorders in children treated with psychotropic drugs. J. Am. Acad. Child Psychiat. *19:* 491–510 (1980).

21   Hall, R.; Feinsilver, D.; Holt, R.E.: Anticholinergic psychosis: differential diagnosis and management. Psychosomatics *22:* 581–587 (1981).

22   Caroff, S.N.: The neuroleptic malignant syndrome. J. clin. Psychiat. *41:* 79 (1980).

23   Rapaport, J.: Childhood behavior and learning problems treated with imipramine. Int. J. Neuropsychiat. *1:* 635 (1965).

24   Huessy, H.R.; Wright, A.L.: The use of imipramine in children's behavior disorders. Acta paedopsychiat. *37:* 194 (1970).

25   Waizer, J.; Hoffman, S.; Polizos, P.: Outpatient treatment of hyperactive school children with imipramine. Am. J. Psychiat. *131:* 587 (1974).

26   Gittelman-Klein, R.; Klein, D.: Controlled imipramine treatment of school phobia. Archs gen. Psychiat. *25:* 204 (1971).

27   Kraft, I.A.; Arddi, C.; Duffy, J.: Use of amitriptyline in childhood behavior disturbances. Int. J. Neuropsychiat. *2:* 611 (1966).

28   Krakowski, A.J.: Amitriptyline in treatment of hyperkinetic children. Psychosomatics *6:* 55 (1965).

29   Lucas, A.R.; Lockett, H.J.; Grimm, F.: Amitriptyline in childhood depressions. Dis. nerv. Syst. *26:* 105 (1965).

30   Campbell, M.; Fish, B.; Shapiro, T.: Imipramine in preschool autistic and schizophrenic children. J. Autism Childh. Schiz. *1:* 267 (1971).

31   Kurtis, L.B.: Clinical study of the response to nortriptyline on autistic children. Int. J. Neuropsychiat. *2:* 298 (1966).

32   Jefferson, J.W.: A review of the cardiovascular effects and toxicity of tricyclic antidepressants. Psychosom. Med. *37:* 160 (1975).

33   Fouron, J.C.; Chicoine, R.: ECG changes in fatal imipramine intoxication. Pediatrics *48:* 777 (1971).

34   Saraf, K.P.; Klein, D.; Gittelman-Klein, R.: Imipramine side effects in children. Psychopharmacologia *37:* 265 (1974).

35   Davis, J.M.; Bartlett, E.; Termini, B.A.: Overdosage of psychotropic drugs: a review. Dis. nerv. Syst. *29:* 246 (1968).

36   Annell, A.L.: Lithium in the treatment of children and adolescents. Acta psychiat. scand., suppl. 207, pp. 19 (1969).

37   Dostal, T.: Antiaggressive effect of lithium salts in mentally retarded adolescents; in Annell, Depressive states in childhood and adolescence, pp. 491–498 (Almquist & Wiksell, Stockholm 1972).

38   Gram, L.F.; Rafaelsen, A.J.: Lithium treatment of psychotic children and adolescents: a controlled clinical trial. Acta psychiat. scand *48:* 253 1972.

39   LaVeck, G.D.; Buckley, P.: The use of psychopharmacologic agents in retarded children with behavior problems. J. chronic Dis. *13:* 174 (1961).

14 The Education of the Retarded
Susan Glor-Scheib

Special education runs the gamut from preschool early identification screening service through school age to vocational and recreational rehabilitation programs for young adults. This article is to help define the educational principles involved in teaching the retarded including assessment, methodology, curriculum and goal planning.

A major influence on the effectiveness of special education has been effectuated by the passing of Public Law 94–142 in November of 1975. This law ensures the handicapped to a free education and other services to enhance and supplement educational services. This article will also highlight some of the aspects of this federal law.

The education of the retarded implies a systematic sequence of specialized teaching which must include assessment, methodology, curriculum and goal planning. All of these aspects of the system are essential to the intellectual and maturational growth of the retarded child and also to maximize the child's potential.

Assessment

The decisions about the curriculum and methodology are guided by the assessment procedure. The direct assessment procedure as outlined by *Peter* [5] is twofold in purpose: (1) to diagnose the child's current level of functioning, and (2) to improve the efficiency of the educational process.

The system itself includes four steps: (a) collect information about the child's background (school and social histories); (b) establish child's levels of functioning; (c) identify educational material to be taught and establish objectives and reinforcers; (d) obtain estimation of child's rate of learning.

One of the most useful tools in the assessment of retarded/multiple handicapped children is a concise developmental checklist outlining the norms of behavior at different ages. Using a method of developmental assessment allows the teacher/therapist to view the child's development as a continuously changing process [1].

The checklist is divided into categories including: motor (fine and gross) functioning; cognitive (perceptual and conceptual) functioning; social and emotional functioning; communication (expressive and receptive language); and self-help areas including feeding, toileting, and dressing. Once levels of functioning are determined (age at which the child successfully passes the developmental items), an educational treatment plan can be established. *Example:* A 5-year-old retarded child, in my classroom, has received no formal education up to this point, but his parents realize that he has developmental problems and does not 'act' like other 5-year-olds. After a week of informal observation in the classroom to ascertain the child's spontaneous repertoire of behaviors, the more formal assessment procedure is performed with a kit of testing materials including:

(1)   Color cubic blocks for tower building, construction imitation, color sorting, and other perceptual skills.
(2)   Assorted size beads and strings for patterning and dexterity.
(3)   Language stimulation picture cards for receptive-expressive communication skills.
(4)   Paper, scissors, pencils and crayons for fine motor abilities and drawing skills.
(5)   Large muscle equipment (stand-in blocks, rugs, tables, etc.) for obstacle course activities to determine coordination, balance, conceptual skills (understanding of on, in, out, up, down, through, etc.)

Once the child's checklist was completed, I had determined that his primary delays are in the areas of perceptual-conceptual development and receptive language. Since the child's motor skills are normal for his age, I can use motor activity to help remediate his weaknesses. An example of such a teaching goal would be:

Goal: Johnny will be able to sort the colors yellow and red while practicing the use of the preposition 'in'.
Activity: Johnny will be given 10 cubic blocks (five red, five yellow) which he will sort by placing them in either a red can on the window sill, or a yellow can under a table.
Evaluation: He will determine his own success by bringing the can to the teacher and

saying aloud the colors of the blocks. His success will be determined by achieving 60% accuracy on the first try and 80% accuracy on the second with the teacher positively reinforcing only his successful attempts.

This activity has incorporated motor activity (which he enjoys) with color sorting and directionality skills (which he needs help with). If this task proves too demanding of him, it should be divided into smaller steps, so that he put only yellow blocks in yellow containers, thereby assuring that he will find success with the activity for the promotion of his feelings of self-esteem and a successful teacher-student rapport.

The importance of an accurate developmental/behavioral diagnostic assessment cannot be overstated. The most effective teaching program reflects the childs' levels of functioning and draws on the strengths to help remediate the weaknesses. One should not try to teach a child to tie his shoes when he is yet unable to unbutton his shirt due to poor digital dexterity. Nor would one attempt to teach a child skills in practical math if he has not yet mastered one to one correspondence.

Many such skill areas must be taught in a developmental sequence to insure understanding and success for the child. Assessment remains a primary responsibility of the teacher or direct care giver for without it, a teaching plan is without a focus. The following are examples of assessment instruments that would be effective for use with a retarded population, and can be adapted for a variety of age ranges. Scoring of these assessment examples is accomplished through observation and interview.

While it should be understood that the establishment of an assessment system for a specific handicapped population may be time consuming at first, the benefits are an excellent record-keeping system and the proof of accountability for continued accreditation. In a hospital or residential school setting, after thorough familiarization with an assessment system, the direct-care staff can play a key role in the implementation of many individual education programs, under the supervision of an educational administrator. Since the major skill areas in the assessment systems are analyzed within the framework of a developmental sequence, with careful planning, the goals for the child will always be relevant and realistic to meet the child's needs.

Once goals are determined the specially trained teacher has then, perhaps, the most emotionally-taxing aspect of the job to perform – teaching the child.

AAMD Adaptive Behavior Scales for Children and Adults
American Association of Mental Deficiency, 5201 Connecticut Avenue, N.W.,
Washington, DC 20014

Areas assessed
Section I
   Personal independence in daily living
Section II
   Maladaptive behavior measures as it relates to personality or behavior disorders

Assessment format
Direct behavioral observation
Standardized

Comments
The instrument is well developed and effective for evaluating the severe/profound range of
mental retardation. However, for more detailed information to develop specific programs,
it should be used with one of the behavioral taxonomies or assessment systems.

Balthazaar Scales of Adaptive Behavior
Research Press, Champaign, Ill.

Areas assessed
Section I
   Functional independence
Section II
   Social adaptation

Assessment format
Sections I and II
   Direct naturalistic observation
   Scoring is individualized
Section II only
   Frequency count per unit of time measurement
Raw scores and percentile ranks can be used

Comments
This is an especially good profile at the severe/profound range of mental retardation. It is
important that the rater become thoroughly familiar with the BSAB as scoring can be
somewhat complex.

Behavior Characteristics Progression Chart (BCP)
VORT Corporation, PO Box 11132, Palo Alto, CA 94306

Areas assessed
Self-help, perceptual-motor, language, social, academic, recreational, vocational
   Skills areas sequenced in developmental intervals
   Mental age range – birth through 7+

Assessment format
Nonstandardized
Behavioral checklist format
System can be used to measure progress and develop new goal for a given instructional
objective

Comments
Independence is the final goal in all behavior sequences. Task analysis of all behaviors is
very finely detailed. This is useful for the severe/profound range up through low EMR.

Camelot Behavioral Checklist Manual and Skill Acquisition Program Bibliography
Camelot Behavioral Systems, PO Box 3447, Lawrence, KS 66044

Areas assessed
Self-help, physical development, home duties, vocational behaviors, economic behaviors,
independent travel, numerical skills, social skills and responsibility
   Mental age range – birth through 9.

Assessment format
Direct observation or interview of caretakers
From checklist data, instructional objective can be developed

Comments
This system is suitable for advanced severe/profound population. The items are too general for a lower functioning population. The bibliography is an outstanding feature of the
system.

Methodology

It would be quite impossible to find two special education teachers whose behavior in the classroom is alike. Teachers bring their own personalities, levels of expectation, personal experience and degree of frustration tolerance into the classroom. Methods of classroom management that may be highly successful for one teacher may be totally inappropriate for another. Possibly the single-most important feature of a successful special education teacher is the effectuation of the appearance of control. It is essential that the children sense the teacher's control of the classroom atmosphere. If a child in the class explodes with an emotional outburst, the other children must feel that their safety is not jeopardized and that the teacher is able to calm the disturbance. As the child's trust in the classroom atmosphere grows, so does the teacher's potential for a successful teaching rapport. While this is important in a regular educational classroom, it is essential for special education. An example of this may be best illustrated by the following vignette.

Ricky has been in my classroom for retarded, disturbed, primary age children for 5 weeks. His spontaneous language is limited to a single phrase, 'I have to go to the bathroom,' and his bizarre mannerisms and level of anxious withdrawal have prevented me from establishing any viable teaching goals. Assessment has been next to impossible. Thoroughly frustrated with him and myself, I sought the expertise of a visiting infant specialist who, I felt, could be much more objective in her observation of my interaction with this child, and perhaps suggest some procedures that might succeed. After observing the child and myself for 20 min then talking to me individually an hour and a half afterwards, she helped me realize that Ricky was not yet ready to see me as his teacher, a person with whom he had to interact, a person he could trust. Her suggestions caused me to realize that being a goal-oriented teacher did not imply only traditional methods to establish rapport. Up to this time, Ricky had made only minimal eye contact with me and his attention span was under 3 s. My knowledgeable advisor had suggested individual intensive 5–10 min interaction sessions where I strip away the layer of directive teacher and interact with him as his entertainer, one who makes funny faces, who hides small objects under cups then gleefully searches for them, who juggles beads before stringing them. I found that within 4 days, Ricky not only gave me eye contact, but he also visibly anticipated the session and particular activities. Within 7 days, he actively participated in the activities and in a couple of weeks I was able to pull away from many of the activities as he was able to perform them independently. The most gratifying aspect of this experience was the teacher-student rapport that resulted from my unorthodox teaching methods. I should also mention that I was then able to successfully assess Ricky's strengths and weaknesses and prescribe educational activities that best suited his needs.

In addition to establishing a successful teacher-student rapport, a teacher must also be able to maintain a classroom environment that is conducive to learning and behavior management principles must be regarded as a necessary component of educational methodology. The key to successful classroom management lies in basic operant conditioning where the child gives a proper response and receives positive reinforcement. The speed of the delivery of the reinforcer is crucial, especially with a retarded population in the severe or profound range. The choice of reinforcers is critical. The reinforcers are selected from six categories: gustatory, olfactory, visualy, auditory, tactile and proprioceptive.

Low functioning populations are usually most responsive to proprioceptive stimuli such as a hug, a swing, a pat on the back or other activities involving movement. *Mager* [4], an educational psychologist, has outlined several conditions for learning including:

(1) Acknowledge student responses, whether correct or incorrect, as attempts to learn and follow the responses with accepting rather than rejecting comments.
(2) Provide feedback that is immediate and specific to the student's response.
(3) Make use of the variables known to be successful in attracting and holding human attention, such as color, variety, contrast and personal preference.
(4) Express genuine delight at seeing the student, and at seeing the student succeed.
(5) Provide instruction in increments that will allow success most of the time.

The last of these conditions is certainly most important for people involved in the education of the retarded.

While behavior principles may increase the effectiveness of the classroom, other considerations must be given to the curriculum of the students within special education for overall program success.

Curriculum

In special education, the curriculum is most often determined by the specific levels of functioning in different areas as ascertained by assessment procedures. The level of retardation is very significant in educational terms and weighs heavily on decisions of future goal planning for children. Since the 1960s, the demarcation line between mildly and moderately retarded has shifted upward toward IQ scores of 55, 60 and 65. Accompanying the trend to integrate 'educable retardates' into general education has come the realization that most children from standard English-speaking homes with

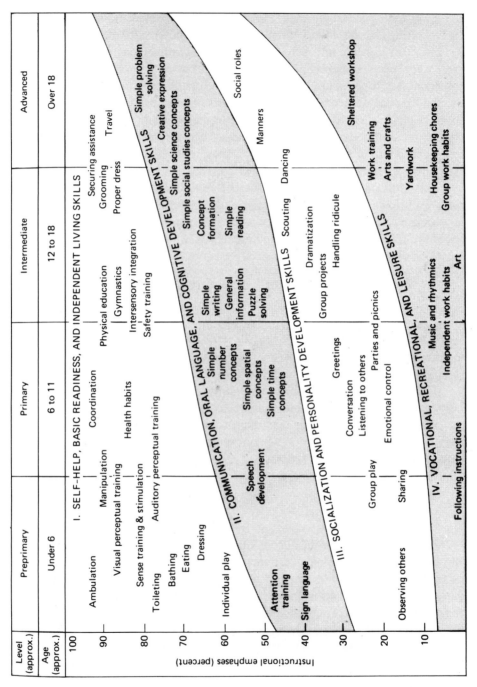

Fig. 1. Specific ingredients in four broad curricular areas by age levels for moderately retarded children and youth. Adapted from *Campbell*, 1968, by *Dunn* [2].

IQs in the 50s cannot function in an academically oriented class. Thus, more of these students are likely to be classified as moderately retarded and placed in self-contained special education facilities. Concurrently, children with IQs in the 20s and low 30s, who are usually unsuccessful in special classes for the moderately retarded, are increasingly being placed in day-care centers and other services for the severely retarded. As a result, instead of calling the moderately retarded 'semi-dependent', they are now referred to as 'semi-independent', reflecting a subtle but important attitudinal change. Therefore, curricular objectives have been broadened considerably to include the following four rather comprehensive goals: (1) self-help, basic readiness and independent living skills development; (2) communication, language and cognitive development; (3) socialization and personality development; (4) vocational-recreational, and leisure skills development.

Figure 1 is a chart of the specific ingredients in the four broad curricular areas by age levels for moderately retarded children and youth [2].

Curriculum for children at the severe and profound ranges of retardation are much more basic in that the areas of stress are most often self-help, living skills development and communication. Behavior modification for such problem areas as self-stimulation and stereotypical behavior is often found to be effective in children at this level of retardation.

Goal Planning

Goal planning for the retarded population is most successful when the decisions are reached by a multidisciplinary staff. The combined expertise is also effective in interagency matters that involve not only the child, but his family and their future, as the child's needs affect it.

A supportive multidisciplinary staff presents varying backgrounds from which parents as well as staff co-workers can draw information. Teachers and social workers often work together for the education of parents who may have antiquated concepts and illusions about the implications of having a retarded child. Psychologists and teachers may plan together various behavior management systems that could be feasible and successful within the classroom. A multidisciplinary staff is particularly effective for interagency meetings whose purpose is to set into motion the long- and short-term goals for a particular child.

Listed below are stages that a multidisciplinary team may cover while identifying and classifying retarded/disturbed children.

I.   *Prevention:* Identification of the child's exceptionality is a first step toward discovering its causes and finding possible preventative and helpful agents.

II. *Identification diagnosis:* Exceptionality of the child must be distinguished from other possible conditions (autism from hearing impairment, retardation from delayed speech) in preparation for differential education [3].

III. *Prescription and prosthesis:* Various devices and treatments may be introduced to lessen the impact of the exceptionality (hearing aids, communication boards, speech therapy, physical therapy, behavior management intervention, etc.).

IV. *Special placement:* The classification of exceptional children often has the result of placing them in a special learning environment and into interaction with specially trained personnel.

V.   *Program implementation:* A continuous program of instruction and remediation can be instituted, which will be based on the individual characteristics of the exceptional child.

VI. *Funding:* The accurate classification of various types of exceptional children enables schools and agencies to apply and qualify for funds from various sources [3].

Certain aspects and legal issues about the rights of the handicapped child and his family must be carefully considered in the proposal of future plans.

References

1   Deppe, P.R.; Sherman, J.L.: The high-risk child (MacMillan, New York 1981).
2   Dunn, L.: Exceptional children in the schools (Holt, Reinhart & Winston, New York 1973).
3   Kirk, S.A.: Gallagher, J.J.: Educating exceptional children; 3rd ed. (Houghton Mifflin, Boston 1979).
4   Mager, R.F.: Developing attitude toward learning (Fearon-Pitman, Belmont 1968).
5   Peter, L.J.: Prescriptive teaching (McGraw-Hill, New York 1965).

15 Education and the Law

Susan Glor-Scheib

With the recent changes regarding the education of the handicapped, it is important that administrators and program directors understand the fine points of Public Law (PL) 94-142. The education of a multiply-handicapped population has become everyone's responsibility with the passing of PL 94-142 ('Right to Education for all Handicapped Act', November 1975; 20 United States Code 1402 as Amended).

This new law basically superimposed on existing federal special education programs without changing them, even though PL 94-142 potentially represents a major revised federal role in both funding and control of special education programming [2].

While problems still lie in the enforcement of the law, growing public awareness of the rights of the handicapped has caused closer scrutiny of the services provided. The law mandates: (1) Free and appropriate education to all handicapped children. (2) The rights of parents to due process in order to assure that the rights of the handicapped and their parents are protected. (3) Federal funding to assist the states and local educational agencies in providing education for all handicapped children.

The term 'handicapped children' refers to people aged 3–21 who have sufficient mental or physical impairment to require significant special educational services. More specifically, the federal definition of handicapped children is ... 'mentally retarded, hard of hearing, deaf, speech impaired, visually handicapped, seriously emotionally disturbed, orthopedically impaired, or other health-impaired children or children with specific learning disabilities who by reason thereof require special education and *related services* (20 United States Code 1402 as Amended).

The term related services means transportation and such developmental, corrective and other supportive services (including speech pathology and audiology, psychological services, except that such medical services shall be for diagnostic and evaluative purposes only) as may be required to assist a handicapped child benefit from special education, and includes early identification and assessment of handicapping conditions in children (PL 94-142).

It should be understood that the *State Education Agency* will have jurisdiction over all education programs for handicapped children within a given state, including those administered by a noneducation agency (a state hospital, for example, or the welfare department).

The law has also stipulated a hierarchy of educational environments that will best serve the needs of each handicapped child. These prototypes of educational environments increase in restrictiveness from the regular education model. (Regular education defined as: The school program for children without needs of special education other than supportive services such as supplemental reading, guidance and possibly speech.)

While the federal law has stipulated that handicapped children shall be educated with nonhandicapped whenever and wherever possible, individual states have determined a hierarchy of educational environments that is similar to the following:

No special needs

Regular education program full time with special education modifications in the classroom

Regular educational program with up to 25% of the time *out* of the regular classroom for special education service

Regular educational program with up to 60% time *out* of the classroom for special education services

Regular educational program with up to 100% of time *out* of regular classroom for special educational services

A day school program: special education program made up entirely of special education children which is substantially separate from the regular education program to the point that it is a facility other than a public school facility

Residential school program: a 24-hour program needed to enable the child to make effective progress educationally

Home or hospital program: provided upon written request of a physician for a child who is to be out of school more than 10 days for medical reasons

This hierarchy is also useful in discharge planning of the child, to determine after careful evaluation, the next placement to best serve the child's needs while also attempting to find a less restrictive environment.

Individual Education Plan

For each handicapped child there will be an 'individualized education plan' (IEP) – a written statement jointly developed by a qualified school official, by the child's teacher and parents/guardian, and if possible by the child himself. This written statement will include an analysis of the child's present achievement level, a listing of both short-term and annual goals, and identification of specific services that will be provided toward meeting those goals and an indication of the extent to which the child will be able to participate in regular school programs (see 'Restrictiveness Codes'). Also included should be a notation of when these services will be provided and how long they will last, and a schedule for checking on the progress being achieved under the plan and for making any revisions in it that may seem called for [3].

The plan is signed by all participants and the 'contract' is established. Involving the parent ensures a better understanding between the educational facility and the family, and the educational facility is then accountable for the progress of the child. The law has built several protections for the handicapped student and for the parents regarding both testing and placement. To insure fair treatment and responsible results, the following must be adhered to:

1   Tests and other evaluation materials must be administered in the child's native language
2   Tests used must have been validated for the purpose for which they are being used in the assessment
3   Tests must be administered by trained personnel as indicated by the producer of the tests
4   Tests and other materials must be used which not only assess general intelligence, but specific needs
5   Tests should best measure the child's aptitude, not simply reflect the basic needs
6   No single procedure shall be used as the sole criterion for determining an appropriate educational program
7   The evaluation shall be made by an interdisciplinary team, including at least one teacher with knowledge in the area of suspected disability
8   Tests should not be racially or culturally discriminating [1]

Parents' Rights

There are procedural safeguards built into the law for the parent's protection. They are: (1) Consent is voluntary and can be revoked at any time in the process by the parent. However, education cannot be denied on the basis of a nonconsent for special services. (2) Parents can *review records*, and can receive a due process hearing if there is incorrect information in the records. (3) A parent can receive an *independent evaluation* of the child if the local educational agency deems it necessary at no cost to the parent. (4) A parent has the right to request a *due process hearing* if any of these rights are denied.

Vocational Rehabilitation

The 'Rehabilitation Act' passed in 1973 established a fund to provide grants to states, with guidelines, for provision of a wide variety of services to physically and mentally handicapped persons so that they may prepare for and engage in gainful employment. The federal government presently funds approximately 80% of the basic vocational rehabilitation (VR) programs and supports employment service to all types of physically or mentally disabled persons with a substantial handicap but with 'high' vocational potential [2]. The States also play a major role as they contribute the other 20% of the funds and *directly* provide VR services. State rehabilitation agencies tailor their programs within guidelines to suit local agency situations. The state personnel are often responsible for diagnostic evaluation, counselling, rehabilitation planning, while private sector personnel perform other services such as medical treatment and vocational training.

Conclusion

Special education has grown remarkably in the last decade through both legislation and public attitude and awareness. Special education has expanded far beyond the walls of a classroom into the home, into alternative living group homes, into mental health facilities, and into long-term residential care institutions. This expansion will continue successfully only with enlightened health care professionals and better trained teachers. The movement of special needs children into public education is currently hindered by public school teachers who lack the proper educational background and expertise to accept and educate these children. The problem lies not with the teachers, but rather the institutions of higher education where they trained and the deficient curriculums for teacher preparation. Until the training of all teachers includes course work and practical experience in the education of special needs children, the public educational sector will perpetuate negative and unjust attitudes towards the 'mainstreaming' of special children into their classrooms. So, therefore, a large part of the solution to a more effective educational process for all children lies in the education of teachers, educational administrators, and others who effect change in childrens' behavior.

References

1   Arena, J.: How to write an IEP (Academic Therapy Productions, Novato 1978).
2   Brever, G.D.; Kakalik, J.S.: Handicapped children strategies for improving services (McGraw-Hill, New York 1979).
3   Goodman, L.V.: 'A Bill of Rights for All Handicapped' in Programs for the Handicapped (HEW, Washington).

16 Social Work with Families in the John Merck Program for the Treatment of Mentally Retarded Emotionally Disturbed Children

Barbara Hanley

Description of the Program

The purpose of this chapter is to describe the John Merck Program in general and to describe in particular, social work treatment with the families of the children who are patients.

The John Merck Program for doubly handicapped emotionally disturbed mentally retarded children at the Department of Psychiatry of the University of Pittsburgh is located at the Western Psychiatric Institute and Clinic. The program has been designed in 1974 by *Irene Jakab,* MD, PhD, Professor of Psychiatry, University of Pittsburgh, and it functioned in the first 3 calendar years as a pilot project directed by Dr. *I. Jakab,* supported partially by grant funds from the John Merck Fund. The original patient census 1975–1978 was 20 (10 inpatients and 10 partially hospitalized children, ages 3–10 years). A multidisciplinary clinical staff of 46 persons cared for the patients.

After the successful pilot phase the John Merck Program in 1979 increased the census to 25 (20 inpatients and 5 partials) and extended the age range (3–12 years). Increases in staff have been made proportionally to the increase in census.

After a child is admitted to the program, evaluation studies are done by the professional in each respective discipline. About 2–3 weeks after the workups, three Diagnostic Conferences are held; first, the John Merck Staff meet and share their findings and recommendations; and then formulate a treatment plan. These findings and the treatment plan are then shared at the Family Diagnostic Conference and an Agency Diagnostic Conference where agency representatives previously working with this child and family are invited to attend.

After the plan has been formulated, a Treatment Review Meeting is held each week, at which time each child's plan is reviewed; one child is reviewed in detail each week for the long- and short-term goals of treatment.

Treatment is formulated on an individual basis; some are short-term care and for some, a longer range of treatment is provided. The average stay is 1 year. The age range is 3–12 years presently.

The populations served are basically low middle class, with patients on both ends of the economic spectrum. All races, creeds and international patients have received treatment through the John Merck Program.

Social Work

Social work practice has as its focus the interactions between people and systems in the social environment.

We are dependent on the resources, services and opportunities in our social environment to realize our aspirations and to help us cope with our life tasks. The life tasks and demands made of the family with a mentally retarded, emotionally disturbed child are far more specialized than the normal stages of crises in the life cycle.

Presently in the John Merck Program there is 1 full-time ACSW worker, 2 full-time MSW staff social workers and 2 MSW students.

Social work intervention with the families of the children in the John Merck Program has as its focus the family system and its individual members as they effect and are effected by the child who has become the patient.

The assets and pathology in the precarious balance of the family system provide the parameters of casework and treatment.

The goals of casework and family treatment are:

(1) relief during acute crises;
(2) maintenance, development and mobilization of adaptive and problem-solving abilities, and
(3) maintenance of family function or reestablishment of disrupted family equilibrium through rehabilitation.

Casework services provided by social workers are:

(1) receiving the initial referral phone calls;
(2) sending out and receiving the application forms and Release of Information Permits;
(3) sending for and receiving records of the previous treatments, testings and/or programs;

(4) setting up preadmission interviews and evaluations and finance interviews;
(5) formulating the waiting list; make some emergency referrals to community services; preschools, public schools; residential care; respite care group homes; MH/MRs, as needed before admission to the John Merck Program;
(6) home visits prior to admission; setting up the admission;
(7) setting up admission and diagnostic conferences and formulating a social work treatment plan;
(8) continuing agency contacts for discharge planning, and
(9) scheduling follow-up appointments.

Treatment provided by the social worker is through counseling and therapy for family and/or primary caretakers.

Parental involvement is a priority in the total treatment plan. The family is seen once a week by the social worker, more often if necessary.

Visiting of the child by the family is usually withheld during the first two weeks. Parental visits are monitored initially and then gradually siblings are included as well as eventual family outings and overnight visits are planned. Parents are encouraged to observe their child in various therapies throughout the hospitalization.

The effect of treatment is the eventual reintegration of the child into the family; however, this requires:

(1) that the child makes sufficient progress in developing socially acceptable behavior on the unit;
(2) has had trial home visits which are satisfactory to both child and family;
(3) methods used by the family to elicit a positive response from the child are satisfactory;
(4) the family cooperates with setting priorities in dealing with the problems they had at home, and
(5) they learned effective methods to deal with those problems.

Not all the children are placed back in the home. If this is the recommendation of the team, the staff of the John Merck Program will visit residential settings and select an appropriate placement for the child and parent. If the child *does* return to the home environment again the John Merck Program staff will visit educational settings and make an appropriate referral for a particular classroom (for example: Pittsburgh Board of Education; Allegheny County Intermediate Unit). Additional family therapy, counseling or play therapy can often be provided through the local Mental Health and Mental Retardation agencies. Follow-up evaluations are done with the child and family every 4–6 months during the first year, at 12 and 18 months and then annually.

Theoretical Frameworks

Family pathology and/or family disequilibrium is often reflected in the child, and a child's social development is not separate from his cognitive abilities. One of the areas to be perceived and accessed from the initial social history interview is the pattern of attachment behaviors between the parents – mostly the mother and the patient. It is important to know the degree of parental bonding initially, as well as over time, until the present hospitalization in order to plan for intervention.

The realization that a child is not only handicapped mentally but is having emotional problems is usually a serious time of crisis in the family. If the mental retardation is not determined immediately following the birth then often it is missed until months later, when developmental delays are noticed by the parent and often, even then, the parents are sometimes told by their doctors 'Let's wait, he is slow in developing and will probably catch up soon'. Most patients are usually evaluated at between 2 or 3 years; some as late as 6 and 7 years.

Whether the crises come shortly after the birth of the child or in later years, according to *Wolfensberger* and *Menolascino,* there are usually three stages experienced by the parents.

The first is labeled *'the novelty shock crisis'* wherein the parent must deal with the loss of the 'wished for healthy child', the expected result of the pregnancy and the actual child. There is the demolition of parental expectancies and the impact of disappointment; feelings of helplessness, failure and fear.

The second stage is considered as *'the crisis of personal values'* during this time the parents deal with their reactions to mental deficit; often mental deficiency is unacceptable to the parents' values and often this child is seen as the extension of the self as well as a representation of self and the family.

The *reality crisis* is the third stage; this is the period wherein the parents experience the everyday impact of their MR/ED child. Similar stages are described by *Solnit and Stark* [25] in the process of mourning the defective child. They describe the grief reaction of mourning, in response to the loss of a valued object or the perfect child, similar to the loss of a loved person, cherished possession, a job, status, home, country, an ideal, body part. The process moves initially into shock-numbness-disbelief-anger. Often parents at this stage blame and/or search for the causes (birth injuries, heredity) then they move to search for the cures, special diets, mega-vitamins, therapies. The next phase described is the period of acute awareness of the loss. There is a realization that this condition cannot be undone; often there is the experience of sorrow, hopelessness, guilt, fear and despair. Grieving reoccurs at other times of disappointment for the parents also; other failures and fears often will bring about another phase of intense reexperiencing of memories and expectations. The wound, so to say, will reopen. The last phase noted is when there is a decrease in the initial intensity around feelings of the loss and unusally with this, there is an adaptation or process toward movement, and the parents are ready for learning different or new aspects for parenting.

According to the Intermountain Newborn Intensive Care Center at the University of Utah, there are certain psychological tasks that parents of defective children need to achieve:

(1) adapting to the hospital environment;
(2) forming and maintaining a reality-based understanding of the child's intellectual, medical and emotional status;
(3) assume a positive parental relationship with the child;
(4) maintain family equilibrium, and
(5) preparing to assume responsibility for the child.

Measurement of parental development can be evaluated by looking at maladaptive and adaptive responses.

Some maladaptive responses are:
 (1) failure to visit or consistently visit;
 (2) emotional withdrawal from the child or overprotection;
 (3) difficulty interacting with the child comfortably during hospitalization;
 (4) resistance to providing minimal caretaking during hospitalization;
 (5) failure to achieve a sense of parenting competence;
 (6) failure to achieve a sense of attachment (bonding);
 (7) distortion of information received; debilitating preoccupation with child's condition;
 (8) ascribing blame for the child's condition;
 (9) fear of taking the child home;
(10) disturbed view of the child and potential needs at the time of discharge;
(11) failure to verbalize needs and concerns to staff and family, and
(12) hostility towards and distrust of staff.

Adaptive responses:
 (1) frequent visits and calls (consistent);
 (2) emotional involvement with the child;
 (3) development of comfortable interaction with the child during hospitalization;
 (4) interest in assuming maximum amount of caretaking during hospitalization;
 (5) growing sense of parenting competence;
 (6) growing sense of attachment to the child;
 (7) objective interpretation of information received regarding the child's status;
 (8) acceptance of and constructive adaptation to the child's condition;
 (9) confidence in assuming total responsibility for the child;
(10) realistic view of the child and potential needs at the time of discharge;
(11) free verbalization of needs and concerns to staff and family, and
(12) realistic view of the staff and its expectations.

Social work intervention with the families helps to decrease the maladaptive and increase adaptive responses.

No matter how the stages of development and acquisition of tasks for parenting the MR/ED child are described, the objective of the services provided by the social workers is to help the parenting persons to help the child to function independently at the highest level he or she is capable of.

There is often an overlapping of the stages described. Mourning is encouraged so that once the grief process progresses, a healthy attachment is formed as opposed to a pathological one. At this point, concrete services can be provided. Throughout the relationship with the parents it is important to listen to their feelings, be supportive and give accurate information to them regarding their child. Often prolonged counseling is needed and sometimes individual therapy is needed for personality reorganization. Most importantly, there is a need to deal with the down to earth issues for maintaining their child 24 h in the home and what this means to total familial relationships. Management programs and various techniques for limit setting are taught according to total family needs. Factors involved are as follows: (1) the family's ability to cope with the impact of the child and stress situations as they occur; (2) the personality needs of the individual family members (parents, siblings, grandparents, and other extended family members), and (3) environmental surroundings and community resource and support systems available.

Formulation of the Casework Treatment Plan

A formulation of the casework treatment plan for the family is made after the following data are collected. A developmental and health history is recorded by the pediatrician, and the child psychiatrist makes a psychiatric assessment of the child. A psychosocial history is noted by the social worker, which includes a full assessment of the family responses to their MR/ED child, inclusive of how they see the problems affecting their present family situation and relationships. The composition of the nuclear family is examined including subsystems and, in particular, the role of the family members. For example:

(1) who parents, leads, makes decisions and how?
(2) who solves problems and how?
(3) who under- and overfunctions and how?
(4) who implements tasks and how?
(5) who takes care of the family's emotional life (hurts, worries) and how?

(6)   who carries a symptom (sick, weak, delinquent) and how?
(7)   who has fun and how?

Another important aspect is the communication patterns in the family. What are the communication styles, verbal vs. non-verbal, overt and covert behaviors, feeling and thinking styles, clearness of messages, meanings of functions, and the degree of assumptions. It is important also to know the flow of communication. Are there triangles, splits, alliances and/or scape-goating themes? An overall picture of family dynamics is needed. It is important to have a sense of how family members relate to the family and to each other. Is there mature self-differentiation or is there unhealthy fusion and lack of self-relatedness? Even though the above elements are seen in most of the families, the quantitative preponderence is what is crucial.

When establishing the psychosocial history of the family it is also significant to relate what the family is experiencing at the time of this child's hospitalization to other turning points or stages of the family's development. Allow the parents to reflect on their first meeting, courtship, marriage, the birth of their children, experiences of children starting school or older children leaving home. The role of the extended family members is also important: who is isolated; who is seen and not seen; who cares for grand-parents and/or ill family members; what family members are deceased and how were these losses coped with; what values and myths have been transmitted and what is the role of religion in the family. What have been the environmental changes the family has experienced? What are the total family's attitudes toward mental retardation in general and the specific characteristics and disabilities of the child who is the patient? What are, if any, the family secrets? All past history has its emotional significance and shows how the family has coped with stresses.

An examination of the family's present social network is also important. What is the family's social and economic status, career involvements, ethnic groups and friends? What relationships do the family members have that are supportive and satisfying? An excellent tool to use with the siblings to elicit this information is family activity drawings using crayons and large sheets of paper.

All of the data collected through the above-mentioned interviews are consolidated and the implications for a treatment plan is developed, with the family strengths and liabilities delineated for long-term and short-term planning.

Types of Social Work Intervention

The following examples are a multidimensional approach to social work treatment with the families of MR/ED children. These treatment modalities approach the family and its subsystems in all the areas which affect the individual members. These modalities are based on the belief that establishing good parent-child relationships as well as healthy sibling relationships are especially problematic when a child is handicapped. It is not only important to sort out the interactional patterns, but also to evaluate the child's particular characteristics and behavioral patterns in the home environment and social-emotional climate. The social worker's knowledge of parental expectations and their techniques of behavior management are essential in treating the entire primary unit. Behavioral changes, environmental manipulations, counseling and education for new approaches to parenting and living with a special needs child are demonstrated in the following case examples.

Short-Term Individual Counseling

One approach to parental treatment is the use of short-term individual counseling.

Example: S. was an 8-year-old boy admitted on September 27, 1977, to the John Merck Program and discharged on December 16, 1977. S.'s diagnosis was as follows: (1) profound mental retardation; (2) over-reaction of childhood, withdrawn, unable to form lasting relationships, self-stimulating alternating with self-abuse, physical aggressiveness, temper tantrums, and destructiveness; (3) epilepsy, and (4) organic brain syndrome of unknown etiology.

Three months of individual counseling with the mother (12 sessions) dealt around the issues of the day-to-day impact of her child in the family. Upon referral her wish was to have S. (who had been in a residential care facility) come back to the family. Counseling sessions revolved around her intellectualizations and feelings regarding the pros and cons of long-term care. Much support and education was given in helping her to look at ways to have quality parenting for S. with the support of a 24-hour residential care facility during the week; and weekends he could visit home. Mrs. S. had recently remarried and also needed to look at the quality of the total relationships in the family, inclusive of one sibling and an expected child. The results were that Mrs. S. was able to formulate some insights about the impact of S.'s needs, and the John Merck Program staff were able to find another residential setting whereby S. could have a higher level of stimulation and attention; which was closer geographically to their home and one where Mrs. S. was better satisfied.

Couple Counseling

Another approach to treatment is couple counseling.

Example: J. was a 3½-year-old boy (twin) admitted to the John Merck Program on August 30, 1977, to the day program and discharged in August 1979. J.'s diagnosis was: (1) severe mental retardation; (2) seizure disorder, and (3) hyperkinesis.

Two years of couple counseling with J.'s parents and siblings dealt primarily with the theme that J. had changed the total family complex in the fact that the two older siblings cared for the two younger ones and J. was playing a significant role in the relationship of these parents. Their overinvestment in him was a result of fear and anxiety that he would die in a seizure. Movement was evidenced prior to discharge by the fact that J. no longer slept with his parents, and the family relationships and roles were redefined with the remaining four siblings receiving the parenting they needed and J., the patient, with seizures controlled, functioning at the EMR level was allowed to function at a higher degree of independence at home.

Counseling Involving the Extended Family Members

Counseling which involves the extended family members and reconstituted units is also needed for different family structures.

Example: T. was a 9-year-old girl admitted to the John Merck Program to residential care. Diagnosis: mildly retarded and disturbed.

Six months of family counseling centered in trying to equalize the adult roles within the family unit, which included the paternal grandmother as well as three step siblings. T.'s new stepmother had 3 children by two previous marriages; T. was a product of the father's first marriage and the youngest sibling was a child of the present marriage. Much work was done with parenting and child management in general as well as instructions for financial resources available to the family. Another emphasis was placed on the reintegration process of T. into the family as well as her sex education. The sleeping arrangements for this family were altered as T. previously was sleeping with the paternal grandmother, which caused rivalry among the siblings.

Intensive Family Therapy

Intensive family therapy is often needed depending on the degree of pathology evidenced in the familial relationship.

Example: L., age 6 years 4 months was admitted to residential care from March 13, 1979, to June 28, 1979, with a diagnosis of profound retardation with emotional components due to self-stimulatory behaviors.

For 3 months family therapy was provided by a child psychiatry resident and the social worker as cotherapist. Sessions over the 3-month period included the parents, the maternal grandparents, and the maternal aunt, each session lasting 1½ h.

Family therapy sessions dealt with the following themes:

(1) maternal overinvolvement with L.;
(2) paternal role in perpetuation of this pattern;
(3) the high-risk situation for sibling K.;
(4) ambivalence regarding separation and residential placement;
(5) parental anger displaced from L. to staff, and passive aggressive modes of expression;
(6) denial of anger and marital tensions;
(7) intellectualization and denial of sadness, anger, and isolation of affect in the grieving process;
(8) overwhelming expectations of self and others;
(9) availability and underuse of the support system within the family unit itself;
(10) patterns of overprotection in the maternal extended family and lack of separation and individuation in maternal family;
(11) apparent pattern of a need for a sick or weak family member to absorb the family's energies, and
(12) patterns of stress and isolation in the paternal extended family.

Movement on the part of the family members in response to therapy has been noted in the following changes:

(1) the decision for placement of L. in a residential setting;
(2) the initiation and search of a setting that family members felt was best for both L. and parents;
(3) an increased ability to express feelings to one another;
(4) an increased expression of some insight into family stresses;
(5) an initial awareness of the grieving process and sadness and anger expressed as a response to this;
(6) an awareness of a need and motivation on the part of Mr. and Mrs. R. to continue in therapy, and
(7) an interest and motivation expressed by Mrs. R. in getting involved in some interior designer work.

Socio-Behavioral Approach

A socio-behavioral approach to treatment for an intact healthy family can also be used. The following is a detailed exploration of one family's treatment.

Example: J.M. III had lived at a residential school for exceptional children for 2½ years prior to his admission to the John Merck Program. His parents made this decision as they felt this would be the best setting to meet J.'s needs. Referral from the school was made on December 4, 1978. Mr. and Mrs. M. and J. were seen by the pediatrician June 1, 1978 for a preadmission evaluation, at which time J. was placed on the waiting list. On December 21, 1978, J. was terminated at school due to his increased behavioral problems. J. was admitted on January 3, 1979, with the residential expansion at John Merck. His diagnosis: mild mental retardation and behavioral disorder of childhood.

J.'s immediate family constellation consists of his parents and two siblings. Mrs. M. presently works as a part-time secretary at a local preschool developmental center. Mr. M. is a carpenter with U.S. Steel. Following their third child, Mrs. M. had a tubal ligation. J.'s brother, age 11, is an average 7th grade student; his sister, age 7, is in 2nd grade and performs above average in her studies.

The M.s present as a highly structured Catholic family unit who experienced a high level of frustration and anxiety regarding J.'s behaviors, regardless of their attempts to set limits and be consistent. Their hope is that J. will be able to be as independent as possible and be able as an adult to work in a sheltered workshop and have friends of his own. This family presented as appropriately involved and workable.

Intervention: one of the intervention methods used with this family was a socio-behavioral approach. Sessions with the family were highly structured therapeutic encounters scheduled on a weekly basis for 8 months from January to September 1979.

The following methodologies were slowly and systematically used:

(1) task-oriented counseling sessions for decision making;
(2) educational sessions with members of the multidisciplinary team (a) for explanations for agreement to the use of diagnostic testing procedures for J., (b) for the use of reinforcement techniques such as social praise for J., (c) for the use of prompting and verbal redirection techniques, (d) for a study of environmental and interactional patterns of the family unit, and
(3) modeling, classroom observations and live demonstrations of behavioral management techniques.

Treatment: decision making and identification. The initial task with this family was to sort out the facts and feelings of each member about J. again becoming a full-time family member. Each member listed the pros and cons of this possible change in their life-style. One main theme that emerged was that they felt incomplete as a family without him and looked forward to their weekends with him because they loved him. The outcome of these initial sessions was a decision to have J. return home if they and J. could learn new ways to make life easier for all of them. The family then identified the issues they saw as needing to be modified and the targets for behavioral intervention were established. The following are direct quotations from the family members:

'J. has to be watched over all the time because of his fascination with plugs, fans, dryers and other appliances.'
'J. never stays in one place.'
'J. doesn't play with toys or enjoy them and doesn't play with other children.'

'J. talks to his hands ... makes strange sounds ... breaks things ... talks out loud in church ... and cries a lot.'

'J. wakes us up too early on Saturday and Sundays and won't go to sleep for hours at night after bedtime, maing strange noises.'

'J. makes my mother nervous because he has to be told over and over to do something and just won't listen.'

'J. wets his pants and bed all the time.'

'J. takes away some attention from the other children.'

Treatment: intervention process. The initiation of the intervention with this family was to have them look at the total environment including issues of control and consequences of present interactional patterns. The workbook text *Living with Children* by *Gerald Patterson* of the Behavioral Research Institute of Oregon was used, with both parents to begin retraining for parenting J. in a new way.

They worked closely with the John Merck Program staff to change some undesirable habits in the family patterns that maintained some of J.'s behaviors. Father increased his limit-setting role and J. as well as his two siblings responded well. Both parents also reflected that they had not reinforced the positive behaviors of any of the children as much as they would accent mistakes or negative performances. A major area of concern that emerged at this time was mother's regime in the house-hold and parenting responsibilities. Father was able to see his minimal involvement was quite controlling and as mother 'let go' of structure and was more relaxed and flexible, he became higher functioning. One example is as follows:

Dinner didn't have to be served at exactly 5:00 p.m. and mother didn't have to constantly superwise J. during dinner preparation; father took responsibility for this time period and they found this most effective.

Another dynamic that surfaced was that these parents learned new ways to compromise, which enhanced their marital relationship. They both expressed feeling somewhat isolated from each other and resentments toward each other regarding responsibilities and not receiving the needed attention from the other, both focusing too much on J. As they began to help each other balance the family needs, they were more able to express and balance their own needs. They then structured more time for themselves. They planned times out together and again enjoyed being with each other. This became so reinforcing, their own motivation was perpetuated for continued change in the family life-style.

J.'s siblings were also involved in sessions. The children were initiated into treatment through the use of family art drawings.

These pictures of family in activities as well as their discussions of their art products reflected the following:

(1)   they felt a need to protect J.
(2)   they didn't know how to play with J.
(3)   they saw J. as a family member, and
(4)   they had a good grasp on the fact that 'J. was a child whose mind was behind other kids his age and that he did do some things that weren't so good'.

After J. learned to play with certain toys and do things like them (such as play ball, play cards and certain games) they had play interaction sessions with J. directed by the therapeutic educator (teacher). They and their parents also involved themselves three Saturday mornings in the preparation for the Special Olympics with J. The physical therapist, also had a session with the children, teaching them physical exercise activities they could do with J. As a result, J. did not spend a lot of his time alone in the basement family room listening to music. The family members increased their play and interactional skills with J. and enjoyed him for longer periods of time.

J.'s reintegration into his family became more natural. Weekend therapeutic home visits were initiated and monitored through the use of the home visit report form which consistently reflected a decrease in J.'s negative behaviors. It was at this point the family requested having J. on Sunday nights also, because they felt things were going so well. Through the use of verbal redirection, J. was able to stay in one place, not talk out loud in church and not break objects. His crying spells also decreased and as his ability to play increased he not only played with them in one place but could also entertain himself with toys for a period of time. J. is able also to share in family outings and activities.

Some environmental changes were necessary also to prevent some of J.'s behaviors. The fan was removed from J.'s reach; a lock was installed in the basement to prevent access to the dryer and other safety measures were established such as plug protectors.

Mr. and Mrs. M. were then instructed in a Bedtime Music Program established by the multidisciplinary team and tried on the unit. It was theorized that J. lying in bed was stimulus-deprived and therefore created his own noise-making. A radio was provided with slow beat music to set him to sleep. The first weekend this was tried at home it was effective within 15 min.

The parents were then instructed in the use of medication in combination with an overcorrection procedure for wet pants and wet bed. J. was placed on Ditropan 5 mg for spastic bladder and because continuous dribbling persisted the overcorrection technique was used. J.'s self-toileting program presently reflects very few accidents at home.

Mr. and Mrs. M. then participated in Modelling Sessions, live demonstrations and classroom observations for the implementation of Behavioral Management Techniques for individually designed programs in the following areas: (1) the program to eliminate auditory-visual self stimulation, through the use of visual screening; (2) the program to increase group play and interactional skills, and (3) the program to improve self-management.

J. was discharged on September 25, 1979, to his home and is attending a classroom for mentally retarded and learning adjustment problem children in his local community.

J. has adjusted well at home. His family is pleased with their changes as well as relieved of their anxiety and pain in parenting this special child.

Group Sessions for Parents

Group sessions for parents in the John Merck Program are also available. One series of parent group sessions guided by the social work staff was held for 8 planned weeks. At each 2-hour session a talk by a representative of each discipline was given by the professional staff including the dentist. This was followed by a period of questions and answers. Then an hour for parental interaction took place whereby parents could share with each other and be supportive. It was a good experience reflected by the fact that they continued for two additional sessions and shared telephone numbers afterward for continued sharing and support.

A second series was set up for evenings so that more of the working parents could have the opportunity for group support also. A series of filmstrips have been developed by *Parents Magazine* on 'Intellectual and Emotional Disabilities', these were used to educate and emphasize the parental roles.

An outcome of these two series is the development of the John Merck Parents Association. This parents' group meets the third Sunday of the month. The purpose of this group is to provide a time to share and receive support from one another.

The parents involved are:

(1) parents of children on the waiting list
(2) parents of children who are presently patients, and

(3) parents of children who have been discharged. The first hour of the session is usually devoted to business-like issues, sometimes a speaker is invited and then the rest of the time is spent in interacting. The parents find this to be a satisfying and rewarding experience for each other in sharing and comfort.

Other Methods

Other methods used with the families and incorporating other professions are modelling, behavior management training, charting, classroom observations and parent-child interaction sessions. The following cases show how these techniques are used.

Case 1. T. is a 9½ year old boy admitted to the John Merck Program on March 14, 1977 as a day patient and on October 25, 1977, to full hospitalization.

Diagnosis: (1) severely mentally retarded; (2) mildly psychotic episodes, and (3) withdrawal reaction of childhood.

Modelling[1] sessions were held on a weekly basis for Mrs. C. with T.'s teacher. The therapeutic educator demonstrated methods of holding T.'s interest in a task and praising him verbally and giving him physical cues. Mrs. C. joined in the sessions at the end with the teacher and T. and increased in her ability to use the techniques in relating to her son. She expressed more enjoyment with T. as she saw him attending and responding for longer periods of time.

Case 2. G. was a 7-year-old boy admitted as a day patient on October 5, 1976, and discharged on March 7, 1978. Diagnosis: (1) moderate retardation; (2) behavioral disorders, and (3) hyperactivity.

These parents (mainly mother) were seen weekly at the John Merck Program. The emphasis was behavioral management training. Many techniques for limit setting and reward systems were taught to the parents for use in the home.

As their confidence increased and the use of firm limit setting was successful, their negative feelings decreased and they became more able to enjoy their relationship with their son. One specific program was geared at being able to have G. go on shopping trips with the family. Initially, he would tantrum. With the management program he would go with the child care worker and mother for a shopping trip and if he behaved he received a reward at the John Merck Program. As time went on he received the reward in the car and finally a reward at home. Eventually he was able to handle the shopping trips.

Case 3. M. is a 9-year-old girl admitted initially to the John Merck Program as a day patient on September 25, 1975, and then to full hospitalization on April 25, 1977. Diagnosis: (1) moderate mental retardation; (2) childhood schizophrenia.

The use of charting with M.'s mother was through the Self-Help Bath Chart. The nurse was accenting hygiene, grooming and dressing for M. It was necessary to make

[1] This type of modelling by professionals and active participation of parents is part of the original design of the John Merck Program by Dr. Jakab and serves as one of the essential treatment tools within the prescribed therapies of most patients.

mother aware of the need to keep M. clean *nightly* so as to help M. with developing a good self-image as well as a means of having her more acceptable by peers and other adults if she looked and smelled clean. Mother was instructed to jot down nightly on charts the time, body parts, as well as the behaviors and the amounts of assistance needed. M. now is totally self-care-oriented for hygiene and dressing except for washing her hair.

Case 4. C. was a 7-year-old boy admitted to the John Merck Program on June 23, 1977, as a day patient and to residential care on August 1, 1977, and discharged on March 31, 1978, against medical advice. Diagnosis: (1) moderate retardation; (2) hyperactivity (distractable and disorganized).

Mrs. H. was encouraged to participate in classroom observations as well as 1:1 task-oriented sessions of C. with his child care worker in order to see how C. was doing in the classroom setting as well as how he interacted on a 1:1 relationship with an adult.

Mrs. H. was unable to focus on the improved behaviors of C. as she really felt he was the same in the home. She would ask questions about other children in order to avoid discussing C. She commented that the 1:1 relationship with the child care worker reflected hers.

Case 5. D. was a 7-year-old girl who was admitted as a day patient to the John Merck Program on July 19, 1976, and discharged on August 12, 1977. Diagnosis: (1) mild to moderate mental retardation; (2) adjustment reaction of childhood.

Both Mr. and Mrs. M. were in individual parent-child interaction sessions. D. had experienced a lot of difficulty in separating from mother; was withdrawn and generally immature and was unwilling to interact with peers and somewhat undisciplined by the parents.

Both parents were more understanding of D.'s abilities and limitations and were able to respond more appropriately to them. The main theme was to help them to allow D. to express herself as an individual rather than them insisting on a level of performance at their expectation, during their play sessions with her. They also learned to set more appropriate limits with D.'s behaviors with the aid of the child care worker.

In conclusion, it is suggested that the following poem be considered for thought:

'Children Learn What They Live'

If a child lives with criticism,
  He learns to condemn.
If a child lives with hostility,
  He learns to fight.
If a child lives with ridicule,
  He learns to be shy.
If a child lives with shame,
  He learns to feel guilty.
If a child lives with tolerance,
  He learns to be patient.
If a child lives with encouragement,
  He learns confidence.

If a child lives with praise,
  He learns to appreciate.
If a child lives with fairness,
  He learns justice.
If a child lives with security,
  He learns to have faith.
If a child lives with approval,
  He learns to like himself.
If a child lives with acceptance and friendship,
  He learns to find love in the world.'

Educational Performance Associates, Inc.

Suggested Reading

1 Anthony, E.J.; Bender, T.: Parenthood its psychology and psychopathology (Little, Brown, Boston 1970).
2 Baum, M.H.: The dynamic factors affecting family adjustment to the handicapped child. Except. Child. *28:* 387–392 (1962).
3 Beck, H.L.: Social services to the mentally retarded (Thomas, Bannerstone House 1969).
4 Begab, M.J.: Casework for the mentally retarded – casework with parents. The mentally retarded child: a guide to the services of social agencies, pp. 58–68 (US Department of HEW, Welfare Administration, Children's Bureau, Washington 1963).
5 Bernal, M.E.; Juel, A.N.: A survey of parent training manuals. J. appl. Behav. Anal. *Winter:* 533 (1978).
6 Carr, J.: The effect of the severely subnormal on their families; in Clarke, Clarke, Mental deficiency: The changing outlook; 3rd ed., pp. 807–839 (Free Press, New York 1974).
7 Cohen, P.D.: The impact of the handicapped child on the family. Soc. Casework *43:* 137–142 (1962).
8 Farber, B.: Effects of a severely mentally retarded child on family integration. Child Dev. *24/2* (1959).
9 Grossman, F.K.: Brothers and sisters of retarded children (Syracuse University Press, Syracuse 1972).
10 Hersh, A.: Changes in family functioning accompanying the placement of a mentally retarded child in a residential school. AAMD Annu. Meet., Boston 1968).
11 Kanner, L.: Parents' feelings about retarded children. Am. J. ment. Defic. *57:* 375–383 (1953).
12 Mahler, M.S.: The psychological birth of the human infant (Basic Books, New York 1975).
13 Mahoney, S.C.: Observations concerning counseling with parents of mentally retarded children. Am. J. ment. Defic. *63:* 81–86 (1958).
14 Nihira, K.; Meyers, C.E.; Mink, I.T.: Home environment, family adjustment, and the development of mentally retarded children. J. appl. Res. ment. Retard. *1:* 5–24 (1980).
15 Olshansky, S.: Chronic sorrow: a response to having a mentally defective child. Soc. Casework *43:* 190–193 (1962).
16 Olshansky, S.: Parent responses to a mentally defective child. Ment. Retard. *4:* 21–23 (1966).
17 Peed, S.; Roberts, M.; Forehand, R.: Evaluating the effectiveness of a standardized parent training program in altering the interaction of mothers and their non-compliant children. Behav. Modif. *1:* 323–349 (1977).
18 Robinson, H.; Robinson, N.: Problems in the family of a retarded child; in The mentally retarded child; 2nd ed., pp. 413–431 (McGraw-Hill, Maidenhead 1976).
19 Ross, P.: Psychological counseling with parents of retarded children. Ment. Retard. *1:* 345–350 (1963).
20 Ryckman, D.B.; Henderson, R.A.: The meaning of a retarded child for his parents: a focus for counselors. Ment. Retard. *4:* 4–7 (1966).

21   Schilds, S.: The family of the retarded child; in Koch, Dobson, The mentally retarded child and his family, pp. 454–465 (Brunner/Mazel, 1976).

22   Seitz, S.; Hoekenga, R.: Modeling as a training tool for retarded children and their parents. Ment. Retard. *12/2:* (1974).

23   Sheimo, S.L.: Problems in helping parents of mentally defective and handicapped children. Am. J. ment. Defic. *56:* 42–47 (1951).

24   Smith, A.D.: Reports of recent research and evaluation in social work with the young handicapped child. Proc. New Concepts in Human Services for the Developing Young Child., pp. 83–93 (1978).

25   Solnit, A.J.; Stark, M.H.: Mourning and the birth of a defective child; in The psychoanalytic history of the child, vol. 16, pp. 523–537 (International Universities Press, New York 1961).

26   Tizard, J.; Grad, J.C.: The mentally handicapped and their families (Oxford University Press, London 1961).

27   Tredgold, R.D.; Soddy, K.: The family and the retarded child; in Mental retardation; 11th ed., pp. 403–433 (1970).

28   Turner, A.: Therapy with families of a mentally retarded child. J. marit. Fam. Ther. *April:* 167 (1980).

29   Wortis, H.: Parent counseling; in Wortis, Mental retardation: An annual review, vol. 4 (Brunner/Mazel, 1972).

30   Wolfensberger, W.: Counseling the parents of the retarded; in Baumeister, Mental retardation, appraisal, education and rehabilitation (Aldine, Chicago 1967).

31   Wolfensberger, W.; Kurtz, R.A.: Management of the family of the mentally retarded (Follett Educational Corp., 1969).

17 Caring for Normal and Developmentally Delayed Infants

Magda Gerber

It is our hope that the professional readers of this book will convey the essence of this message to the parents whose children are under their care.

This paper deals with two important but often misunderstood elements of raising children: quality time and discipline.

Quality Time

Quality time! We all talk about it. We all want it, both for our children and for ourselves. But, do we really know what it is all about?

It is full unhurried attention. Under the right circumstances it is a peaceful rewarding time for *both* parties because, ideally, it is a time of no ambivalence, one for open listening, taking in the other person, trying to fully understand the other's point of view. This unique time can happen under many circumstances, but we divide it into two themes:

The 'Wants Nothing' Quality Time

That is when the parent does not want to *do* anything with the child, has no plans other than wanting to simply *be* with the child. Just floor-sitting, being available, being there with all the senses awakened to the child; watching, listening, thinking of only that child. It sounds easy, but few can truly do it.

Most of us are used to and conditioned to *doing* something. This is not 'I've-got-to-do-this' kind of time. It is more a time for taking in and waiting. We fully accept the child's beingness just by our own receptive beingness. We are telling the child that we are really there and aware. (Not what shall I cook, clean, or whom to call). The child should not feel he has to perform, because the parent is not sending out the kind of demanding vibes that say,

'I am here now, what would you like to do?' Most relationships are based on performance. We tend to stimulate our children to produce something. This should not happen during this time of quality listening and watching. If the child feels like doing something completely on his own, do not leave. It is very comforting to know that the parent is there, really *there* without the little person under pressure to have to do something to keep the parent's attention.

For an infant it is a peaceful presence – a quiet assurance in this being-ness. This separate play from the parent teaches the child to depend on his own inner security. If you do this with a newborn, you see the child fully, you really observe and discover a person unfolding.

Quality time is like an investment in the future of your child as well as in the present, you are available, waiting; the child is the initiator.

The 'Wants Something' Quality Time
This is when you *do* have a goal to accomplish something together, such as dressing, bathing, feeding, etc. This too should be regarded as quality time. You can make sure the child knows that this time is different from your 'wants nothing time' by actually saying 'now I want to diaper you. Now it is time to get dressed, etc.'

This is a time when you work for cooperation. If you think in terms of quality, you use the time for learning to do a task together when you expect the child to cooperate. It should become something you both enjoy doing together. Your *availability* is still there, except during this time you *also* have expectations. This is the beginning of introducing and reinforcing discipline.

Teaching is not a separate function. It is an everyday life experience. Too many educators put pressure on parents to try to teach their infants earlier and earlier.

A safe environment in which the baby can move and explore is the kind of learning experience the child profits from the most. Teaching is one thing and learning is another. What the parents teach are themselves, as models of being human, their moods, their reactions, their facial expressions and actions. If the mother always tells the child what she is doing, the baby is learning about the real world around him.

Quality time is a time of growth, movement, ebb and flow. If you can give these two kinds of quality time ('wants nothing' and 'wants something' themes), then you are really growing with your children. The child never feels manipulated. What you do with your child is an investment for the

Table I. Guidelines to make all care activities optimal learning experiences; the dialogue

Carer	Infant	Process of learning through
Greets child: 'you seem to be having a good time with your rubber giraffe', tells and shows what she is going to do; 'but I want to pick you up and diaper you'	pays attention	anticipation attention awareness
Waits for infant's reaction:'you're not quite ready so I'll wait a little; one or two minutes later: 'now you seem ready'	responds to the initiations of carer (positively or negatively)	responsiveness to each other expectations
Asks for cooperation or follows child's lead: 'first we have to remove your overall, you pull out your foot'	cooperates and participates	the joy of pleasing
Encourages mastery: 'you helped with this (touches foot), now pull out the other one'	achieves mastery, becomes playful, teasing; doing the opposite of what is asked	and actively participating mastery
Enters the game (smiling): 'this doesn't look like a foot, but more like a hand to me', but eventually gets back to (business) task	enjoys the process (laughs)	autonomy security
Enjoys the process		challenge

future. Quality time is what everybody really wants – a gift of time and attention. For guidelines to make all care activities optimal learning experiences see table I.

Discipline

Close your eyes and mentally clarify how you feel about discipline. Open your eyes and write down your own definition of it. You may be surprised as was I after reading this dictionary definition of discipline: 'training that develops self-control, character'.

If one would think of what is to be accomplished, what is to be achieved by discipline, there would be an entirely different feeling for what it is. With discipline, you must have a certain goal in mind. Basically, most parents are afraid of the power struggle. They are afraid of overpowering the child, afraid they will destroy the child's free will and personality. This is a terribly erroneous attitude. Lack of discipline is not kindness, it is neglect.

Confusion over discipline arises when you lose sight of what is important and what is not. The idea of discipline is like the red, yellow, and green light: The *red light* is when the baby crawls on the floor right over to a big, sharp knife. Watching this, you do not stop to ponder about the effect of taking the knife away will have on the child's psyche. You just cleanly reach and pick up the knife. With the red light there are no guilt-weighing, ambivalent thoughts. You just do what you must do immediately.

With the *yellow light* the situation can be negotiated. For example, the child wants you to be with him and at the moment you want to do something else. Should you sacrifice your moment for the child's demands or is that not realistic just then? Sacrificing your own needs for the child's only creates inward anger within both of you. If it is important that you finish reading the newspaper before you play with your little person, then clearly convey that message. Let the child know what it is you want to do for yourself and what you expect the child to do, so that playing quietly while you read can later grow into hours of secure separateness; both of you doing something independent of the other and still feeling good about your relationship.

The *green light* is when you want what the child wants. You give the child a few choices of something to do, and you are ready to do any of them. We all need many green lights in life to be able to accept the reds and yellows, too.

It is not always easy for parents to say 'no'. A parent's ambivalences, guilt feelings, and areas of confusion in his or her role will be picked up and used amazingly fast by children. They seem to have a sixth sense for it. Any ambivalence from a parent will produce a nagging child.

One misconception most parents share is that children must be happy all the time. That is an unrealistic expectation. Many goals involve pain to get there. When children find this out too late in life, after being sheltered and buffered unrealistically, they will find things difficult and frightening to cope with. There is no way over indulged children are going to be happy, because they seldom get direct honest responses from their parents. These are basically neglecting parents. Children are begging for discipline and for structure. A child has a difficult time growing up with ambivalent parents. When you say 'no', really mean it. Let your face and posture reflect 'no' as well.

Once the external disciplinary lessons are learned, the child begins to internalize – to learn the lessons on his own, and even realize that some things that are desired are not always good for us or the other person. Structure, expectations, predictability – all add to responsibly raising and loving our children. How free we all feel deep within ourselves once we understand where we stand in the scheme of things.

Postscript: Wishes for Parents and Babies

First, my wishes for children, I wish they could grow according to their natural pace, sleep when sleepy, eat when hungry, cry when upset, play and explore without being unnecessarily interrupted. To be allowed to grow and blossom as each was meant to be and not molded or shoved into some mode of faddism that confines like a violin case. And I wish children would *not* have to: (1) perform for their parents, sit up when ready for rolling, walk when ready for crawling. A child can be pushed to these things, but physiologically may not be really ready. In our culture we push to attain these states faster than they should be reached. (2) I wish children would not have to reassure parents of their effectiveness, i.e., smile when frustrated, clap hands when sleepy – 'if my child smiles at me this shows I am a good parent.' (3) Not be Ping-Pong balls between parents. (4) Not be experimental subjects of toy manufacturers, cereal makers, new fads and theories in child care. Please, parents, the next holiday season do not succumb to the pressure of buying expensive, complex toys designed to be used certain ways. They rarely give children opportunities to explore and use them in their own way. Toys designed to entertain create passive onlookers, future TV addicts, rather than curious, actively learning children. Pressures from commercials are especially strong at the holiday time of year. So think. Think of the many children who are lost and bored unless entertained and who keep asking, 'what shall I do now?'

And my last wish to children would be that they could communicate to their parents this poem (author anonymous):

Please let me grow as I be,
And try to understand why I want to grow like me,
Not like my mother wants me to be,
Not like my father hopes I'll be,
Or like my teacher thinks I should be,
Please understand and help me grow
Just like me!

For parents, I wish a lot of things too. I wish they would: (1) feel secure but not rigid; (2) accepting, but setting limits; (3) be available, but not intruding; (4) be patient, but 'true to thine own self'; (5) be realistic, but consistent in their expectations; (6) have the wisdom to resist new fads; (7) achieve a balance in giving quality time to their children and to themselves and, (8) achieve a state of self-respect and give equal respect to their children.

And I have a special wish for fathers too. I wish that fathers could assume a new role of fatherhood based on human relationship rather than believing that being warm and gentle is not 'manly' or that a father is expected to be tough – to throw the children into the air, or blow cigarette smoke in their faces (yes, I have seen this done 'playfully'). Rough-housing scares babies. What I am saying is that playful pummeling is okay as long as it is not forced by father and hard on the child. I would like fathers to not be afraid to be their own drummer, to be themselves, to know that just because they are men, being 'macho' is not really expected of them by their infants. They can be tender and soothing and quiet and still be 'manly'.

I wish above all else that parents do not lose sight of laughter. That through all of the pain we might see and feel around us we maintain our sense of humor. People who take life too seriously are terrible to live with!

Disorders Frequently Associated with Mental Retardation

18 Development of Communication Skills as Related to Early Psychosocial Development

Lawrence A. Bloom

The purpose of this paper is to explore certain aspects of language acquisition which are of major significance to anyone attempting to understand some of the reasons why the retarded child encounters difficulties in language acquisition, and some of the reasons why speech-language pathologists encounter difficulties in developing effective treatment strategies for retarded persons.

This chapter is not intended to encompass all aspects of the development of communication skills. Subjects such as the relationship of language and the brain, the required integrity of the organism, perception, stages of language acquisition, language and cognition, language and hearing, etc. have been dealt with extensively in the literature [1, 3, 5, 7, 10, 12, 13, 17]. A suggested reading list follows the references.

This chapter will explore the relationship between psychosocial development and the acquisition of communication skills, as well as the implications of this relationship for the understanding of communication problems of retarded persons and their treatment needs.

Psychosocial Communication Development

Communication skills evolve as an integral part of total development. The major requisites for the development of human communication skills fall into two broad categories. The first relates to the integrity of the organism. In order to learn to communicate the infant must be reasonably intact organically. The extent of the required intactness is not fully understood. One sees children with documented major brain damage who learn to communicate, and children with suspected 'minimal' brain damage who do not. The second category of requisites relates to the integrity of relationships. If the child is to develop communication, he must be able to relate to a primary caregiver, or a psychological 'mother.' This person must engage with the child in an intense relationship, integral to which she furnishes a communication system and a high level of expectancy that the child will learn the system and use it.

The child learns language in order to organize his experiences [4], and in order to communicate with others. In a sense, he learns to 'talk' in order to talk to himself and talk to others. These are interdependent tasks. The most significant 'other' for the child in the early language learning years is the mother. It is she who furnishes the model for the use of language for organization and use of communication in relating, the impetus for the use of communication, and the expectancy that the child will do all of this. The manner in which all of this takes place will be the subject of the remainder of this section.

The relationship between psychosocial development and communication development will be reviewed in a framework of *Margaret Mahler's* concepts [8, 9]. Stages of development discussed here will be those described in detail by *Mahler* et al. [8] in The Psychological Birth of the Human Infant. References to concomitant language development will be primarily those of this author.

Mahler described the first few weeks of extra-uterine life as an undifferentiated period during which there is no discernable distinction for the infant between inner and outer reality and no distinction for him between himself and his inanimate surroundings. There is even a lack of awareness of a mothering agent. *Mahler* designates this as the stage of 'normal autism.'

From approximately the second month on, a dim awareness develops as to the fact that what relieves the infant's instinctual tensions (hunger, etc.), comes from the outside world. A rudimentary perception of the need-satisfying object (person) marks the beginning of this phase of normal symbiosis, 'in which the infant behaves and functions as though he and his mother were an omnipotent system – a dual unity within one common boundary' [8]. This phase lasts through approximately the 5th month.

It is generally agreed that the sound production engaged in during the first few months of the infant's life is primarily reflexive in nature. Thus, the infant who does not differentiate between self and surroundings, or between symbiotic self-mother and surroundings does not appear to engage in sound production which has any communicative investment. The infant produces all the sounds which the human mechanism is capable of producing, and does not appear to be influenced, in the first few months, by the more selected sounds presented from the linguistic environment. An essential feature of the symbiotic state is the delusion of the omnipotent fusion and common boundary between the infant and the mother. The omnipotence implies that there is nothing of significance outside this shared core, thus there is no significance of communication to or from that which is outside the shared boundary.

There is, however, a major communicative experience being shared within the common boundary. The infant and mother engaged in a highly complex exchange of information which *Mahler* has referred to as 'mutual cuing.' Within this process, all sense modalities are involved, and a gradual evolution of mutual response takes place. In a sense, this is a process of total communication. The spoken word is often included in the process, though it is not necessary, and in the early months it is probably not the most important element in the mutual exchange. This is a continuous process of stimulus-response, which becomes increasingly complex and sophisticated over the period of months. It is probably this process, which is inclusive of but not exclusive to vocal sound production, which has resulted in the assumption of mothers that they can distinguish between different cries of their infants. The cry is probably only one of the multitude of cues to which the mother is responding. Inasmuch as these cues are taking place within the symbiotic boundary, it is unlikely that these cues will be appreciated by others in the environment.

This exclusive interaction pattern between infant and mother is the early, primitive origin of pleasurable communication for the child. This aspect of bonding is also a source of pleasure for the mother.

Throughout the next few months, as the infant's sensoriperceptive skills increase, he very gradually develops a primitive awareness of 'self' and 'non-self.' This developing awareness is essential to the development of a body concept, a concept of differentiation, and the onset of the normal separation-individuation process. This origin of early discrimination between one thing and another, which develops and evolves through the symbiotic relationship, may be considered the precursor of the kinds of discrimination abilities which will become increasingly important to the linguistic and cognitive development of the child.

During the early symbiotic months, the young infant has familiarized himself with the mothering half of his symbiotic self. *Mahler* indicates that this familiarization is accompanied by the unspecific, social smile. This gradually becomes the specific smiling response to the mother. This may be interpreted as a crucial sign that the specific bond between the infant and mother has been established. The social smile, and particularly the preferential smiling response to mother are usually a source of great pleasure to the mother. This constitutes another step forward in the mutual communication process, with the pleasure implied in and derived from the specific smiling response acting as a catalyst for a positive circular exchange of 'cuing.' Thus, the pleasurable aspects of communication are further reinforced for the infant.

Approximately by the end of the 5th month, which is the peak of the symbiotic stage, the beginnings of the next phase can be observed. This following stage is called separation-individuation by Mahler, and consists of four subphases. Each of these subphases has significance in the development of communication skills.

The first of *Mahler's* subphases is termed differentiation. It begins at approximately the age of 5 of 6 months and lasts for the next 4 or 5 months.

Obviously, the ability to differentiate and to perceive differences evolves and becomes heightened during this subphase. At first, this process centers around the mother. The infant familiarizes himself more thoroughly with all aspects of mother, including feel, taste, smell, look, and the total of that which is 'mother.' The child then perceives more clearly the differences between mother and those who are other than mother. It is during the latter part of this subphase that the child demonstrates what is sometimes referred to as 'stranger anxiety,' but which might better be described as a differential response to persons who are other than mother. Clearly, the differentiation can be expanded to more and more distant objects. Integral to this process is the additional differentiation of self from mother and others.

During this time span in the developing child's life, a change in oral sound production is usually noted. Sounds which are not heard by the child in his linguistic environment are likely to fade out of the child's production repertoire, and he is likely to restrict his oral sound production to those sounds produced by his mother and significant others in his environment. Careful listening reveals that the child is essentially babbling in the language of his environment. In addition, the child's overall oral sound gradually incorporates the 'melodic' aspects of the language he hears around him. Intonation and stress patterns of the environment will be recognized in the child's production. This incorporation of the phonemic and melodic patterns of the community may be summarized in the statement that the English child babbles in English, the French child babbles in French, etc.

All of this behavior is prelinguistic in nature, but appears to be a part of the ongoing development of the communication process which leads to the use of true language. Obviously, differentiation is dependent upon both organic and psychosocial development.

Mahler states that it is at the end of the first year and the early months of the second year that one can see clearly that the process of separation-individuation have two developmental tracks. One is the track of individuation, which is the evolution of intrapsychic autonomy, perception, memory, cognition, and reality testing. The other is separation, which involves differentiation, distancing, boundary formation, and disengagement from mother. Optimal situations are those in which the child progresses along both tracks at a similar rate of speed.

The second subphase of separation-individuation, as described by *Mahler,* is the practicing period.

> *Mahler* separates this subphase into two segments, the early practicing period, and the practicing period proper. She states that the early practicing phase is ushered in by the infant's ability to move away from the mother by crawling, righting himself, climbing, etc. The proper practicing period is characterized by free, upright locomotion. She states that at least three interrelated developments contribute to the child's early movement toward awareness of separateness and toward individuation. These are the establishment of a specific bond with mother, rapid body differentiation from mother, and growth and functioning of the perceptual apparatuses in close proximity to the mother.

During this second subphase, one is able to observe in the child a further movement along the line of developing communication skills. The child often begins to demonstrate some simple 'understanding' of the spoken word of others. He will continue to incorporate the linguistic sounds of the environment into his utterances, so that his utterances sound even more like the true language of his environment. He demonstrates awareness and interest in the communication of others, and is likely to incorporate increasingly more utterances in his communication to others, particularly to mother. Clearly he has begun to develop both receptively and expressively a 'communicative set.' However, the child's periodic need for refueling through direct physical contact with mother indicates that this phase of development is still highly dependent upon the relationship with and availability of mother.

The third subphase is referred to by *Mahler* as rapprochement. She states that this begins as the child becomes able to walk, and lasts from about 14 to about 22 months.

> 'A seemingly constant concern with mother's whereabout characterizes the third subphase. As he becomes aware of his ability to move away from mother, the toddler seems to have increased need and desire for his mother to share with him every new acquisition of skill and experience. For this reason we call the third subphase the period of rapprochement ...' 'Another important characterization of this subphase is the beginning replacement of vocalization and preverbal gestural language with verbal communication. The words

"me" and "mine" have great affective significance' [8]. Signals of potential danger are several: unusually great separation anxiety or 'shadowing' of the mother, or the opposite, a continual impulse-driven darting away from her with the aim of provoking her pursuit, and excessive disturbances of sleep.

This is a period of the expansion of social relationships for the child, with particular emphasis on the expanded role of the father. This child is able to include others into the hitherto small group of significant persons in his world, and will use many means by which to include these additional persons. The development of true expressive language, which is usually noted during this period, along with the emergence of early symbolic play, is inextricably entwined with this subphase. Much of the behavior described just above is dependent on and enhanced by a means of communication. Physical distance is relatively easily mediated by the spoken word. It is easier for the child to gain confidence in separation if he has available to him a flexible means of communicating to and maintaining a tie with mother. On the other hand, it is most helpful to the mother, who must deal with her own ambivalence regarding this phase, to know that both she and the child share a system of communication which will mediate this complex process for her. In essence, it is hard for the child to move very far away if he cannot verbally summon help or verbally engage his mother in the sharing of his new experiences. It is difficult for the mother to tolerate and foster this separated process if she feels she cannot depend upon the child to use communication skills in a manner which assures her that he is safe and that he can master this major step.

Mahler refers to a rapprochement crisis, which takes place between approximately the ages of 18 and 21 months.

She states that conflicts arise in the child that hinge upon his desire to be separate, grand, and omnipotent, and on the other hand to have mother magically fulfill his every wish, without having to recognize that help was actually coming from the outside. She describes a change in the prevalent mood to one of general dissatisfaction, insatiability, and proneness to rapid swings of mood and to temper tantrums. She characterizes this period as including rapidly alternating desire to push mother away and to cling to her.

Mahler states that one of the major aspects of development which supports the resolution of this crisis is the development of language. The ability to name objects and express desires with specific words seems to provide the toddler with a greater sense of ability to control his environment. The ability to express whishes and fantasies through symbolic play and the use of play for mastery appear to be additional, related aids in the resolution of the crisis. If mother and child cannot work their way reasonably smoothly through this complex rapprochement dilemma, further aspects of development may be significantly impaired. To some extent, the child may be at least partially fixated at a stage in which he is constantly caught up in the crisis. When this is the case, communication development is likely to be as firmly fixated as is the child.

It is during this developmental stage that one sees a tremendous spurt in the development of many parameters of communication skills. By 24 months of age, most children are considered to be 'talking.' With the child for whom organic factors prevent or delay the development of communication skills, negotiation through the rapprochement phase will be extremely difficult.

The fourth subphase of separation-individuation is called the consolidation of individuality and the beginning of emotional object constancy. The main task of the fourth subphase is twofold: (1) the achievement of a definite, in certain aspects life long, individuality and (2) the attainment of a certain degree of object constancy.

Having developed an ability to differentiate himself from others and a concept of himself as an individual, separate and different from mother, the child has the impetus to interact and communicate with others on behalf of himself. As long as the child existed in a state of symbiotic tie with mother, there was little need to communicate with others. The 'I,' which emerges at this point in the language of the individual, finds it necessary and desirable to develop ever more complex means by which to communicate with the 'others'.

Application of the Developmental Model to the
Communication Acquisition Problems of Retarded Persons

The required integrity of relationships is obviously a significant category in the development of communication skills, along with the category related to the integrity of the organism. In dealing with retarded persons, there is a tendency to focus on the 'retardation,' on the integrity and potential of the organism, and to treat lightly the issues of psychosocial development, particularly the impact of these latter issues upon communication development. This approach to only one-half of the human equation has led to many years of frustration on the part of those who attempt to help retarded persons. Although 'break throughs' are frequently made, we struggle with considerable lack of understanding of the causes and treatment of communication problems in the retarded.

It is the contention of this author that an application of the material discussed in the above section II of this paper would prove beneficial in the exploration of the retarded person's communication problem. Clearly, the mother-child interaction patterns must be given major considerations. In order to understand the evolving relationship between a mother and her retarded child, one must understand both the mourning process through which a mother must go, having given birth to a defective child [15], and the adaptation of the parent to such a birth [6].

Solnit and Stark [15] likened the task of the mother who gives birth to a defective child to the crisis following the death of a child. They state that the mother must mourn the loss of her expected, normal infant. However, while this long and intense mourning process is taking place, she must undertake the additional task of forming an attachment to her actual living child. This presents the mother with still another stress, inasmuch as the defective child is likely to require extraordinary means of child rearing. *Drotar* et al. [6], stressed these extra demands placed upon the mother because of the special needs of the child which occupy a considerable amount of the parent's energy. Altough they state that the initiation of the mother's relationship with her child serves to aid in the reduction of her own anxiety, they indicate that the parents must work their way through several stages of reaction, which take varying amounts of time for individual parents. These stages are shock, denial, sadness, anger and anxiety, adaptation and attachment, and reorganization. The task of work through these intense stages is quite likely to interfere with or at least modify the processes described by *Mahler*. In addition, those processes may necessarily be altered by the fact that the defective child may not be ready for or capable of participating in the separation-individuation process along the same time schedule as delineated by *Mahler,* or in concert with the mother's time schedule.

The mother who brings home a defective infant is likely to be in a very active stage of mourning, and will spend a considerable amount of the following months dealing with her shock, denial, sadness, anger and anxiety. She may also be required to spend extraordinary amounts of energy on the process of caretaking for the infant. The odds are stacked against her being able to make the same kind of commitment and attachment with the infant as she might have been able to make had the child been 'normal.' Her ability to engage in the process of mutual cuing may be significantly impaired, and she may not be able to bring to the symbiotic relationship all that is required of her. Indeed, her defective infant may suffer from the same inabilities to bring appropriate behavior to the process. The retarded child is likely to appear to remain in a state resembling 'normal autism' for a period far longer than the expected 3 or 4 weeks. This may cause the mother further stress, and require that she continue to participate in this rather onesided relationship for an inordinate amount of time. If this experience clashes with her expectations based upon observation of other infants or her own experiences with mothering other children, her stress may be even greater. The delay of the infant's psycho-social development, which may in part by his organic problems and in part be caused by the mother's diminished ability to relate, is likely to significantly delay such important landmarks as the social smile, thus further diminishing the mother's pleasure with the infant. It is not difficult to understand how the problems may become self-perpetuating and self-determining.

At this point it is important to explore another issue faced by the mother of the defective child. Clinical experience indicates that the mothers of retarded children experience problems in receiving appropriate emotional support for themselves. As described by the mothers, this difficulty obtaining support seems to fall into two broad categories: problems of the mother with a child whose defects are known, and problems of the mother with a child whose defects are unknown.

Many mothers of children whose retardation is known or strongly suspected soon after birth describe significant difficulties in obtaining adequate support from significant others. From their descriptions, it would appear that some of this difficulty, particularly with the children's fathers, may be due to the fact that the fathers are working through the adaptational stages along a time schedule which is dissynchronous with the mothers'. But some of the difficulty, as described, appears to be the result of a stronger need on the part of the fathers, grandparents, and even professional persons in contact with the mother to deny either the defect, its severity, or the impact upon the mother-child relationship. Many of these mothers describe themselves as essentially parenting alone, relying heavily upon their own, presently highly taxed resources.

The second group of mothers are those who give birth to a child who appears to be intact, but whose retardation will not be confirmed until many months or even years later. According to their descriptions, many of these mothers begin to suspect that there is 'something wrong' with their child, long before anyone else does. They struggle with their own shock and denial, and the need to obtain support from others. They state that, when they broach the subject to their spouse, family members, or professionals, they are usually accused of being 'overanxious.' They often describe themselves as being terrified by their suspicions and ashamed at the same time.

They, too, describe themselves as parenting with a feeling of loneness and lack of support. They dread the day when 'the ax will fall' and the diagnosis will be made. Their problems are further complicated by the fact that the diagnosis is not easily made, seldom clear cut, and may require the opinion of more than one specialist.

Both groups of mothers often indicate that the problems of obtaining support for themselves result in an even greater inability to relate well with their infant.

Although such lack of support is not necessarily experienced by all mothers of retarded children, it is a fairly common experience. All of the stresses described in this section, together with many others too numerous to explore in this paper, are likely to have a negative impact on the psycho-social-communication development of the retarded child. The subphases of separation-individuation, if and when they are entered into, are likely to be considerably distorted by the child's basic deficits and the interactional deficits described above.

The first subphase of differentiation, with its decrease in bodily dependence on mother and maturational growth of locomotor functions, sensori-motor investigation of mother and interest in his own bodily movement, is quite obviously in jeopardy for the retarded child. The second subphase of practicing with the increase of exploration of the environment and greater perfection of motor skills resulting in the ability to venture further from mother's feet, as well as to return for emotional refueling, may be unobtainable or at least greatly delayed for such a child. The third subphase, rapprochement, with increasing ability to physically separate from mother, the constant concern with mother's whereabouts, the need to have communication skills available to aid in negotiation through this subphase, are all at high risk for the retarded child. Depending on the degree of the child's retardation, and the resources available to mother in dealing with a child's developmental process, the ability of the retarded child to enter into and work his way through such an advanced phase as the rapprochement crisis will be in jeopardy. Many children never reach or pass through this phase, and many others experience significant delays in this respect, together with unresolved residuals of earlier phases, greater than those seen in 'normal' children. By the age of 24 months, the average child is moving into the fourth subphase of separation-individuation. It should be noted that many retarded children are first seen by the speech-language pathologist for evaluation and/or treatment sometime between the ages of 2 or 4 years. In evaluating these children, and particularly in planning treatment strategies, it is common to explore the organic half of the equation to measure many aspects of perceptual and motoric development, as well as to ascertain the highest level of cognitive development achieved by the child. It is rather unlikely that an additional attempt will be made to measure issues related to the other half of the equation – the level of psycho-social development. For this reason, it may be very difficult to determine whether or not the child is ready to 'learn language' or to determine what aspect of language should be 'taught.'

We often find ourselves tempted to begin 'language training' with material which we would expect to be mastered by the child's chronological age, or to begin the training with material we expect to be mastered by the child's 'mental age'. In avoiding the question of the child's stage of psycho-social development, we tend to make many mistakes.

Planning for the retarded child must include an evaluation of the psycho-social development of the child, and a treatment strategy which accounts for the attained phase. Treatment should then include strategies designed to help move the child to his highest potential of attainable psycho-social development. In many instances this will require that the professional person engage in a mutual cuing kind of activity with the child, or that the parents be instructed in and, importantly, supported in engaging in mutual cuing with the child. It should be remembered that mutual cuing is not exclusively, and may not even be predominantly verbal in nature [2, 11, 14, 16].

When all aspects of the child's development and needs are taken into account while planning treatment strategies, the retarded child (or adult) is more likely to experience movement toward the acquisition of useful communication skills.

References

1   Benedict, H.: Language comprehension in 9–15 month old infants; in Campbell, Smith, Recent advances in the psychology of language. NATO Conf. Ser. III: 4a (Plenum Press, New York 1978).
2   Bradtke, L.M.; Kirkpatrick, W.J., Jr.; Rosenblatt, K.P.: Intensive play: a technique for building affective behaviors in profoundly mentally retarded young children. Educ. Train. ment. Retard. 7: 8–13 (1972).
3   Bradtke, L.M.: From communication to language – a psychological perspective. Cognition 3; 55–287 (1978).
4   Church, J.: Language and the discovery of reality (Random House, New York 1961).

5   Darley, F.: Evaluation of appraisal techniques in speech and language pathology (Addison-Wesley Publishing, Reading 1979).

6   Drotar, D.; Ochs, E.; Schiefflin, B.: The adaptation of parents to the birth of an infant with a congenital malformation: a hypothetical model. Pediatrics *56:* (1975).

7   Folger, K.M.; Leonard, L.B.: Language and sensorimotor development during the early period of referential speech. J. Speech Hear. Res. *21:* 519–527 (1978).

8   Mahler, M.; Pine, F.; Bergman, A.: The psychological birth of the human infant (Basic Books, New York 1975).

9   Mahler, M.; La Perriere, K.: Mother-child interaction during separation-individuation. Annu. Meet. Am. Orthopsychiat. Ass, Chicago 1964.

10   Miller, J.; Chapman, R.; Branston, M.; Reichle, J.: Language comprehension in sensorimotor stages V and VI. J. Speech Hear. Res. *23:* 284–311 (1980).

11   Reich, R.: Gestural facilitation of expressive language in moderately/severely retarded preschoolers. Ment. Retard. *16:* 113–117 (1978).

12   Robinson, R.O.: Equal recovery in child and adult brain. Devl Med. Child Neur. *23:* 379–383 (1981).

13   Schiefelbusch, R.; Lloyd, L.: Language perspectives – acquisition, retardation, and intervention (University Park Press, Baltimore 1974).

14   Silverman, F.H.: Communication for the speechless (Prentice-Hall, Englewood Cliffs 1980).

15   Solnit, A.; Stark, M.: Mourning and the birth of a defective child. Psychoanal. Study Child *16:* 523 (1961).

16   Vanderheiden, G.C.; Grilley, K.: Non-vocal communication techniques and aids for the severely physically handicapped (University Park Press, Baltimore 1977).

17   Westby, C.E.: Assessment of cognitive and language abilities through play. Lang. Speech Hear. Serv. Schools *11:* 154–168 (1980).

Suggested Reading

1   Bangs, T.: Evaluating children with language delay. J. Speech hear. Disorders *26:* 6–18 (1960).

2   Bloom, L.; Lahey, M.: Language development and language disorders. (Wiley, New York 1978).

3   Buddenhagen, R.G.: Establishing vocal verbalization in mute mongoloid children (Research Press, Champaign 1971).

4   Clark, R.: The transition from action to gesture; Lock, Action, gesture and symbol: the emergency of language (Academic Press, New York 1978).

5   Condon, W.S.; Sander, L.W.: Neonate movement is synchronized with adult speech: interactional participation and language acquisition. Science *183:* 99–101 (1974).

6   Corsaro, W.: Sociolinguistic patterns in adult-child interaction; in Ochs, Schiefflin, Developmental pragmatics (Academic Press, New York 1979).

7   Cunningham, M.A.: A comparison of the language of psychotic and nonpsychotic children who are mentally retarded. J. Child Psychol. Psychiat. *9* 229–244 (1968).

8   Doll, E.A.: Diagnosis and appraisal of communication disorders (Englewood Cliffs, Prentice-Hall 1964).

9   Dunn, L.M.: Peabody picture vocabulary test: manual (American Guidance Service
    Minneapolis 1959).

10 Eveloff, H.H.: Some cognitive and affective aspects of early language development.
    Child Dev. *42:* 1895–1907 (1971).

11 Fraiberg, S.: Intervention in infancy: a program for blind infants. J. Am. Acad. Child
    Psychiat. *10:* 381–405 (1971).

12 Friedlander, G.: A rationale for speech and language development for the young
    retarded child. Train. School Bull. *59:* 9–14 (1967).

13 Geschwind, N.: The organization of language and the brain. Science *1970:* 940–
    944.

14 Goldfarb, W.; Goldfarb, N.; Braunstein, P.; Scholl, H.: Speech and language faults of
    schizophrenic children. J. Autism Child. Schizophrenia *2:* 219–233 (1972).

15 Goldman, R.; Fristoe, M.: Goldman-Fristoe test of articulation (American Guidance
    Service, Minnesota 1969).

16 Irwin, J.; Marge, M.: Principles of childhood language disorders (Appleton Century
    Crofts, New York 1972).

17 Johnson, W.; Darley, S.; Spriestersbach, D.S.: Diagnostic methods in speech pathol-
    ogy (Harper & Row, New York 1963).

18 Kahn, J.V.: Relationship of Piaget's sensorimotor period to language acquisition of
    profoundly retarded children. Am. ment. Defic. *79:* 640–643 (1975).

19 Katan, A.: Some thoughts about the role of verbalization in early childhood. Psy-
    choanal. Study Child *16:* 184–188 (1961).

20 Leiter, R.G.: Part I of the Mannual for the 1948 Revision of The Leiter International
    Performance Scale. (Psychological Service Center, New Jersey 1959).

21 Lenneberg, E.H.: On explaining language. Science *164:* 635–643 (1969).

22 Lenneberg, E.H.; Nichols, I.A.; Rosenberger, E.F.: Primitive stages of language devel-
    opment in mongolism; in Rioch, Disorders of communication, vol. 42: Res. Publ.
    ARN MD (Association for Research in Nervous and Mental Disorders, 1964).

23 Leonard, L.B.: Meaning in child language (Grune & Stratton, New York 1976).

24 Mahler, M.: On human vicissitudes of individuation (International University Press,
    New York 1968).

25 Matthews, J.: Communication disorders in the mentally retarded; in Travis, Hand-
    book on speech pathology and audiology (Appleton Century Crofts, New York
    1971).

26 McCarthy, D.: Language disorders and parent-child relationships. J. Speech Hear.
    Disorders *19:* 514–523 (1954).

27 McCarthy, S.; McCarthy, J.J.; Kirk, W.D.: Illinois test of psycholinguistic abilities
    (University of Illinois Press, Urbana 1965).

28 Myklebust, H.: Auditory disorders in children (Grune & Stratton, New York
    1954).

29 Nelson, K.; Bonvillian, J.: Early language development: conceptual growth and
    related process between 2 and 4 ½ years of age; in Nelson, Children's language, vol. 1
    (Garden Press, New York, 1978).

30 Peins, M.: Bibliography on speech, hearing and language in relation to mental retar-
    dation: 1900–1968. PHS Publ. No. 2022, (Dept. HEW US Public Health Services,
    Washington 1969).

31 Ringler, N.M.; Kennell, J.H.; Jarvella, R.; Navojosky, B.J.; Klaus, M.H.: Mother-

to-child speech at 2 years – effects of early postnatal contact. Behav. Pediat. *86:* 141–144.

32   Rosenberg, S.: Problems of language development in the retarded; in Haywood, Social-cultural aspects of mental retardation, pp. 203–216 (Appleton Century Crofts, New York 1970).

33   Rutter, M.; Rutter, J.A.M.: The child with delayed speech (Spastics International Medical Publications, London 1972).

34   Schiefelbusch, R.: Language of the mentally retarded (University Park Press, Baltimore 1972).

35   Schiefelbusch, R.; Copeland, R.; Smith, J.: The development of communication skills; in Language and mental retardation, pp. 92–109 (Holt, Rinehart & Winston, New York 1967).

36   Schlanger, B.: Mental retardation (Bobs-Merrill Co., Indianapolis 1973).

37   Snow, C.E.: Mothers' speech research: an overview; in Snow, Ferguson, Talking to children: language input and acquisition (Cambridge University Press, Cambridge 1977).

38   Staver, N.: The child's learning difficulty as related to the emotional problem of the mother. Am. J. Orthopsychiat. *23:* 131–141 (1953).

39   Wing, L.J.; Yeats, S.; Brierley, L.: Symbolic play in severely mentally retarded and in autistic children. J. Child Psychol. Psychiat. *18:* 167–178 (1977).

40   Zisk, P.K.; Bialer, I.: Speech and language problems in mongolism: a review of the literature. J. Speech Hear. Disorders *32:* 228–241 (1967).

19 Physical Therapy for the Handicapped Retardate

Dorothy Linn

Physical therapy is a form of direct patient care that can be applied to most disciplines of medicine and plays a vital role in the total care of patients who have a permanent or temporary disability due to injury, disease or birth defects.

Mental retardation has been defined as an intellectual deficit which is present from birth and is characterized by a state of arrested or incomplete development of the mind [26]. It involves approximately 1–3% of the total population and is possibly as high as 10% of the school-aged population in the United States [4, 17b]. Mental retardation is frequently associated with considerable delay in motor development; therefore, physical therapists have traditionally been a part of the total care, education, habilitation and guidance of the mentally retarded person in order to insure his individual rights to proper medical care and to enable him to develop his abilities and potentials to the fullest possible extent.

To support an individual's growth to its fullest potential is indeed a high and somewhat altruistic goal. It is a goal that reflects a special combination of values and attitudes within the health care system that strives for accountability in services, calls for the assurance of quality care and demands equal opportunity for all of its citizens.

The multiple needs of the retarded population, in conjunction with the demands of society for excellence and accountability, places a heavy responsibility on those of us who are advocates for, as well as providers of, services to the mentally retarded.

It is a responsibility that is greater than providing intensive treatment programs to the select few. For the physical therapist it is a responsibility that challenges the entire profession as well as its individual members.

In order to meet this challenge, physical therapists are at this time taking action at the university level by expanding the curriculum to include care of the mentally retarded. However, several unresolved issues will influence the adequacy of that care. Issues such as manpower, understanding the reasons for motor delay, developing more effective treatment methods and investigating the system of delivery of services, must be resolved so that therapist time can be used more efficiently to benefit the greatest number of persons who have need of services.

Manpower

The profession of physical therapy has grown dramatically in number and in scope of practice during its first 62 years.

In 1926 the American Physical Therapy Association (APTA) boasted an active national membership of 287 with a student affiliation of 14. By 1956 the membership had grown to 5,000 and in 1978 the figures totaled 23,189 active members with a student affiliation of 4,248. There are 82 physical therapy schools in the United States graduating approximately 2,500 physical therapists annually [14].

Along with growing numbers of practicing physical therapists, there has been a gradual change and expansion of the scope of practice as well as a general trend toward specialization. Currently there are 14 areas of specialization in the APTA, such as neurology, rheumatology, surgery, orthopedics, cardiopulmonary, pediatrics, etc. Each section is working toward the development of curriculum guidelines and competencies within its own area of expertise.

In recognition of the changing role of the physical therapist, the American Association of Mental Deficiency officially recognized physical and occupational therapy as a division at the 103rd annual meeting in 1979. There are 276 members in this new division. Hopefully this nucleus of interested therapists will stimulate others to provide services for the retarded as they begin to review issues surrounding specialty training, peer review, quality control and the role of the therapist in the public schools.

Manpower is an issue that will greatly influence the amount and the quality of care to all who fall within the broad category of the developmentally delayed. Statisticians project that the passing of the Education for All Handicapped Children Act (PL-94-142) has created immediate job opportunities for 15,000 physical therapists across the United States.

Given the annual growth rate of the APTA, 2,500, along with the combined number of therapists interested in mental retardation, 276, there is no realistic way demands for physical therapy services can be met in the near future. Physical therapists will be forced to move more toward methods of indirect care and/or consultation.

Growing demands for physical therapy services will challenge therapists to develop efficient methods in order to provide adequate care for those who are handicapped by the multiple problems related to mental retardation.

Understanding the Problem

Delays in motor development, regardless of the presence of a related neuromuscular deficit, is frequently associated with mental retardation [12].

Neligan and Prudham [20] found delayed walking and talking to be a reliable predictor of mental retardation. Smiling and sitting has been suggested as the earliest sensitive indicator of an intellectual deficit [25].

While the incidence for slow motor development is high among retardates, the mechanism of deviant motor functioning is not clearly understood. Delayed motor accomplishments in the retarded may reflect a lack of interest and self-initiated desire for exploration or the delay may be a consequence of a subtle impairment of the neuromotor system itself [19].

Gubbay [11] believed that clumsiness in children was related to the lack of ability to motor plan. He defined clumsiness as a comparative term contingent upon normally accepted standards which increase with chronological age. He stated that the integrity of many differing neurological functions were necessary for the execution of skilled movement, but the most fundamental factors were consciousness, intelligence and the ability to plan a motor activity. Consciousness depends on the alerting effect of the reticular formation upon cerebral cortical functions. Depression of consciousness results in inferior intellectual performance. Because motor planning itself is an intellectual function, according to *Gubbay* the retarded child will be clumsy even when there is no neurological basis for delay. The mentally deficient child will exhibit increasing degrees of awkwardness as physical tasks become more complex and intellectually challenging.

Kelso et al. [16] designed a study to investigate the underlying mechanisms involved in the acquisition of motor skills and precision in movement in educably retarded children in relation to movement coding and memory. He noted the role of the kinesthetic system in relaying information to the central nervous system (CNS) for the detection and correction of errors of movement. Synchrony developed between an intended action signaled within the CNS and the kinesthetic information arising as a result of the action is a major determinant of skilled performance [6]. *Kelso* et al. [16] looked at the ability of retarded children to utilize preselection (the child selects the movement) to remember movement more effectively and whether or not this information could be retained over a period of time. They found that educably retarded children were deficient in their rehearsal processes to aid short-term memory. Kinesthetic information could be retained for a 7-second interval and rehearsal processes were active for that period of time. The inability to retain kinesthetic information for longer than 7 s was thought to be related to lack of precision in motor skills in retarded children.

Molnar [19] proposed that the mechanism for delayed motor accomplishments in retarded infants and young children might be related to a disorder of postural adjustment controls. Early research in neurophysiology suggests that a complex hierarchy of reflexes and postural adjustment reactions laid down in the central nervous system provides the underlying substrata for muscular tone, posture and movement. These reflexes have been observed repeatedly and their time table described [22]. Their purpose is to provide a supportive background for the development of skill in precise coordinated motor performance [18, 23, 27a].

Normal development is dependent on the orderly appearance and dissolution of infantile reflexes as automatic postural reactions emerge [7]. However, *Molnar* [19] found in an analysis of 53 retarded infants and young children with slow motor development that while primitive reflexes did not persist beyond the expected age, the appearance of postural adjustment reactions was considerably delayed and showed marked temporal variability. She proposed that the slow motor development in retarded infants and children may be related to a disordered postural adjustment reaction control rather than inability in learning. Physical therapy measures were suggested as a remedial method to facilitate the development of postural reactions and to enhance the achievement of motor milestones along normal developmental lines.

Keshner [17a] reevaluates the theoretical model underlying the neurodevelopmental theory based on a review of the literature and calls for more research in the area.

Treatment Methods

Methods of providing physical therapy for the handicapped retarded are dependent upon a variety of factors. The therapist must give primary consideration to the designated reason for referral and recommendations of the physician prescribing treatment. Age, level of retardation, severity of the handicapping condition, ratio of patients to staff within a given setting and relevance of physical therapy to overall goals of treatment, determined frequently by a multidisciplinary team, will also influence goals set for physical therapy. Programs may be designed for the physical therapist to provide direct patient care on an individual basis, within the context of small groups, or to provide services indirectly through supportive personnel trained to implement programs with supervision.

Indirect Care

In treatment facilities where there is a high ratio of patients to staff, the role of the physical therapist may be to provide services indirectly through staff education and training. For example, programs designed for feeding, positioning and handling severely involved, profoundly retarded residents of state institutions can be managed most effectively by the direct care workers.

Severely involved, profoundly retarded persons are frequently restricted in mobility and may engage in stereotyped patterns of movement that predispose them to deformity and impede forward progress [15]. For those who are not ambulatory or are unable to sit independently, it is particularly important to train staff in proper handling techniques, adequate positioning methods, and the correct use of adaptive equipment. Adequate positioning reduces the danger of deformity and provides improved body alignment so that scoliosis, hip dislocation, pressure areas and contractures can be avoided. Adaptive equipment can be designed to assist positional changes that stimulate the subject's interest in the environment and provide support for special functions such as feeding. Proper positioning is fundamental to a successful feeding program. Adequate head and trunk alignment for feeding reduces danger of choking, gagging, or aspirating food into the lungs, a frequent source of chronic infection.

Feeding, positioning and handling techniques have been managed quite adequately by direct care staff with the supervision of competent physical therapists.

Mueller [21], Campbell [8], Keen and Sullivan [15], Bergan [5] and Fraser, Galka and Hensinger [10a], provide useful information for the care of those who are severely handicapped by developmental delay.

Direct Care

Physical therapy is frequently prescribed for remediation of a specific neuromotor dysfunction or to stimulate the attainment of developmental milestones where there is a motor delay as so often noted in the handicapped retarded. Several methods of treatment have been developed to inhibit atypical neuromuscular activity and to enhance normal patterns of movement. The theoretical base for these therapeutic techniques is grounded in traditional neurophysiological principles.

Sherrington's [27b] investigation regarding spinal reflex physiology and the modulating influence of the spinal alpha motorneurons (ventral horn cells) that innervate voluntary musculature provides sound rationale for physical therapy techniques. *Sherrington* showed that stimulation of peripheral nerves and sensory receptors affected the excitability of alpha motorneurons, caused outright impulse discharge in targeted areas of motorneurons and subliminally excited others in anatomical proximity [2]. *Rood's* [24] system of physical therapy is one technique that builds on *Sherrington's* theories and attempts to modify muscle tone and to promote active contraction of muscles through the application of cutaneous stimuli to discrete areas of the skin. Mechanical or thermal stimuli such as ice, heat, brushing, vibration, quick stretch and deep pressure can be used successfully to change the excitability of motorneurons, muscle tone and the strength of volitional effort in the contraction of specified muscles of muscle groups.

A second theoretical basis for treatment grows out of the concept that various parts of the central nervous system, from the spinal cord through the higher centers, will respond to sensory stimuli with crude unrefined motor patterns. These motor responses are inherent in the CNS and are thought to be unlearned automatic phenomena that exert a continuous influence on muscular tone, posture and movement and operate as a supportive background for skilled purposeful function [22].

Neurodevelopmental treatment (NDT) is an approach that is directed toward normalizing muscle tone, inhibiting abnormal patterns of movement and applying peripheral stimulation to facilitate the development of the automatic postural responses that are presumed to provide the supporting substrate for the development of motor milestones. NDT techniques are reported to be effective with young children and the mentally retarded because they do not require that the patient be particularly attentive. Propping responses, as well as, righting and equilibrium reactions are developed along with components of normal movement patterns. The patient is progressed along normal developmental lines.

Denhoff [10] suggests more critical reviews of treatment methods.

Ziegler [29], in a more recent paper, emphasizes his former view shared by *Sparrow* [28] that patterning is not recommended for severely disturbed children.

Specific physical therapy techniques require a basic understanding of neurophysiological principles and developmental theories. They should be used in direct patient care by a qualified therapist with expertise in this particular area of treatment.

Group Physical Therapy

Physical therapy services may be provided within the context of group activities where peer interaction and mutual support is desirable and thought to be beneficial for the patient. For example, the children in the John Merck Program have been observed to make consistant progress within small group therapy sessions. Goals of treatment are designed to expand developmental skills, to increase levels of physical fitness, to develop perceptual motor and body image concepts and to provide opportunity for positive peer and adult interaction through play experiences.

For the retarded child, developmental gains in motor skills are concrete experiences of mastery. Motor masteries enhance the development of a positive self-concept in these children who so often experience frustration and failure in all areas of learning. Perceptual motor tasks are selectively programmed to reinforce current academic goals. For example, children who are learning the colors yellow and red in the classroom frequently perform a task in group motor sessions learning the same colors in a different environment using different cues. Directionality concepts, such as in, out, over, under, around, and through, become more meaningful to a retarded child when incorporated into a movement experience. [13, p. 72].

Retarded, disturbed children are seldom able to enjoy play experiences because they lack the necessary skills and frequently cannot interact appropriately with their peers. *Curry* [9] pointed out that play in deprived or disadvantaged children more typically involves manipulative or gross motor skills. She further noted that these children need the active participation of an instructor to maintain the intensity of the play. Still it is desirable to provide opportunities for play in the handicapped retarded. Play by virtue of its pleasurable qualities can be a major vehicle for constructive socialization, widening empathy with others, lessening egocentricism and alleviating the emotional turmoil disruptive to learning [1].

Delivery of Services

No comprehensive system has been developed for delivering physical therapy services to the handicapped retarded. Physical therapists are employed by state institutions. The Department of Public Health provides physical therapy services in rural areas of many states. Agencies such as the Association of Retarded Citizens, Easter Seal Society and United Cerebral

Palsy provide therapy for infants, young children, and adults. School districts may employ physical therapists independently or contract services through a providing agency.

Certainly there are geographic considerations. Therapists working in the area of mental retardation are few in number and tend to be clustered near the larger cities and medical centers. Limited services are available in rural communities.

Legal restrictions are also a factor in the delivery of physical therapy services. Physical therapists cannot legally provide treatment without a physician's written prescription. Physical therapy assistants cannot provide care unless a licensed physical therapist is on the premises. The significance of these laws will be heightened as physical therapists move away from the traditional clinical setting to provide treatment in the public school system as mandated by Public Law 94-142. The resolution of these issues must be addressed and a comprehensive method of delivering services developed in the near future.

Economic factors impact on delivery of services to retarded persons. *Batshaw and Perret* [3] advocate public discussion in the selections of funding various services.

Physical therapy plays a vital role in the total health care, habilitation, and guidance of the handicapped retarded. Therapists provide direct care and consultation services in parent-child early development programs, school and pre-school programs, adult programs, community living arrangements and in residential care facilities. Equally important, therapists are actively working to meet the needs of retarded persons through the development and improvement of physical therapy education, practice and research. Together with related health professionals, physical therapists work within multidisciplinary teams to insure rights to proper medical care and full development of potential for the recipients of that care – the mentally retarded.

References

1   Arnaud, S.: Polish for play's tarnished reputation; in Engstrom, Play: the child strives for self-realization. Proceedings of a conference (University of Pittsburgh, Pittsburgh 1971).
2   Basmajian, J.: Therapeutic exercise; 3rd ed. (William & Wilkins, Baltimore 1978).
3   Batshaw, M.L.; Perret, Y.M.: Children with handicaps (Brookes, Baltimore 1981).
4   Begab, J.: The development of emotional disorders in the handicapped. Conference on innovative treatment for the developmentally disabled, Pittsburgh (1976).
5   Bergan, A.: Selected equipment for pediatric rehabilitation (Blythedale Children's Hospital, Valhalla 1977).
6   Bruner, J.: Organization of early skilled action. Child Dev. *44:* 1–11 (1973).
7   Bobath, B.; Bobath, K.: Motor development in the different types of cerebral palsy (Heinemann Medical Books, London 1975).

8 Campbell, S.: Program guidelines for children with feeding problems (Childcraft, New Jersey 1977).

9 Curry, N.E.: Consideration of basic current issues on play; in Engstrom, Play: the child strives for self-realization. Proceedings of a Conference (University of Pittsburgh, Pittsburgh 1971).

10 Denhoff, E.: Current status of infant stimulation or enrichment programs for children with developmental disabilities. Pediatrics, Springfield 67: 32–37 (1981).

10a Fraser, B.; Galka, G.; Hensinger, R.: Gross motor management of severely multiply impaired students, vol. 1 and 2 (University Park Press, Baltimore, Md., 1980).

11 Gubbay, S.: The clumsy child (Saunders, Philadelphia 1975).

12 Illingworth, R.S.: The development of the infant and the young child, normal and abnormal (Livingstone, Edinburgh 1960).

13 Isaacs, S.: The children we teach (University of London Press, London 1932).

14 Journal of the American Physical Therapy Association 11: 59 (1979).

15 Keen, R.; Sullivan, S.: Feeding, positioning, and handling. Pennsylvania training model (Pennsylvania Department of Public Health, Harrisburg 1974).

16 Kelso, J.A.C.; Goodman, D.; Stamm, C.; Hayes, C.: Movement coding and memory in retarded children. Am. J. ment. Defic. 83: 601–611 (1979).

17a Keshner, E.A.: Reevaluating the theoretical model underlying the neurodevelopmental theory: a literature review. Phys. Ther. 61: 1035–1040 (1981).

17b Khanna, J.L.: Brain damage and mental retardation (Thomas, Springfield 1968).

18 Magnus, R.: Physiology of posture. Lancet ii: 531–536, 585–588 (1926).

19 Molnar, G.E.: Analysis of motor disorder in retarded infants and young children. Am. J. ment. Defic. 83: 213–222 (1978).

20 Neligan, G.E.; Prudham, D.: Potential value of four early developmental milestones in screening children for increased risk of later retardation. Devl Med. Child Neur. 11: 423–432 (1969).

21 Mueller, H.: Facilitating, feeding and prespeech. Physical therapy services in the developmental disabilities (Thomas, Springfield 1979).

22 Peiper, A.: Cerebral function in infancy and early childhood (Consultants Bureau, New York 1963).

23 Rademaker, G.G.J.: Das Stehen (Springer, Berlin 1931).

24 Rood, M.: The use of sensory receptors to activate, facilitate, and inhibit motor response, autonomic and somatic in developmental sequence; in Sattley, Approaches to treatment of patients with neuromuscular dysfunction (Brown, Dubuque 1962).

25 Schmitt, R.; Erickson, M.T.: Early predictors of mental retardation. Ment. Retard. dev. Disabil. 11: 27–29 (1973).

26 Shepherd, R.: Physiotherapy in pediatrics (Heinemann Medical Books, London 1974).

27a Sherrington, C.: The integrative action of the central nervous system (Yale University Press, New Haven 1961).

27b Sherrington, C.S.: The integrative action of the central nervous system (Cambridge University Press, London 1947).

28 Sparrow, S.; Zigler, E.: Evaluation of a patterning treatment for retarded children. Pediatrics, Springfield 62: 137 (1978).

29 Zigler, E.: A plea to end the use of patterning. Am. J. Orthopsychiat. 31: 388–390 (1981).

20 Dental Prevention Program for the Institutionalized Person

George H. Bentz

Normal social interactions are hindered if severe oral conditions are offensive or cause pain when a person tries to smile, speak or eat. But such conditions are common among people from institutions. The problem of oral neglect has exacerbated to the point where frequently the limited existing dental resources are insufficient to attend to the critical needs of residents.

Unfortunately, society has been inclined to believe that oral health is unimportant to the institutionalized person and that, as a priority, it rates low in relation to overall individual well-being. It is also assumed that many of the institutional residents do not have the capacity to be concerned about oral health or its implications of well-being, function and appearance.

Residents of institutions have, for years, been the victims of needless pain and suffering as a result of poor dental therapeutic services [1–5].

It would then seem appropriate to explore alternative methods to deliver care if the present mechanisms are inadequate due to the limited allocation of resources and a traditional crisis care orientation. If, through a constructive, well-programmed, preventive approach to oral health, the incidence of oral disease can be decreased, the magnitude of the active dental disease can, in turn, be reduced. In time, this reduction in workload will enable the dental profession to distribute its resources adequately in such a way as to treat the amount of active dental disease and return all institutionalized people to a status of good oral health.

But to construct such a planned approach requires an understanding of the etiological factors which are responsible for the disease process itself. This can be best portrayed by the graphic shown in figure 1. Each of the four contributing factors, when considered independently, cannot initiate oral disease. It is only when the bacteria or plaque have adequate nutritional or dietary resources, acting over a period of time on the tooth and oral structures that dental disease will result. Altering any of the variables totally is extremely difficult – if not impossible. Thus, a viable alternative involving

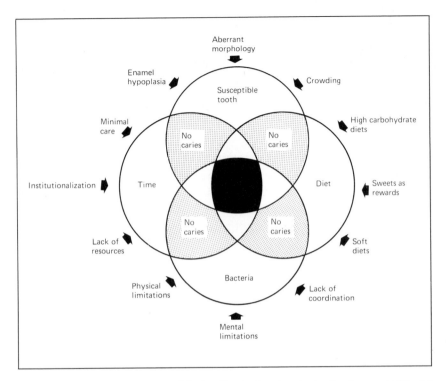

Fig. 1. Complicating factors of the handicapped patient in the development of dental caries. Modified from *Newbrun* [14].

alteration of each variable recognizes that the multifaceted interruption of the disease process will significantly inhibit or, in many cases, stop the process. Understanding this, it becomes relatively easy to change the environment of the institutionalized individual in such a way as to reduce the etiological factors contributing to decay and periodontal disease.

Resources Available

It is essential in all facilities to inventory the resources available for the establishment of a preventive dental program. Such inventories will vary greatly due to the nature of the facility. Sheltered workshop environments will differ from community-based living arrangements which will vary from the traditional institutional setting.

It should also be mentioned that innovative approaches to motivation should be sought, thus, extending the resources which might be available in a particular setting. For example, a record could be played to regulate the time of brushing; disposable toothbrushes can be added to lunches of working residents. Items associated with poor oral health habits should also be identified and eliminated from the environment. Improper or worn toothbrushes, cosmetic mouth rinses and toothpicks should be sought out and disposed of, indicating to residents the reasons for such actions.

Program Initiation

After compiling resources, the staff and dental personnel or consultant should establish a purpose for the preventive dental program. This purpose should clearly state the reasons for program establishment, how the program will apply to the specific setting, and the limits or boundaries placed on the program. Objectives or 'action plans' can then be constructed to insure the fulfillment of the formulated purpose. Once established, responsibilities must be assigned in conjunction with the appointment of a single individual to supervise the overall program. Resources can then be dispersed to aid in the execution of the program. As an aid in the preparation of this portion of the program, a guideline is available from the National Foundation of Dentistry for the Handicapped on Quality Dental Health Care (based in Denver, Colo.) in large residential facilities for the developmentally disabled.

Once the program is administratively established, attention and efforts should be turned toward the etiological factors contributing to the disease process. Each of these elements will be discussed with steps for institutional implementation and the preventive dental orientation.

Susceptible Tooth

The decay process cannot occur if there is no tooth present for the other elements to act upon. But in consideration of the tooth itself, certain variables augment susceptibility to decay. Numerous studies have been done which show a relationship between various handicapping conditions and the morphology or shape of teeth [7–13]. Frequently, the biting surfaces of mentally retarded people are 'wrinkle' or show an excessive number of deep grooves which facilitate food impaction. Given the diets and poor health conditions frequently encountered with retarded or otherwise institutionalized handicapped people, decay is a more probable result.

Fluoride has been shown to be, and now enjoys a wide acceptance as an effective therapeutic method of reducing dental decay. It is a means by which a susceptible tooth can be made more resistent to decay. There are presently three methods of incorporating fluoride into the tooth: (1) systematic incorporation in the developing tooth; (2) topical or surface application by a dental professional, and (3) topical or surface application by the individual, a staff member, or homecare giver.

Only two of these methods will be discussed here since application of the fluoride by a dental professional is not germaine to the establishment of a meaningful dental program run by the staff of an institution or provided by care givers in the home.

Systematic incorporation of fluoride is the best fluoridation method for protecting teeth from decay. This method of incorporation is limited to children from birth until the teeth are completely developed, usually about age 12. Caution needs to be exercised in this area since the formation and eruption of teeth is delayed in some disabling conditions. For example, the Down's syndrome individual may not have all permanent teeth until late teens or the early twenties. In this situation, systemic fluoride should be continued for a longer period of time. Institutions which have fluoridated water supplies need not be concerned about this fact; however, in places where fluoride is not naturally occurring or is not added to the water supply, supplements should be prescribed by a dental professional and administered by the staff or parent in the home. This can take the form of fluoride included in vitamins or as a separate tablet taken or ingested in the rinse taken daily by the handicapped person.

Toothpastes now contain fluorides which are of aid in the reduction of dental decay. The type of toothpaste is of significance in that some toothpastes form a heavy foam which can cause gagging in people with a sensitive or compromised gag reflex. Monitoring by care givers can facilitate the selection of a fluoridated toothpaste to minimize this problem.

Recently mouthwashes containing fluoride have become available without prescription. Presently, two types are available – a liquid and a tablet which is dissolved in water. The time it takes the tablet to dissolve has been regulated to 2 min, which equals the time that the individual should be brushing. Thus, the tablet provides a time measure for brushing by being the visual display of elapsed time while the resident brushes.

Other preventive services such as sealants or conservative restorations in teeth with anatomical defects are therapies provided by the dental staff and will not be discussed here. It suffices that such services should be available and residents should be seen regularly by a dentist so that decisions concerning this element of prevention can be made in an efficient and timely manner.

Diet

Perhaps the most difficult factor to control is diet. Society has established norms which include the consumption of large quantities of sugar and carbohydrates which contribute significantly to the caries and periodontal disease process. In those settings where meals are provided for residents, dietitian consultations with dental professionals or staff should evolve a dietary program which is low in sugar and carbohydrates. Substitution should be accomplished, particularly in the area of desserts, utilizing fruits, nuts, yogurts or other less cariogenic products. Breakfast menus should eliminate the use of presweetened cereals, pancake and waffle syrups, and substitute such items as nonsweetened cereals or toppings of cream soups, fresh fruit or fruit canned in its own juices.

Usually institutionalized food is of a consistency which readily adheres to the teeth, thus promoting oral disease. Detergent foods such as carrots, apples and oranges are avoided because of the fear of choking from the compromised ability of the resident to masticate the food properly. This situation must be carefully reviewed by a team of professionals. The goal should be a normal diet eaten under normal conditions.

A frequent source of sweets for residents are food gifts from parents or loved ones. Letters should be distributed to families and friends outlining the detrimental effects of such food gifts and offering lists of appropriate substitute items which are nonperishable.

Vending machines are available in the community and have become an integral part of most institutional environments. These also offer a significant source of sugar – frequently substituting for meals where the menu is not appealing to individual tastes. Contacting the vending agency and requesting a list of sugar-free items will reveal a sizeable selection of less cariogenic snack foods. These changes should be supported by display of nutritional posters in the areas of the vending machines and be reinforced by the educational programs which facilitate the making of unguided choice by residents.

Time

The factor of time is critical in the process of oral disease. Decay and periodontal disease are not rapidly advancing processes, but rather take a significant amount of time to occur. Thus, the more often the process is interrupted, the longer the time necessary until decay or periodontol disease are present at a significantly destructive level in the oral cavity. The time between interruption in the process is significant. Each individual should interrupt the destructive process once each 24-hour period with adequate oral hygiene. It is also important to see a dentist as least twice each year or more for those with natural teeth when the individual situation warrants. People who have full dentures should be examined once each year. Information concerning the results of these dental examinations should be provided to parents and staff.

Bacteria

The bacteria or plaque involved in the decay process and periodontal disease is a primary contributing etiological factor. The plaque or material formed by (1) the bacteria, (2) the food, and (3) the by-products of the bacteria are also the focal point of periodontal disease. Regular and systematic removal of this plaque is essential if the incidence of oral disease is to be reduced. No matter how well protected the teeth are with fluoride or other similar preventive measures, no matter how frequently the individual sees a dentist, or how careful the individual is with diet, if plaque is not adequately and routinely removed by daily brushing, the incidence of oral disease will be higher.

Establishing the Program

The establishment of any program, means the assignment of responsibility to staff within a manageable subdivision of the institution. The number of residents should be no greater than 30 per supervisor, who in turn assigns specifically named staff people to each resident. Dentists or dental hygienists should be available for consultation. A check list for program development should be of assistance (table I).

In-service programs for staff should be held prior to implementation

Table I. Check list for program development

1 Assign responsibilities for the program (administrative discussion)
2 Inventory resources available – see resource list suggestions
3 Assign responsibilities for the program (administrative discussion)
4 Set up brushing kits for units of the institution containing:
   a   Individual plaque evaluation sheets
   b   Unit report to dental personnel on individual plaque evaluations
   c   Disclosing solution or tablets
   d   Cotton tipped applicators (if liquid disclosing solution used)
   e   Multi-tufted soft nylon bristle brushes with polished ends in appropriate sizes –
       child, adolescent, adult – and marked with the resident's name
   f   Fluoridated toothpaste
   g   Dental floss and holder if applicable
   h   Fluoridated mouthwash
   i   Timing device to regulate brushing time – record, egg-timer, etc.
   j   Tongue depressors to aid in opening the mouth (if needed)
   k   Items to modify or bend toothbrush handles.
5 Establish monthly reports of resident performance to be sent to supervisor of project
6 Develop a dental examination and treatment strategy for all residents
7 Evaluate system after implementation at 6 months _____ (date to be performed)
8 Establish times to present educational programs:
   1   For staff _____ (date to be performed)
   2   For residents _____ (date to be performed)
   3   For parents and loved ones _____ (date to be performed)
9 Establish a date for program initiation on the units in the institution _____
   (date to be implemented)
10 Establish times and dates for on-site in-service, administering the program with residents:
      A Unit _____ date
      B Unit _____ date
      C Unit _____ date
11 After successful implementation of brushing programs for people with and without
   natural teeth, develop fluoride mouth rinse program. Use same strategies as that
   used for brushing program
12 Evaluate the integrated system of brushing and fluoridated mouth rinse 6 months
   after implementation _____ (date to be performed)
13 After successful development, implementation and integration of mouth-rinse program with brushing programs, develop a dental-flossing program.
14 Evaluate total dental prevention program integration of all three elements
   _____ (date to be performed)

and resident education classes should be started during the same period of time. Staff classes should be taught by a dentist or dental hygienist who is overall in charge of the program. This in-service program should include:

1 Basic ethiology of oral disease
2 Assessment of oral conditions
3 Assignment of responsibilities
4 Outline and responsibilities in the program
5 Other activities at the institution related to the dental program, i.e., dietary vending machines, parent information and participation, resident education
6 Demonstration of techniques
7 Participation in mock program by staff
8 Review and questions on the program

At this time, supplies for the program should be distributed along with information on utilization and integration of resources previously inventoried into the total program scheme.

During this same period of time, resident evaluation and instruction should begin. An assessment of each resident's capabilities and level of performance at the onset of the program should be completed. Performance goals should be constructed and a personalized instructional program established. Steps should be taken in such a program to establish observable, measurable tasks in the accomplishment of these goals.

Additional educational classes should be conducted for families and concerned individuals. During periods away from the institutional setting and during which residents are under the care and supervision of others, continuity should exist in the dental prevention program. Education of these 'significant others' can help promote this continuity.

Monitoring and evaluation of the program becomes essential if the program goals are to be attained. In an effort to effectively perform this evaluation, a system of individual performance evaluation should be established.

Resident Evaluation

A complete program of oral hygiene evaluation should be established at the facility. Such a program has been evolved by the National Foundation of Dentistry for the Handicapped. Dental consultants should be available to assist with tailoring such an evaluation program to the facility.

Procedure for Evaluation

The person working with the resident paints the liquid disclosing solution on all surfaces of the teeth. The resident is told to 'brush the red off all the teeth'. Upon completion of brushing, the mouth and prosthetic appliances, if applicable, are evaluated and the staff person completes the grading sheet. Establishment of an acceptable percentage level for oral hygiene is difficult. In the normal population a percentage of cleanliness between 85 and 90% could be expected. However, there are numerous individual resident limitations. It is, therefore, more realistic to measure individual performance in terms of improvement and capabilities rather than utilizing data established for the normal population. Such an assessment should be part of the basic skills training program for residents. Those individuals with low scores who had not shown significant improvement could then be designated as needing additional assistance in performing oral hygiene. This can be provided by actual staff assistance or additional instruction until a level of hygiene reflecting the normal population is attained.

Records must also be kept which indicate the last visit to a dental professional for oral disease evaluation. This should be performed at least twice yearly for those individuals having natural teeth and once each year for people who have no natural teeth. If direct care services are needed, referral must be made. While many institutions have medical staff facilities and personnel for dental care, some others are dependent on community resources. In the absence of professional dental staff, the program director should have knowledge of community resources so direct care can be obtained. Aggressive follow-up is necessary to insure that dental deficiences are corrected.

This program would provide a cost-effective method of care, with a built-in factor of re-evaluation in order to remain dynamic rather than static in meeting the varied and changing needs of retarded persons.

References

1 Bentz, G.H.: The forgotten patients. J. Acad. gen. Dent. *26:* 1 (1978).
2 Gullickson, S.: Oral findings of mentally retarded children. J. Dent. Child. *34:* 56–64 (1969).
3 Horowitz, H.S.; Greek, W.J.; Hoag, O.: Study of the provision of dental care for handicapped children. J. Am. dent. Ass. *71:* 1398–1410 (1965).

4   Miller, J.; Taylor, P.: A survey of the oral health of a group of orthopedically hand-
    icapped children. J. Dent. Child. *37:* 331–343 (1970).
5   Rosenstein, S.N.; Bush, C.R.; Gorlick, J.C.: Dental and oral conditions in a group of
    mental retardates attending day centers. N.Y. St. dent. J. *37:* 416–421 (1971).
6   Nowak, A.J.: Dentistry for the handicapped patient (Mosby, St Louis 1976).
7   Kraus, B.S.; Clark, G.R.; Oka, S.W.: Mental retardation and abnormalities of the
    dentition. Am. J. ment. Defic. *72:* 905 (1968).
8   Kraus, B.S.; Gottlieb, M.A.; Meliton, H.R.: The dentition in Rothmund's syndrome.
    J. Am. dent. Ass. *81:* 894 (1970).
9   Kraus, B.S.; Jordon, R.E.; Abrams, L.: Dental anatomy and occlusion (Williams &
    Wilkins, Baltimore 1969).
10 Kraus, B.S.; Jordon, R.E.; Nery, E.B.; Kaplan, S.: Abnormalities of dental morphol-
    ogy on mentally retarded individuals: a preliminary report. Am. J. ment. Defic. *71:*
    828 (1967).
11 Kraus, B.S.; Oka, S.W.: Wrinkling of molar crowns: new evidence. Science *157:* 328
    · (1967).
12 Goodwin, W.C.; Erickson, M.T.: Developmental problems and dental morphology.
    Am. J. ment. Defic. *78:* 199 (1973).
13 Bentz, G.H.: Frequency of abnormal tooth morphology in children with learning
    disabilities: a pilot study; thesis Pittsburgh (1978).
14 Newbrun, E.: Cardiology (Williams & Wilkins, Baltimore 1978).

Community Services and Administrative Aspects

21 Deinstitutionalization of the Developmentally Disabled[1]

Valerie J. Bradley, Mary Ann Allard

Introduction and Background

The Last Two Decades

The increasing emphasis on community-based services for the developmentally disabled is a direct challenge to traditional assumptions regarding the care and treatment of such persons. For years, it was an accepted fact that persons with disabilities such as mental illness, epilepsy, cerebral palsy, and other mental and neurological handicaps were best served in remote institutions where they could be protected from the pressures of daily living and the insensitivity of the community. It was also assumed that such persons had little potential for habilitation or rehabilitation and that their prime needs were for care and supervision. In many ways, the rejection of these notions represents a revolution in public policy and service delivery.

Unlike many other social reform movements, the changes which have taken place in the field of developmental disabilities have a relatively short history. In less than two decades, the principles which guided the system of care for developmentally disabled persons have undergone major shifts. These changes in orientation have resulted in increased expectations for developmentally disabled persons, a multidisciplinary approach to the problems of developmentally disabled persons, an acknowledgment of the civil and human rights of such persons, and a recognition that individuals with developmental disabilities fare better in smaller, more normal living environments.

The general acceptance of these principles, however, has not been sufficient to guarantee the efficient and expeditious implementation of reforms in the service delivery system. Funding has been inadequate, planning has been haphazard and uncoordinated, and the specific objectives of an alternative system have been ill-defined. Though the development of the general

[1] This paper is an abstract of the book by *Bradley* et al. [1].

philosophical outline of the system has not proved difficult, making the system work in practice has been a much more elusive task.

In many ways, the problems currently being encountered in the move to reduce the populations of large, congregate care institutions for developmentally disabled persons can be attributed to the rapid evolution and acceptance of the principles of normalization. This is not to say that the goals and objectives of the movement are ill-founded, but rather that the rush to implementation which followed such acceptance caused dislocations in the system which a longer view might have precluded.

A review of the political, social, and economic factors, which influenced the direction of the service system for developmentally disabled individuals and which continue to have an impact on deinstitutionalization efforts, is helpful to an understanding of the appropriate direction for planning. Reform efforts in the field of developmental disabilities coincided with a variety of events which coalesced in the 1960s:

(1) the growth of the civil rights movement which increased the publics awareness of the plight of a number of disenfranchised and neglected groups (i.e., the elderly, poor, developmentally disabled, mentally ill, etc.);

(2) an increasing outrage regarding the inhumane conditions in publicly administered institutions;

(3) the validation of research findings regarding the debilitating effects of institutionalization;

(4) the spread of the consumer movement coupled with an increasing militance among parents and families of developmentally disabled persons;

(5) the documentation of new program approaches and their positive impact on even the most severely disabled;

(6) a recognition of the importance of early intervention and the role of parents in providing stimulation and assistance in the development of cognitive skills, and

(7) the articulation of the theory of 'normalization' which asserts that developmentally disabled persons can best be served in programs and in facilities which deemphasize the stigma and isolation of such persons.

This optimism which characterized the decade of the 60s made it possible for advocates of the developmentally disabled to secure legal and programmatic changes in a number of states and localities. However, though this zeal extended to the early 70s other forces came into play which hampered the efficient and expeditious implementation of deinstitutionalization efforts. These pressures included:

(1) increasing inflation which escalated the costs of public services for the developmentally disabled and, in a relative sense, decreased the availability of public funds for the expansion of community-based services;

(2) a growing disaffection with the massive public human services programs which grew up in the great society era of the 60s;

(3) a backlash against the abuses of deinstitutionalization articulated by institutional employee organizations, the media, and others;

(4) expressions of concern and trepidation by some parents of institutionalized developmentally disabled children who feared that deinstitutionalization was commensurate with an abandonment of the states responsibility for the welfare of their children;

(5) the advent of litigation as a tool of system change which preempted funding priorities in many states and redirected planning efforts toward the improvement of conditions in specific state facilities, and

(6) an increasing competition for scarce resources which pitted many organized interests representing the handicapped against one another.

Lessons

There are lessons to learn regarding the conduct of deinstitutionalization efforts in the past. Given that it is always easier to criticize in hindsight, the critique is necessary in order to define a course of action for the future.

Termination versus Policy Development

Regarding the thrust of deinstitutionalization efforts, it is increasingly clear that early reformers of the system of care for developmentally disabled persons spent too much energy discrediting the institutional system and fighting for its eventual termination and not enough on the documentation of the benefits of community alternatives nor on the creation of statutory and budgetary mechanisms which would assure the development of community services.

Institutional Inertia

As in many attempts to discredit or change bureaucratic systems, the institution, which is the target of reform, has a resilience and 'staying' power which is sometimes underestimated by those who seek to overhaul it. This has certainly been the case in moves to phase down or alter institutional delivery systems. Several factors have been responsible for prolonging the implementation of any major changes – employee opposition, continued pressure for increased appropriations to upgrade the quality of care in institutions, changes in state administration, etc.

Flexibility of Funding

One of the major objectives of deinstitutionalization was to shift funds from the institutional system to community alternatives as the populations of state schools and hospitals declined. Since the majority of public funds for the developmentally disabled have traditionally been allocated to the institutional system, this tactic seemed reasonable in the absence of significant new allocations of funds for community programs. However, shifts in funds were stalled by escalating institutional costs which eliminated any savings from declining caseloads. Increased federal standards under the Medicaid program also forced states to, in many instances, *increase* institutional appropriations. As a result, funds did *not* necessarily follow clients into the community, and the anticipated start-up and operational funds which had been anticipated for community services were not forthcoming. Without the transfer of anticipated institutional savings, many states had only meager grant-in-aid funds to stimulate the development of services.

Faith in the Marketplace

Some states – most prominently California – established purchase of service mechanisms to reimburse the costs of community programs for the developmentally disabled. Of necessity, these mechanisms relied heavily on the ability of private vendors to generate needed services. This approach had two problems. First, it ignored the importance of 'seed money' or start-up funds for the initiation of new services. Short of that, it also ignored the value of building amortization factors into the service rate structure, so that development costs could be offset over time. Second, though this mechanism puts the purchaser of services in a position to choose among competing vendors, it does not allow for the initiation of services – even on a temporary basis – where no vendors exist in a particular program area (i.e., respite care). Though there is a value in removing the purchasing agent from the conflicting role of provider of service, it has meant that the development of community services is potentially erratic and not necessarily responsive to actual need.

Locus of Responsibility

In many states, the assignment of responsibility for the system of services for the developmentally disabled did not coincide with the requisite budgeting and monitoring authority necessary to mount a comprehensive program. In most instances, the state authority had little or no access to the policies governing the expenditure of crucial health, welfare, and rehabilitation resources for persons with developmental disabilities. State plans setting the guidelines for the allocation of such funds were prepared by other state officials, and only through formal or informal interagency agreements was any coordination secured. In addition to the lack of viable budgetary control, the state developmental disability authority was often separated from the standard-setting function and thereby had diminished control over the content of services being provided to the developmentally disabled. As more and more developmentally disabled individuals were released or diverted from institutions, it became increasingly clear that their needs could no longer be met solely by the developmental disability authority. Other generic and specialized services, such as housing, income maintenance, job training, and health care, were necessary and in most instances were provided by other state agencies. This left the developmental disability authority with statutory responsibility, but little or no power to assure that appropriate services were delivered.

Continuity of Responsibility

In addition to the lack of coordination at the state level, many states also overlooked the necessity of designating specific points of accountability at the community level. As institutional residents returned to the community, there was rarely a mechanism available to prepare a comprehensive plan for the resident or to link him or her to appropriate services.

Developmentally disabled persons were thus forced to negotiate a complex system of agencies – each only able to meet a portion of their needs. As a result of this discontinuity, many developmental disabled individuals were underserved or not served at all. Monitoring and follow-up suffered, and many persons were forced back into institutions and into inappropriate facilities.

Public Attitudes

Resistance to the development of community facilities has been a major stumbling block in the development of alternative community living arrangements for the developmentally disabled. Many of them remain inapropriately institutionalized because zoning and other barriers related to community resistance have delayed the creation of residential programs.

None of these miscalculations should be viewed as irrevocable. Rather, they should be seen as lessons which can provide a basis for future planning and implementation efforts. Specifically, this delineation of problems serves as a backdrop for the conduct of any conceptual analysis of state efforts to reorganize the system of care for the developmentally disabled.

Imperatives for the Future

After a period of intense and at times controversial activity in the field of developmental disabilities, it is clearly time to solidify the gains which have been made in the past two decades and to develop standardized approaches to the solution of the problems which remain. Some of the tasks which must be undertaken in any systematic state planning, budgeting, and administrative process include:

(1) The short and long-term roles of public institutions should be defined and justified.

(2) Characteristics of current and potential recipients of services in both institutional and community-based services should be assessed in order to assure that service development coincides with actual need.

(3) Discriminatory zoning practices should be assessed to determine the feasibility of state legislative or regulatory reforms.

(4) Mechanisms should be developed which assure that developmentally disabled individuals receive attention and services from generic agencies in the community (i.e., recreation, education, welfare, etc.).

(5) Sufficient information should be made available to identify and replicate model programs for developmentally disabled persons.

(6) Information systems should be developed which aid in assessing program effectiveness.

(7) State statutes and regulations should be reviewed to identify any changes necessary to promote general system goals.

(8) Systematic public information campaigns should be mounted to explain the aims and benefits (both fiscal and humanitarian) of community alternatives to institutional care.

(9) Continuity of responsibility should be guaranteed through the designation of accountable agencies in the community.

(10) System priorities should be built into the budgeting process.

(11) Consumer participation should be built into the system at all stages of planning and implementation.

Summarizing Remarks

Reviewing the context, in which changes have taken place, and pointing out the lessons which can be learned from past oversights are preliminary steps in the process of building a conceptual framework for analyzing state deinstitutionalization and service reorganization efforts. With this information in mind, it is now possible to examine the basic assumptions, which form the rationale for the system, and to further analyze those external and internal policy considerations which should be included in any systematic analysis of state deinstitutionalization efforts.

Basic Assumptions

Institutionalization versus Community Alternatives

Several recent studies of state developmental disability programs have indicated that many residents of state facilities could benefit from alternative placements in community residential programs such as group homes, foster homes, sheltered apartments, etc. These studies have relied on both institutional staff and outside review teams to assess the appropriateness of continuing institutional placement. In both instances, raters discovered significant numbers of people whose functional levels were sufficient to justify placement in a variety of more independent and less restrictive community-living arrangements. Recent institutional surveys commissioned as a result of litigation in New York, Alabama, and Washington, D.C., have also revealed substantial numbers of persons placed inappropriately in institutional settings.

The fact that developmentally disabled individuals are placed inappropriately in state schools and hospitals – or remain in institutions beyond the time necessary to complete a program of habilitation – is no longer a point at issue. The task at hand is to develop the assessment and evaluation tools necessary to determine the individual needs of current and potential residents, and to match these characteristics with tested models and programs. This will entail a substantial improvement in most state information systems – both in terms of the individual characteristics of clients of services and the performance levels of developmentally disabled persons in specific service modalities.

Another assumption regarding the service system is that alternative community programs will prove less costly than institutionalization. This assumption remains in contention. Though the per diem rates of many alternative programs are substantially lower than institutional rates, potential cost savings of deinstitutionalization will probably not be evident for some time. During the period of transition, most states will be forced to run two systems simultaneously – on the one hand maintaining the fixed overhead costs of state institutions, while expanding support for a burgeoning community program. Other factors also will increase the costs of transition:

(1) Legitimate demands of institutional employees, whose jobs may be terminated or phased out, for retraining, transfer of state benefits, etc., will require increased expenditures to satisfy.

(2) Initial capital and operational 'start-up' costs will be required to develop many community services.

(3) In order to develop the expertise required to provide the consultation, monitoring, and quality control necessary to adequately oversee community-based programs, many states have to expand staff at the central office level.

This is not to say that substantial savings cannot be realized over the lifetime of any one developmentally disabled individual, but it is to suggest that the general cost-saving assumption is subject to reexamination. Clearly, the savings in human potential which will result from more individualized and intensive habilitation efforts are unarguable. This may in the long run be a firmer basis for policy development and a more realistic view of the impact of system change. Arguments based on cost savings may prove to be true in the long run, but in the short-term they ignore the complicated fiscal and budgetary issues which must be contended with.

Factors which Influence the System

Fiscal Incentives
In most state systems, current fiscal incentives are tipped in the direction of institutional and/or medically oriented treatment. Most localities fare better financially if they place developmentally disabled individuals in state facilities or nursing care institutions, since they are rarely assessed for

any contribution to the cost of such care. If they choose to serve developmentally disabled persons in locally based programs, many can only expect that a percentage of the costs will be borne by the state. Thus, it is to their financial benefit to continue to rely on state-run programs.

Federal financing, specifically the Medicaid program, provides strong incentives for state and local utilization of skilled nursing or intermediate care facilities for the developmentally disabled. This has made many states heavily reliant on Medicaid reimbursement to offset institutional cost, and in some areas Medicaid funding has been utilized to fund deinstitutionalization efforts.

Because of the strong fiscal incentives held out by the Medicaid program, many developmentally disabled persons may have been placed in nursing care units as an expedient rather than as a result of a careful assessment of their individual needs.

State/Local Organizational Structure

The development of a conceptual approach to the state budgeting and planning process for community-based services must take into account the variations in the ways states and localities are organized to provide developmental disability services. At the state level, the developmental disability authority may exist as a separate department (Illinois) as a subagency within a department of mental health and mental retardation (Virginia) or as an entity within an umbrella human services agency (Pennsylvania). The line and program authority delegated to the developmental disability agency may also differ from state to state. In Pennsylvania, for example, the Office of Mental Retardation has no direct line or program authority over the states institutions for developmentally disabled persons.

At the local level, several patterns exist: (1) state/local government partnership (Pennsylvania); (2) regional nonprofit agency under contract with the state (California); (3) state administration/local planning bodies (Massachusetts); (4) state grants-in-aid to local providers (Illinois), and (5) regional nonprofit agency/local governmental partnership (Nebraska). Each pattern has been evolved as a result of political and organization traditions within the state, and any conceptual plan must be sufficiently flexible to accommodate these differences in organization.

Whether any one state or local organizational model is better than another is something which should be explored during the course of any analysis – keeping in mind that variations in the social and political cultures of the 50 states may hamper the replication of specific approaches.

Fragmentation

Fragmentation in the current system of services for developmentally disabled persons continues to hamper the development of comprehensive and coordinated services for such persons. Recognition of this fact in the developmental disability program – and in other human services – has stimulated many states to develop integrated human service agencies combining the majority of such programs under one umbrella. This and other models of integration should be explored during the course of an analysis. The analysis must be guided by the assumption that successful integration in any structure is contingent on the development of joint goals and priorities and accountability mechanisms which assure that each functional unit performs according to such jointly established objectives.

Consumer Awareness

Consumer awareness and participation are two increasingly important aspects of the delivery system for developmentally disabled persons. The term 'consumer' extends to both the recipient of services and to the family and friends of the recipient. Recognition of consumer interests can be seen in the expansion of right to education programs which bestow on parents and the developmentally disabled person rights of appeal and due process. Consumer participation in the development of habilitation plans and the choice of service options is also a growing trend.

Consumer advocacy in the area of developmental disabilities has perhaps had more influence on the development and expansion of needed services than in any other human service field. The desire of and ability of such advocates to play an oversight role in the delivery system must be recognized in any conceptual framework, and realistic and meaningful opportunities must be developed to that end.

Advocacy

The term 'advocacy' has almost lost its identity, since it is now being used in such a wide variety of contexts. Advocacy may be construed as legal representation; it may refer to *Wolf Wolfensberger's* concept of 'citizen advocacy'; it may extend to case management or purchase of service agencies which are responsible for assuring that the client's needs are met, etc. Developing 'advocacy programs' is currently a popular objective in many states, and this is probably a healthy sign. However, if services do not exist and the advocate has little or no power to generate their development, then such programs may prove disappointing – and worse yet, they may have falsely raised the expectations of consumers.

Referral Patterns

An inspection of such patterns can illuminate problems and discontinuities in the system. Such questions as:

(1) Is there a single entry point in the community for all developmental disability services?

(2) Are continuing relationships maintained between institutional and community-based programs?

(3) Is any one agency responsible for assuring that referrals are in fact consummated and that appropriate services are provided?

(4) Are referrals based on a comprehensive plan for services or are they simply made on a routine basis?

All of these issues should be taken into account in the development of any conceptual framework.

Custodial Responsibility

This element of the system is particularly important since it determines accountability. It should also be assessed in two ways: (1) Who has the *legal* responsibility for the individual insofar as guardianship is concerned, and is this individual or agency the most appropriate guardian to assure that the interests of the developmentally disabled individual are represented? (2) Who has the *programmatic* responsibility to assure that the needs of the developmentally disabled person are met in the most appropriate fashion possible?

Both of these spheres of responsibility are important in the organization of services and should be treated in tandem in the conceptual development.

Other Considerations

In addition to the factors mentioned above, other issues will also influence the functioning of the system:

(1) integration of funding sources and budgets for all developmental disability services;

(2) the flexibility and responsiveness of state standards for developmental disability services;

(3) the resiliency of the system (both fiscally and structurally) and its ability to adapt to changing administrations, economic decline, etc.;

(4) the nature of any ongoing litigation in the state, and

(5) the effectiveness of evaluation and monitoring techniques.

Difficulties in System Change

As mentioned previously, though a great deal of rhetoric has been advanced on the side of system reorganization and the development of community alternatives, the fact remains that in most states, the bulk of funds are still being allocated to the institutional system. An initial list of some of the factors which have hampered the transition include:

(1) In many states, the local program structure has not been strong enough to provide a countervailing political force to offset vested institutional interests.

(2) Federal funding through the Medicaid program has allowed many states to maintain and even expand the level of institutional services.

(3) Legislators in many states are not well enough acquainted with the principles underlying community programs and are still more attuned to line-item institutional appropriations.

(4) The director of the developmental disability agency in most states controls only a small portion of the funds needed to support developmental disability services.

(5) Communities ready and willing to develop alternative programs are often given little or no technical assistance and direction from the central office.

(6) Deinstitutionalization of the developmentally disabled has not been a priority at the federal level, and, therefore, little direction has been given to states either through regulation or technical assistance.

(7) Institutional programs have been inadequately integrated with community-based programs.

(8) Fiscal and other crises have prevented state administrators from proceeding with the expansion of community services in a methodical and thoughtful fashion.

All of these factors have made many state developmental disability systems vulnerable to political shifts and forces, and unable to establish the type of concrete foundation necessary for rational growth and development.

State Models

There is now sufficient experience in many state developmental disability programs to allow for the isolation of successful and unsuccessful approaches to systematic service delivery. These so-called 'pioneers' provide useful documentation for the formulation of model conceptual systems for use by developmental disability administrators [1, p. 56].

California

Instead of state or local government administration of community programs, California developed a system which combines a regional nonprofit assessment and purchase of service entity with private providers of service. The system of local agencies is also directly linked to the state institution, since it screens institutional admissions and is responsible for discharges from state hospitals. There have been two major problems in the model. First, there is no 'seed money' available for the development of services, and the regional purchase of service entity is legally precluded from initiating services. This has meant that, in some instances, funds allocated for specific services have reverted to the state general fund when no vendor could be located to provide the service. Second, the rate structure, which governs the level of reimbursement for services, has been criticized as being too rigid and inadequate to support a decent level of care.

Pennsylvania

The Pennsylvania system is a county/state partnership with the state reimbursing counties from 90 to 100% of the costs of services for developmentally disabled persons. Pennsylvania has developed a special line-item appropriation which provides start-up funds for the development of group homes for developmentally disabled persons. The availability of these funds has resulted in a dramatic increase in such facilities. Consultation and direction provided by the Office of Mental Retardation has helped to guide the development of these community alternatives. The Pennsylvania system also has drawbacks, however. The administration of institutional programs is carried out by an agency which is separated from the developmental disability program office. This makes coordinated planning and policy direction difficult. In addition, institutional and community services budgets are developed separately, thereby making it difficult to transfer funds from one system to another.

Massachusetts

The Massachusetts system is essentially state administered and is broken down into regional and area organizations. Local boards of consumer and other representatives help to determine area priorities. Massachusetts is constrained by a variety of factors: (1) a threatened loss of federal Medicaid funds in its state institutions; (2) a militant employee group which has made demands for relocation, retraining, etc., as institutional programs are phased down; (3) a confusion in roles between the state developmental disability authority and the special education authority administering the state's comprehensive right to education program, and (4) a general fiscal crisis. State leadership, however, is cognizant of these problems and appear to be systematically seeking reasonable solutions.

Nebraska

The ENCOR program in the eastern region of Nebraska has been held up as an early model of community services for the developmentally disabled. The ENCOR system, unlike the California model, initiates and operates services. The ENCOR philosophy is that this is the best method to guarantee quality programming and continuity. The ENCOR program has been particularly successful in 'mainstreaming' developmentally disabled individuals in generic services in the community. The major criticism of ENCOR, however, is the high costs per recipient of services. Perhaps as more generic services are utilized and additional federal funds are indentified, the costs per person will diminish.

Each of these models – and others – must be explored during the course of an analysis. Understanding the strengths and weaknesses of each approach and the context in which these approaches have proven to be successful will facilitate the development of optional conceptual systems.

External Catalysts

In addition to the internal dynamics of the system, there are several external contingencies which must be taken into account in any systematic assessment of state organization and planning for developmental disability services. Some of these factors include:

(1) changes in federal regulations governing federal funding – such as the impact of the new ICF/MR regulations;

(2) the effect of right-to-education litigation and the Education Of All

Handicapped Children's Act (PL 94–142) on program funding and organizational auspices;

(3) the impact of the pending Government Accounting Office study regarding deinstitutionalization of the mentally disabled in five states on Congressional and Executive policy in the field of developmental disabilities;

(4) the content of judicial orders in current and future litigation directed at the rights of the mentally retarded.

The whole field of deinstitutionalization is presently under scrutiny by several agencies and the American Medical Association. Further research may clarify the details of this process and help meet the needs of the clients as well as the needs of the community designated to absorb the deinstitutionalized retarded persons.

Reference

1   Bradley, V.J.; Ashbaugh, J.W.; Allard, M.A.: Deinstitutionalization of developmentally disabled persons (University Park Press, Baltimore 1978).

22 Administration of Facilities for the Treatment and Rehabilitation of Retarded Persons

Irene Jakab

This chapter provides an overview of the administrator's role in clinical services, staff management, architectural environmental design and finances. All these components of a treatment facility are interdependent and neither one can exist without the other. Prevention, treatment or habilitation are each people-to-people direct 'helping' services. The finances and the environment (space) where the treatment (help) takes place can encompass extreme variations, from the most abysmal poverty and 'no-walls space' of missionary work – like that of Mother Theresa in India – to the most expensive European or North American small private hospitals with their period architecture and furniture, fine linen and silverware. The essence of the treatment and rehabilitation is, nonetheless, the interaction between the staff and the patients (clients); they have to meet emotionally at some point in space and time. A good administrator will foster this meeting of staff and patients by providing the optimal space and optimal staff-patient ratio, within the budget.

The quality of staff interaction and the motivation of the staff are both intangible elements which require the art of administration and management. The therapeutic atmosphere can be fostered by architectural space design and by a high staff-patient ratio (high budget), but the quality of interaction must be elicited and enhanced by the artful choice of staff and by sustaining the motivation of the staff members within their roles.

It is not hard to understand (but it is hard to keep in mind) that without patients no program can be managed. Administrators are frequently too enmeshed in details of financial nature and staff management, while at the same time they are missing to realize the needs of the patients as a group and even more importantly, as individuals. The quality of care is the administrator's business whether he/she is a physician or the graduate of a school of administration.

The first task of a director, or administrator of a program or facility for retarded persons is to identify his/her categories of responsibilities. The following categories are elements of any service delivery system: *(1) Patients (clients); (2) staff; (3) space (environment), and (4) funding.* Additional aspects of a project may include: *(5) professional education, and (6) research.* A review of the administrative tasks related to each of these categories follows.

Patients

Administrative Responsibilities Related to the Client-Patient

Mentally retarded persons of all ages require some services of habilitation, special education, job training, sheltered workshops, and different levels of supervision and guidance by professionals, in community living facilities or in the family home. Some retarded children and adults need rehabilitation and treatment for complications and conditions associated with their mental retardation. The administrator is responsible for the selection of the client-patient population to be served by a given facility. This will depend on several factors:

(1) Patient-related factors such as age, the level of retardation and the type of associated disorders. Children require different staff and different environment for habilitation or treatment than adult retardates. A relatively healthy retarded population can be served by a small staff with few specialists, for instance in the following situations: supervision of independent living; group homes; halfway houses, or homebound services to children and older retardates and their families. On the other hand, a larger staff and more specialists must be available for the diagnosis and treatment of the multihandicapped. More space is also needed to deliver the necessary specialty treatments.

(2) The number of staff (staff-patient ratio) and the type of specialists available on the staff, or as consultants, are further factors in selecting the type of patient-client population to be served.

(3) The size and architectural characteristics of the space available will also influence the proposed program – and therefore, the selection of clients who can be served in a facility.

(4) The cost. The staff-patient ratio, the size, and the equipment of the rehabilitation and treatment areas are ultimately translated into financial figures. The available funds will determine the number and type of clients (patients) who can be served, since the original investment and the operat-

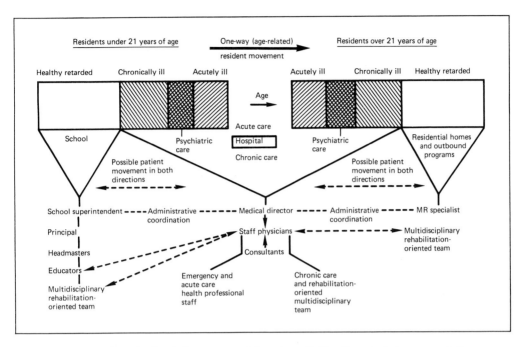

Fig. 1. Organizational chart suggested for a large facility for retarded persons of all ages. The physically and psychiatrically healthy retardates are managed in the least restrictive environment. The acutely and chronically ill are provided with different levels of hospital care. The psychiatric cases are treated in a special unit. Transfer within these units is made according to the need for care or treatment. The school superintendent, medical director and MR specialist will report to the institute's director.

ing costs related to the type of services provided will differ greatly from program to program.

Supervision and facilitation of client-patient processing from the referral through the diagnostic work-up and the treatment to the discharge is the next patient-related responsibility of the director-administrator of a program or facility. This job requires management tools and skills.

Management Tools
Division of Clinical Services

This is relevant and needed for larger institutes and programs serving multihandicapped retarded persons of all ages and with different associated conditions. Figure 1 is a sample of the grouping of patients according to

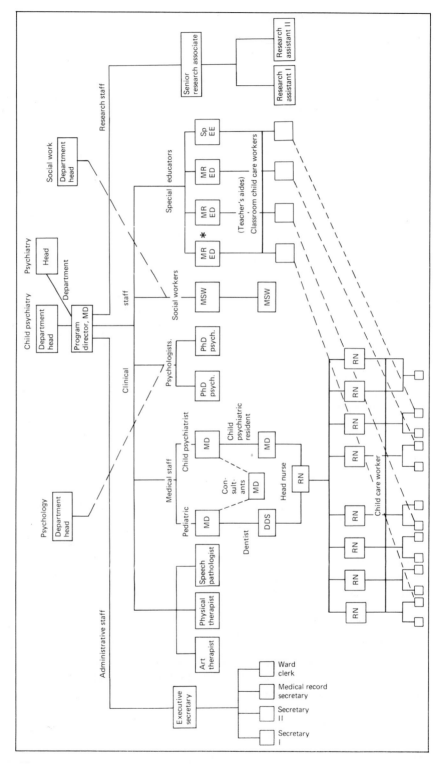

Fig. 2. Table of organization. Staffing pattern sample used at the John Merck Pilot Project (1975–1978) directed by the author. This project served 20 severely emotionally disturbed retarded children (Department of Psychiatry, University of Pittsburgh). * = Teachers specialized both in mental retardation (MR) and emotional disturbance (ED).

their needs, determined by age and the type of handicap. Acute and chronic conditions, medical, psychiatric, educational and rehabilitation needs are taken into consideration in this layout in order to provide a functional and economical staff and space assignment for the delivery of specialized services. There is a built-in flexibility in this system for long-term care patients who can move from one service to another and back again according to their condition. Patients (clients) may be admitted to any of these sections and discharged from any of them to the community.

Table of Organization

The staff responsibilities and lines of supervision reflect the functional aspect of the clinical services. Figure 2 is a sample of staff asignment in a psychiatric treatment program for doubly handicapped, emotionally disturbed retarded children (designed by this writer for the John Merck Program at the Department of Psychiatry, University of Pittsburgh). One of the innovative factors in this staff utilization is the crossing of specialty lines between nursing staff and educators. Members of the nursing staff are assigned to function, part of the day, as classroom aides under the supervision of the therapeutic educators, while on the other hand the therapeutic educators participate in the milieu therapy whenever they are not in the classroom or tutoring. In the milieu, the activities designed by team decision are supervised and carried out by nursing staff with the participation of educators.

Procedure Manual

The development of a comprehensive procedure manual is also an administrative organizational tool. It serves as a reference book in the day-to-day operation as well as a source of information for new staff. It has to be updated regularly, each time when procedures are improved or changed, or new ones are adopted. The procedure manual should contain in its body or as an appendix a complete set of the job descriptions pertinent to the staffing pattern of the facility. This is useful in recruitment and in the ongoing supervision of staff members. The knowledge of different job descriptions may serve as an incentive to young staff aiming at the 'next level', on their way up. If they know what qualifications are required (job description) to reach a higher level or enter an altogether different job category, they will be more likely to work for this reachable goal by improving their skills through practice and/or formal education. Unclear or unavailable job descriptions cause tension between staff members and make objective supervision very difficult. By linking the procedure manual with the job descriptions it becomes a tool, of fostering accountability by making it clear who is expected to do what within a given procedure. This manual, through its different chapters, will provide an understanding of the total facility and its services. For example, the procedures may be organized under clinical services (admission, diagnosis, treatment, and/or schooling, rehabilitation), administrative services (purchasing, accounting, management and supervision of nonclinical services), safety procedures, etc.

The procedure manual should be easily available to all staff all the time. Staff should be encouraged to use it, look through it, often and most of all to suggest improvements and changes as they may be necessary to upgrade a given procedure or the function of the whole program. The administrator should recognize receipt of every suggestion, it means that the staff cares about improving the system. Some suggestions may appear impractical while others look promising. Recommendations in this latter category should be presented from time to time for staff discussion and if accepted by the majority, they should be incorporated into the manual. Most suggestions aim at improving client-patient services. Some suggestions, however, may appear to aim only at making the staff's work more comfortable. The administrator should not dismiss these lightly as 'nonproductive investments'. The 'creature comforts' provided for the staff are the key to their loyalty and to increased quantity and improved quality of work. The opposite of this is frequently experienced, namely, staff uncomfortable with the job conditions becomes impatient with the clients due to the subliminal, but persistent feeling of frustration with some minor environmental factors. For instance, the lack of a staff lounge for those who do not have an office makes it virtually impossible for them to get away from clients during their break time, to relax in privacy for 10–15 min and renew their energies for the difficult people-to-people work they are doing 8 hours a day or more. Staff burnout and fast turnover may be the price.

Record Keeping

A program philosophy of considering both the assets and the pathology in the treatment plan helps avoid the pitfalls of the problem-oriented record keeping, which essentially disregards the healthy aspects of the patient. It is, however, the strength in a given area of functioning (physical, emotional, educational, intellectual), which can be used to overcome the deficits.

The Diagnostic and Treatment Data Chart. This consists of a concise listing of assets and pathology in each sphere of functioning. It is an instrument of planning treatment goals and methods. It is useful both for staff and patient information, since it serves as an indicator of progress at regular treatment review checkpoints.

Progress Notes. This is a constant source of administrator's headache. There is, it seems, an 'inborn' aversion in most people in the area of health care work against 'paperwork'. I have often speculated about the reasons for this negative attitude toward record keeping as compared with the practices in other professions. I have seen architects keeping very accurate progress notes on the step-by-step process of building. I have seen lawyers writing detailed notes on every aspect of their contact with their clients or agencies or the court. Of course, I have also seen physicians and other health professionals writing regular notes on their patient's status or progress. The difference is that the architect or the lawyer did not complain while the physician (especially the psychiatrist) has more often than not resented the requirement to write daily progress notes. It is felt that today institutions are drowned in a swamp of paperwork [62].

The difference in the type of work may determine the difference in attitude toward writing progress notes and especially about the required frequency of such notes, determined usually by the administration and not by the clinician. In medical and mental health work changes occur slowly, the interaction has many intangible aspects hard to measure, and the occurrence of changes (progress) does not follow an accurately predictable schedule. On the other hand, an architect can record the 'growth of a building' in each stage and predict that if the work (service) is provided as 'prescribed', the building will 'stand' and possibly on the date predicted for completion. The lawyer creates 'documents' by recording facts, and the document itself may be the goal of his activity. The goal of the physician and of the other health professionals is to 'heal' or rehabilitate. The work is done by direct interaction, regardless whether details are recorded or not. Often the staff has a feeling of 'wasting their time' whenever they are not actually 'working with the client-patient', i.e. when they are writing progress notes. The administrator can lessen the staff resistance to writing notes by specifying the type and frequency of note required, and by the use of progress report forms with preprinted outlines. The two types of progress notes are the medical model progress report and the contact sheet.

(1) Medical Model Progress Report. For good professional practice the progress note follows usually the traditional medical model including the following details: (a) The problem for which treatment or intervention has been needed; (b) the intervention (physical therapy exercise, drug prescription, art therapy, psychotherapy, etc.) provided, and (c) the patient's (client's) subjective reaction, or the objective changes achieved (improvement) as a consequence of the intervention. This is a step-by-step documentation of the rehabilitation or treatment process. This type of note is written more frequently in acute cases than in cases which require a long time to achieve changes. Certainly, daily or even more frequent progress notes are indicated in a case of alcoholic delirium in the detoxication phase, while in the case of a neglected depressed and anxious child, where the goal is to build trust and change the low self-esteem, nobody can expect daily measurable changes, i.e., 'progress'. Therefore, progress notes at less frequent intervals (weekly or monthly) should be sufficient.

(2) Contact Sheet. The fact that visible, measurable progress cannot be recorded every day does not exclude the need to record the intervention provided (every day in some cases) toward reaching the progress as expected. This is a different progress note. It is required by administrators as proof of services delivered. The progress note which does not necessarily account for 'progress' in the clinical sense is actually a contact report. Its aim is to prove that the professional has had face-to-face contact with the patient-client and has provided the service for which he or she, or the facility which employs him or her, has generated a bill. The contact report does not have to include measured progress each day and it may be quite brief. This contact documentation is required by most third-party payors. It is also a management tool, assuring staff accountability.

In summary: The medical model progress note is a documentation of the patient's status and progress as well as of the treatment methods. It serves also as a communication tool informing other staff working with the same patient, and of course it is an important collection of facts about the treatment which may be needed in the future for medical-rehabilitational or even legal purposes. The contact report is a documentation (for billing purposes) of the services actually provided by the staff. The difference in the progress notes' ultimate use will help the professionals realize that while a brief note must be submitted for each staff contact, the frequency of com-

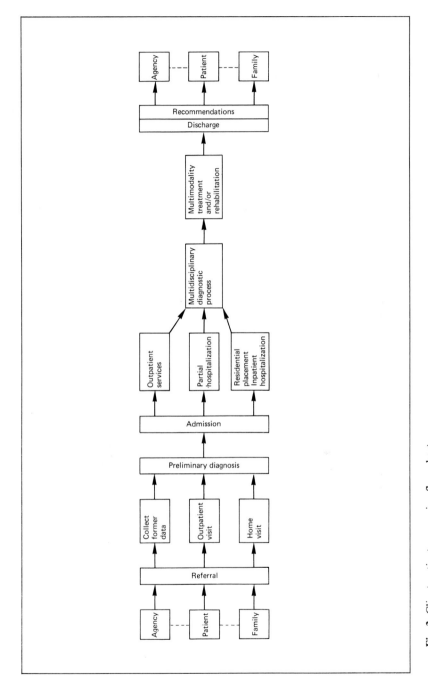

Fig. 3. Client-patient processing flow chart.

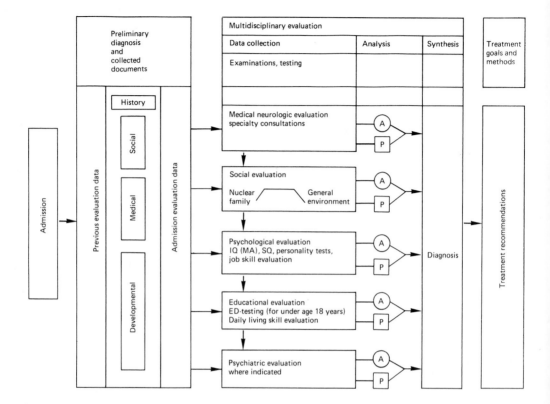

Fig. 4. Diagnostic process flow chart. A = Assets; P = pathology.

prehensive progress notes about the patient's status is to be based on their clinical judgment.

Flow Charts. The use of a flow chart is an administrative tool for assuring smooth service delivery and keeping up-to-date on the cost of services. The staff should participate in designing the different details and the sequences incorporated into the flow charts related to services provided by the program or facility. Samples of general purpose flow charts are provided in figures 3–6 and tables I and II. These can be adapted to the needs of the client-patient type and the services provided by a given facility.

Questionnaires and Progress Report Forms. The time-consuming narrative progress reports can be substituted by standard or specially designed report forms at regular intervals, as an alternative. Examples of progress

Treatment process flow chart

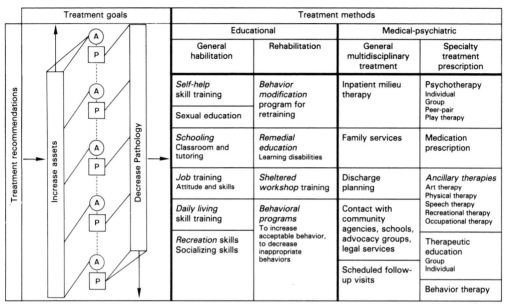

Fig. 5

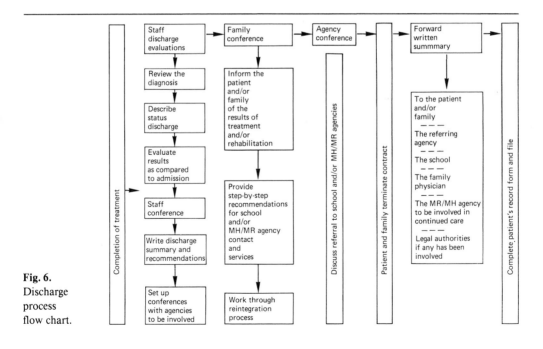

Fig. 6.
Discharge
process
flow chart.

Table I. Detailed treatment process description

Educational methods		Medical-psychiatric methods	
General habilitation	Rehabilitation	General multidisciplinary treatment	Specialty treatment prescriptions
Self-help skill training	*Remedial education*	*Inpatient milieu*	*Psychotherapy*
Eating habits	Learning disorders	*therapy*	Individual
Dressing skills	Academic tutoring	Attitude therapy	Group
Toilet training		Monitored visits	Peer-pair therapy
		Therapeutic home	Play therapy
Schooling,	*Sheltered workshop*	visits	
Classroom education	Job attitude and	Community outings	*Medication*
Trainable level	job skill	Recreational therapy	Anticonvulsants
Educable level	Remedial training	Socializing skill	Neuroleptics
		training	Other
Academic tutoring,	*Behavioral*		
Job training	*modification*	Fostering ego	*Art therapy*
Job habits	*to decrease*	development and trust	*Physical therapy*
Job skills	Socially unacceptable	by consistent and	*Speech therapy*
Volunteering	habits	predictable schedule	*Sign language*
Job interview in	Messy eating	of events	Developing verbal
competitive market	Ruminating		language
	Disrobing	*Family services*	Remedial therapy for
		Parent counseling	stuttering,
Sexual education	*Uncensored sexual*	Referrals to support	articulation disorder,
Menstrual hygiene	*habits*	groups	aphasias
The need for privacy	Inappropriate sexual	Contact with	
Masturbation	curiosity	advocacy groups	*Behavior therapy*
Intercourse	Inappropriate touching		For symptoms of
Pregnancy	of people	*Discharge planning*	Aggression
VD	Public masturbation	Contact community	Self-abuse
Marriage, genetics	Exhibitionism	agencies for continued	Stereotype behavior
		care if needed	Short attention span
Daily living skills	Other behavioral		Negativism
Group living	adaptation deficits	*Gradual discharge to*	
Living alone	Obnoxious attention	Family	*Therapeutic education*
Commuting skills	demanding	School	*and tutoring*
Financial management	Overtalkative and	Independent living	Trust building
	overfriendly behavior	Job	Social skill training
Recreational skills	Hugging and kissing		Increase frustration
Hobbies	relatives and strangers	*Schedule next follow-*	tolerance
The use of community	indiscriminately	*up visit*	Teach to give and take
facilities:	Unsafe smoking habits		
Movies	Unsafe commuting		*Occupational therapy*
Lectures	habits		To increase self-esteem
Sports			To gain confidence for
Restaurants			job training and
			collaboration
			To learn discipline and
			responsibility

Table II. The program director's administrative responsibilities, quality care and financial accountability

Balance					
Income accounting					
Prorated staff time accounting for services				Cost	
Diagnostic		Treatment		Direct	Indirect
Staff	Function	Staff	Function		
SW	Intake contact with referral source, patient, family	RN, LPN, aides, child care workers	Milieu therapy (hours per day, days per week)	Face-to-face services / Staff salary / Fringe benefits	Administration staff / Secretarial staff
SW	Collect data of previous evaluations	Staff specialists and Consultants MD, PhD	Specialty treatments / Length of session / Number of sessions per week	Supervisor's fees	Medical record librarian
SW, MD, ED	Screening meeting, schedule outpatient office visit		Total sessions	Consultant's fees	Dietary staff
SW, MD, ED, administrator	Outpatient visit / Financial interview / Preliminary diagnosis / Schedule of admission	Staff: Art therapist / Physical therapist / Speech therapist / Occupational therapist / Recreational therapist / Job training specialist	Ancillary therapies / Length of session / Frequency per week / Total sessions	Pharmacy / Equipment / Supplies	Housekeeping / Security
SW, MD, other staff, administrator	Admission to: / Outpatient clinic services / Partial hospitalization / Inpatient hospitalization			Mail / Telephone	Maintenance
SW, RN	*Home visit*	*Assign staff duties*		Food / Transportation for patient or staff (home visit)	Public relation staff / Audiovisual staff
SW, MD, psychiatrist, psychologist, legal counsel	Court hearing where required, before or at the time of the admission process	*Assign therapy space, tools, supplies*	Provide staff with printed forms for diagnostic data collection and for progress reports: standard questionnaires and reporting forms, specially adapted, modified and newly designed forms		Utilities / Staff time spent in meetings and writing reports

SW = Social worker; ED = educator; RN = registered nurse; LPN = licensed practical nurse.

Progress report on play therapy

Patient: _____ Therapist: _____

Date and time:				
Location:				
Observers (if any):				
Child's attitude towards entering the playroom:				
Child's mood during the session:				
Child's spontaneous motor activity:				
Child's spontaneous verbal activity:				
Child's general attitude towards the therapist:				
Child's response to therapist's verbal intervention:				
Child's response to therapist's physical intervention:				
Child's activity in relation to toys and other physical objects: Content of play a) manifest b) symbolic				
Interpretation (if any) a) by therapist b) by patient				

Fig. 7

report forms are provided here for play therapy (fig. 7), art therapy (fig. 8), speech therapy (fig. 9), and therapeutic tutoring (fig. 10). This type of format is best arrived at by a collaboration of the administrator with the specialists in each field making the reporting format both time-saving and meaningful for monitoring the treatment. A specially designed questionnaire may be used to substitute lengthy interviews. For example, the 'visit report' form (fig. 11) designed by the staff of the John Merck Program provides information to staff, while at the same time it assists the family to be more observant in recording interactions.

The administrator-director is responsible for the quality of services and their proper documentation. An in-house peer-review system, as a first line

Progress report on art therapy

Chronological age	Mental age	Art therapist
Diagnosis	Diagnosis	*Sessions*
6 months	6 months	No./week
12 months	12 months	Time

Name: _____ Recommended for art therapy treatment _____

Date treatment begins _____

	Diagnostic evaluation	Sessions		
Date:				
Characteristics of art work				
Relationship of art products to clinical pathology				
Behavior during sessions				
Relationship to therapist				
Goals				

Supervisor's comment: _____   Signature: _____

Fig. 8

of quality control, should be established by assigning the staff members in rotation for these duties. In addition to the content review by specialists it is useful to have a monthly review of the records of each client for completeness including the necessary progress notes. A model of procedures and filing system should be used for these reviews and the missing items are to be recorded by the reviewer. The staff responsible for the missing item is then contacted by the reviewer through administrative channels. The date of receipt of the missing item is to be recorded on the reviewer's form with any comments deemed necessary. These frequent reviews will alert supervisors of some staff members who are habitually missing deadlines and the problems can be discussed and solved. The staff taking part in rotation in

Progress report speech and language therapy

Patient's name _____   Therapist: _____

Intermediate goal: _____   Beginning date: _____

Date and objectives	Procedures	Material	Criterion	Met	Un-met	Met	Un-met	Met	Un-met

Supervisor's comments: _____   Signature: _____

Fig. 9

these reviews will become more aware of the total operation and record system of the program. A sample patient record review form is given in figure 12.

The Management of Deinstitutionalization. By definition this means discharging a retarded person who has been 'institutionalized'. The concept has psychological connotations which must be understood before the process of deinstitutionalization can be accomplished. The term 'institutionalized' means: (a) that the person has been a resident for several years (or lifelong) in an institute for retardates; (b) that he or she became overly dependent on the staff and the care provided, and (c) that he or she has not

Progress note on tutoring

Patient's name: _____   Tutoring teacher _____

Language

Assessment tool: _____   Level of functioning: _____

Skills: _____

Session number and date	Goals	Method	Materials	Progress

Comments of supervisor: _____   Date: _____

_____   Signature: _____

Fig. 10

acquired daily living skills required for independent living in the community. The trend (and often mandated process) of decreasing the size of institutes by discharging the residents to various community facilities providing different levels of care has led to the social phenomenon of 'deinstitutionalization'.

The planning for the discharge of the institutionalized retarded (deinstitutionalization) starts usually by assuming that the candidate's level of intelligence is sufficient to learn the necessary daily living skills. Unfortunately in many cases, an IQ level may be the only criterion considered for initiating the action of discharge. The psychological factors often overlooked are related to the exacerbation of adaptive deficiencies in the new

Home visit report

Name of Child: _____   Date: _____

Parent: _____

Based on your own experience with your child (this visit), please fill in the following:

1. How did you enjoy your visit? _____

_____

2. What did your child do (hobbies, painting, chat, etc.)? _____

   Indicate: _____

3. Did your child take medication? _____

4. Eat well? Please describe skills: _____

_____

5. Dressing? Please describe skills: _____

_____

6. Toileting? Please describe skills (accidents?): _____

_____

Additional comments: _____

_____

Did your child ...   *Mark one answer for each question*

	Often	Sometimes	Not at all
7. Appear restless or overactive			
8. Look unhappy or sad			
9. Become quarrelsome			
10. Steal			
11. Lie			
12. Have temper outbursts			
13. Show destructive behavior (what did child do?)			
14. Disturb other children (describe) for example: hit, bite, push, or in any other way hurt or attack children:			

_____

_____

_____

	Often	Sometimes	Not at all
15. Become excessively tired or lethargic			
16. Self-stimulate			
17. Isolate himself from others			
18. Become stubborn			
19. Become uncooperative			
20. Refuse to do what is asked of him/her			
21. Express concern about physical health (i.e., headaches, pains, etc.)			
22. Show interest in violence, death?			
23. Express ideas about himself/herself which are extremely strange?			
24. Hear voices and/or talk to imaginary people?			
25. Wet his/her pants			

26. Have you noticed any changes in your child since receiving care at the hospital? Please describe.

_____

_____

_____

27. Have you noticed any changes in yourself, or any other member of the household since hospitalization? Please describe.

_____

_____

_____

28. Is there anything you can think of that might be done to help your child or family? Describe.

_____

_____

_____

29. How is your child doing with his/her behavioral program at home?

_____

_____

30. What difficulties do you experience in following the behavioral program in the home? Please describe.

_____

_____

Fig. 11

Peer review form: medical record review

Patient's name:

Date: Reviewer:

Missing items	Who is responsible	Date completed	Comments

Signature of Reviewer: Signature of program director:

Fig. 12

life situation. The intellectual potential may be useless if motivation is lacking while the discharged resident is struggling with the loss of the emotional ties with the 'institute'. This stage can be compared to the leaving of the family by growing-up children. For the institutionalized person the staff and fellow residents were the source and recipients of essentially all emotional experiences. Love, hate, respect, fear, and support, anxiety and security were all played out in the confines of the 'institute'-home. All this is lost with one stroke of the administrator's pen. The identity of residents is that of being a member of the 'family' of staff and residents under the same roof where basic needs of food, shelter, clothing and more were provided 'unearned'. With discharge they lose their identity. They are not anymore a member of the 'institute family'. This is very different from teenagers or young adults leaving the family and keeping their identity as members of the family regardless of where they settle. It is irrelevant whether they love or hate the family, their identity is not lost by the move. The loss of emotional ties and of 'family identity' causes depression and/or anger against (and increased anxiety of) any new situations. Even the resident who says that he or she hates the staff and the other residents will 'wake up' to the surprise of 'missing those to be hated'. It is a loss, no matter how optimistic a picture is painted by the staff of the expected independence after discharge.

The success or failure of deinstitutionalization depends for the most part on the administrative management of this process. Some factors enhancing the chances of successful deinstitutionalization are the following:

(1) Matching the actual level of functioning with the community placement's requirements instead of 'hoping' that the resident will integrate into a higher level of functioning just because he or she has the intellectual capacity to learn the necessary skills.

(2) Providing emotional continuity and support for a time for minimal expenses of scheduled brief (5 min) telephone contacts with an assigned staff member (in the first month weekly, after that once a month for a few months), and by sending occasional postcards (about five in the first year) with brief messages written by a staff member about 'life in the family' of the residents still in the institute and expressing their care about the one who left ('I hope you are well, let me know how things are going').

(3) Wherever possible an occasional invitation to return to the familiar ward for a holiday or a recreational function (a dance, or bowling evening) will also be an expression of 'belonging' and not being 'kicked out', just graduated to a different level of life-style. The memory of having been at one time a member of an institute should not be erased or qualified as 'bad' or shameful, but understood as the past which made it possible to reach the present level of functioning. This attitude will help in adjusting to future moves upwards to less and less sheltered conditions, while understanding the need for each phase of 'individuation and separation' lived through in the process of becoming as independent as possible. Being deinstitutionalized is always a 'cultural shock'. This can be decreased by educational methods of training the resident in many of the daily life skills required in the new environment. Some examples are: commuting independently; shopping; keeping a personal level of self-care, grooming, and social manners customary in the new environment. The adjustment can be fostered by visits to the new place and meeting (in recreational conditions) the members of group homes or halfway houses before joining their living quarters. Methods of role playing were also suggested for exit training [39, 72].

(4) Setting up and managing the type of transition described above does cost staff time and energy but in the long run it may be cost-efficient by preventing readmission or the need for more expensive community mental health services to treat the symptoms of maladjustment. Dealing with the realities of the need for 'decreasing the census' should not be disguised as an 'altruistic act of discharging a resident to make him or her happier'. It is best to inform the resident matter-of-factly that the staff believes that he or she can function in a different setting and therefore discharge plans are made. Do not tell them that it is done 'to make them happy', instead provide support to cope with the difficulties. There is no need to add guilt for 'not being happy' when losing the shelter and the human ties of the institute.

Freedom and independence may well be the ultimate goal in the pursuit of happiness from the point of view of the administrator or social worker, but not necessarily of each resident. Some residents would, indeed, be happier by keeping their dependency level of being taken care of in an institute. Sometimes discharged residents have to face not only a prejudiced community, but the opposition of their own families [27, 40, 46, 74]. Most authors writing on deinstitutionalization recommend it [8, 10, 11, 15, 20, 40, 56, 61, 68] in spite of examples of failure due to inappropriate planning [14], high cost [34] and somewhat limited success [12, 18, 41, 42, 48, 58]. Others report no improvement in community settings [9, 28, 50, 56].

Staff

Staff management includes the following areas:

Recruitment
The treatment of mentally retarded patients requires exceptional energy from the staff. They must give their best for minimal return, knowing fully that the goals are limited and the progress is very slow. Trying to recruit persons of high energy with excellent academic preparation and a broad background in working with retarded or disturbed patients is only half of the work. The administrator has to be aware of the applicant's own preferences and professional needs and therefore, it is only fair to inform fully each applicant at the job interview of the difficulties of treating retarded patients and of expecting slow progress, even within the limited goals. The applicant is the best judge for determining whether he or she plans to embark on the job under these conditions as they are candidly

disclosed. For instance, the job descriptions tailored to the special interaction styles required in contact with the mentally retarded, emotionally disturbed patients help in finding the best match of the applicants and the position openings in this difficult field. A natural consequence of a good staff-patient match is a low staff turnover.

Team Work

Well-selected staff will benefit from training in working together smoothly as a team, which includes the readiness to accept and carry out the team's decisions. In larger programs, the communication between teams must be open and frequent in order to operate the total program successfully. As *Jones* [37] puts it, teamwork is the key to success.

The number and type of staff of a facility, or program, depends on the type of client to be served and the budget of the facility. In modern management the team concept is predominant. Depending on the size of staff one or more teams will be organized, each composed of at least one representative of each specialty. Some specialists may have responsibility to more than one team. For instance, if there are four teams and only one pediatrician and two psychiatrists, then the pediatrician will attend all four team meetings and provide services to the patients of all four teams while each psychiatrist will be responsible to two teams. Team assignment by definition crosses specialty lines of authority and therefore causes a stress factor in staff management. The vertical lines of authority within each specialty are crossed by horizontal lines of responsibility to the 'team' as a functioning organizational unit. Within the team the vertical authority lines are temporarily suspended when decisions are worked out based on the equal weight of each member's contribution regardless of the level in the specialty hierarchy of a given team member. Repeated administrative clarification of roles and responsibilities is necessary in this dual mesh of authority lines. For example, in team meeting it is reported that a patient becomes very agitated and sometimes aggressive at community outings. Two suggestions are made: One, by a nursing aide to revoke privileges for a week and increase participation in supervised group activities on the wards; the second suggestion made by the charge nurse (also a member of the same team) is to increase the patient's tranquilizer and keep his participation in community outings. The team as a body may decide to accept the suggestion of the nursing aide. The tension starts outside of the team's frame, when until the next team meeting the charge nurse has to 'enforce' and supervise the program which she felt is not the optimal one. She 'orders' the aides to provide the activities as decided in team, based on an aide's proposal. Naturally, at the next meeting, when evaluating the results, the team will take into consideration several independent reports and the decision may be in favor or against continuing the previous program prescription. In-service training should deal from time to time with the philosophy of teamwork, in addition to the ongoing administrative support provided to the staff.

Staff Utilization

Nurses, attendants and child care workers can increase their clinical efficiency by involvement in delivering specialized services under the supervision of the respective specialist (speech and language stimulation, gross motor activities, exercises for eye-hand coordination, etc.). This very rewarding extension of the clinical role of nursing provides continuity of treatment. It leads to a great increase in the number of specialty treatment hours provided under the guidance and supervision of the professional staff or consultants. In the treatment facilities where therapeutic interventions are provided only by the specialists themselves, whose time is, of course, very limited, the patient gets less exposure to the therapeutic intervention.

Efficient use of the consultant's time includes diagnostic evaluations, staff training and supervision of staff to whom the details of specialty work can be delegated. The consultants reevaluate from time to time the ongoing specialty program and set appropriate new goals for the patient. The results of this structure are seen in the following areas: (1) Economical use of consultant time; (2) the emphasis on the professional training aspects of the consultations is enjoyed by the consultant and consultees; (3) paraprofessional staff receives challenging assignments and opportunities to widen and refine their skills in new areas of the total treatment program; (4) the patient receives excellent evaluations from professional staff and consultants; (5) the patients receive two to three times as many sessions per week as would be feasible even under optimal conditions if all sessions had to be delivered by the specialists themselves. This is an essential factor in treatment, since due to the slow progress and the need for more repetition of each training phase, the retarded patients require substantially more sessions in rehabilitation than nonretarded persons; (6) it is an advantage that the same person, generally a member of the nursing staff, provides the special training as well as other daily activities. In the case of retarded children the nurses and aides in residential facilities while interacting with the patients, are also assuming a parental role of 'raising the child' and helping them to master daily tasks. The child will generally work well with a trusted, parenting staff member with whom he or she has many successful experiences in various daily activities.

Staff Morale

The difficulties experienced in working with multidisciplinary mentally retarded patients and their families are recurring problems inherent in the patient selection. It is difficult to accept that all the energy investment leads ultimately to a 'defective end product', not a fully normal person but one who is still retarded. Of course, keeping in mind limited goals, the results can be very encouraging. For example, admitting a psychotic retarded child and discharging a nonpsychotic retarded child who is happier, healthier, and better adjusted is a very rewarding experience.

Sustaining staff motivation and staff morale require active administrative attention to working out the treatment goals through team decision, where each member's input is essential and listened to by all other team members. Based on their professional background each member can add a specific aspect to the total treatment plan and its implementation. It is the administrator's duty to help staff to feel needed and appreciated by being considered an important factor in decision making. Those who have a voice in the planning of patient management will be proud of the work done by co-workers as well as of their own work. Setting limited, thus reachable goals, is one of the clinical management tools of keeping up the staff motivation during their tedious work to achieve small changes at a slow pace.

Staff Turnover

The administrative task is to keep down the cost of hiring and training new staff by keeping the unplanned staff turnover at a minimum. At the same time one must realize that a planned turnover of staff, especially in a teaching hospital, is an excellent balancing factor of staff motivation. Planned staff turnover provides a replenishment of energy, fresh outlook and new motivation in the group as a whole, while the skills are passed on by the staff who has already established working methods with the patient population of the facility. An example of planned staff turnover is the hiring of persons who are enrolled in higher education and who plan to leave in about 2–3 years in order to embark on a higher-level job. These young staff members, who know that they do not have to do the same tedious work forever, invest more energy and are still shielded from becoming victims of burnout.

A well-managed staff becomes a stable and cohesive group, whose members are of mutual support to each other in their work with the client-patients.

Staff-Patient Interaction Management

In general it is advisable to remind staff of the need for expressing their respect for the client as a person. All too frequently retarded adults are treated in an infantilizing way, and even called 'children' or 'boys/girls' when they have long passed middle age. It is hard to build self-esteem and a healthy self-image of being equal to the rest of the people unless one is treated equally. If John Doe just broke a leg and needs treatment, he will be addressed as Mister Doe while the history of this injury is taken and while he is treated. If he were a retarded person it is very likely that he would be addressed by first name already by the receptionist and by most other persons in the clinic or hospital. 'Talking down' to a retarded person is even more frequent in institutes, it leads to overdependent behavior and it may become a license to act immaturely. A change in staff attitude through good management practices will change the behavior of the residents to a more mature and responsible attitude.

A specific interaction which may require management policy is the giving of gifts. Gifts given by the patients to their parents and relatives or to each other is a learning experience. To be able to give is a great achievement especially for emotionally disturbed mentally retarded patients who generally do not socialize or interact and who have so many unmet needs which must be filled before they can give to others, either psychologically or materially. These patients should be encouraged and helped by staff to produce gift items themselves and to donate those to their parents, siblings, or other family members. In an exchange of gifts on special occasions, they may surprise their fellow patients with a gift item. It is a normalizing experience 'to give' and not just always receive.

A management policy may be needed to deal with the giving of gifts by staff to patients. A word of caution is in order: Gifts should be given collectively, although staff members may express a great wish to give individual gifts to 'their' patient. The rationale for collectively giving is the following: A patient receiving a gift from a particular staff member will be very happy with it, but (a) he or she may assume that 'the others (who did not bring a gift) do not love him or her', (b) may feel envy towards other patients who get a gift from the same staff member. This policy may be flexible in the case of children who have no family and where a staff member literally assumes individual parenting role, although even in those cases it is advisable to delegate this role as soon as possible to foster parents or visiting volunteers.

Staff Training

'No specific guidelines are available with respect to the kind of personnel and the number of staff necessary to conduct comprehensive community retardation programs. Nor are there any federal guidelines for staffing retardation programs which could be used for guidance. Certain national sources, such as the American Psychiatric Association, the American Association on Mental Deficiency, the Child Welfare League of America, the National Advisory Committee on Sheltered Workshops, and the National Association for Retarded Children, have developed some material on staffing requirements with respect to their own specific concerns' [43]. It is essential to train the staff through formal staff in-service education and on-the-job close supervision. Senior staff members should be ready to act as a nucleus for the training of new staff members in their respective fields, and for providing professional education to the staff of other agencies and future programs in the community. Staff members should be encouraged and sponsored to attend meetings, fostering exchange of ideas through direct contact with other programs and agencies or by attending conventions of a larger national scale. Young paraprofessional staff members and aides, child care workers should be encouraged to engage in formal college and graduate school education. This is a continuous source of improving the quality of the staff and it leads also to the planned turnover as mentioned above.

In some special programs staff members from different fields of expertise have to become familiar with each other's specialty methods in order to treat the whole patient. An example is the treatment of emotionally disturbed retarded children. The children served by such a program are unique in the sense that they have two handicaps, any one of which is usually sufficient to impair their social adjustment, personal happiness, growth and maturation. The psychiatric treatment required to alleviate the emotional disturbance and the special education techniques necessary to provide appropriate learning experiences must both be provided. It is evident that these two programs (treatment and education) must be intertwined. The staff implementing the psychiatric and the educational programs must deal with the whole child. The requirement for staff qualifications and job descriptions for those working with the emotionally disturbed mentally retarded child must be based both on models of child psychiatry and special education. The double handicap of the patients makes it necessary that all staff members be trained in the therapeutic value of special education methods, including behavioral therapy, as well as in the psychodynamic understanding of emotional disturbance and its social and educational consequences. All staff must understand the special psychiatric therapeutic interventions including the psychopharmacological aspects of the multimodality treatment. There is a need to provide indices for understanding the treatment program [1].

An administrative strategy to facilitate communication among staff members is to schedule a 30-min staff meeting to be held each morning, serving the purpose of briefly sharing overall information about each patient. About 25–30 patients can be covered in 30 min in a prepared condensed report. In larger institutes the morning report meetings may have to be decentralized in order to give sufficient time to mention each patient.

The following schedule of meetings is a sample of ongoing staff training activities related to the clinical work in an inpatient facility:

Daily. General staff meeting, 30 min. The morning report to be given by the head nurse on each patient consists of a brief summary of all nursing and other reports regarding the previous day or weekend. This is followed by a brief discussion of case management and general policies. The social workers report on new applicants and preadmission decisions are made. Teachers give school report. Members of any other profession may bring up subjects related to treatment, management, or research.

Weekly. Treatment review meetings conducted by each multidisciplinary team. Staff communications meeting on policies and procedures, with representation of the administration.

Monthly. Grand rounds and case presentations to consultants, and teaching faculty. Other meetings with built-in staff educational aspects are the scheduled case conferences on each patient related to the diagnostic workup and treatment planning, annual reevaluation and discharge planning.

Environment

The environment in which rehabilitation or treatment takes place consists of the following elements: (1) The land surrounding the facility and its general location within the community; (2) the building(s) with both its exterior and interior architectural design and the use of colors; (3) the type and arrangement of furniture, equipment and decorative elements, and (4) the human environment – clients (patients), staff and the neighboring community.

General Environment

The location in which facilities for retardates are situated has undergone a change in the course of this century from out-laying wooded or farm areas which were supposed to have a 'calming effect' to more urban locations. With this change, the size of institutes has continuously decreased and ultimately the modern trend is community housing and 'store-front clinics'. Both the human therapeutic aspects and the financial advantages of one setting versus the other are debatable although more and more publications support the advantages of community living [3, 14, 17, 25, 44, 59, 69, 79].

The Architectural Design as a Treatment Tool

Ideally the available space should be created or adapted to the planned rehabilitation education or treatment functions to be carried out in it. For example, the size of the institute, the size of inner spaces, window levels and furniture should be scaled down for programs for children. Referring to the building design of older institutes *Wolfensberger* [77] points out how it provides an insight into the attitudes toward retardates (barred windows, TV out of reach, etc.).

The literature on the environmental impact on patient behavior can be divided into three categories:

(a) Papers containing theoretical prescriptions of how an ideal institute should be designed. The authors of most of these papers are hospital directors or superintendents of institutes, in other words in a peer position. The content of these papers in many cases is actually identical to the instruction to the architect who is commissioned to build the facility. They do not provide follow-up evaluations to validate the hypothesis and the rationale given for the specific prescriptions. Some of the authors of theoretical prescriptions suggest both interior and structural changes [5, 22, 52, 53, 60, 70, 73], others restrict their prescription to interior design changes only [30, 31, 54, 63]. Some of these papers contain additional suggestions of staffing pattern and treatment methods [36, 65, 80].

(b) Some publications based on staff questionnaires and on patient behavioral observations provide prescriptive suggestions for improving the

Percentage of occurrence

	L	P	C
Before structural changes all three areas without window	33	21	46
After structural changes with window in the playroom	25	39	36
Mean change	-8	+18	-10

Fig. 13. Percentage of occupancy during free play with a choice of three interconnected areas (L = living room; P = playroom; C = corridor). Subjects: 14 hospitalized, 3- to 12-year-old, emotionally disturbed mentally retarded children. Number of sessions: ten consecutive day sessions before structural changes and ten sessions after the changes (window access in the playroom). Results: increase of playroom choice from 21 to 39% after structural changes.

architectural environment based on the assumption that the suggested changes would improve the treatment results [2, 46, 49]. These authors are mostly ward physicians who have lived with the consequences of changes ordered by the administration. There are no follow-up data on the actual implementation of any of their suggestions.

(c) Publications with validated research observations and quantitative data regarding the results of architectural changes on patient behaviors are few. These studies provide a set of observations as baseline before the changes are made and complete the data with observations after the changes [6, 32]. The environmental changes may include painting and new furniture [32] or new location of partitions [55]. The size of space was found to be relevant in terms of promoting interaction rather than as an element in a numerical density factor [35, 76]. Most experimental studies used behavior mapping for sampling the patient's reaction to the environmental changes.

It was also suggested by *Spivack* [66] to use the architect's design log as a guide to postoccupancy evaluation by transforming the design log into a questionnaire. The number of validated empirical studies is still very small although in the past decade several authors have expressed their views on the desirability of surveys on the effect of the physical environment on behavior [23, 26, 29, 54].

In a controlled empirical study carried out on the John Merck Program by this author, a correlation has been found between the structural change in one area and the time spent in that area, based on the spontaneous choice of space from among three available areas during free play time by a group of 14 emotionally disturbed retarded, 3- to 12-year-old children. Behavioral mapping techniques were used. During the first observation phase all three areas living room, playroom, and corridor, were windowless inner spaces. The structural change consisted in providing window access in the play room. Following this change the occupancy during free play has increased in the playroom from 21 to 39% (fig. 13).

The complexity of environmental factors and their combined impact on the patient's behavior is to be considered on an administrative level. It is the administrator's role to coordinate the suggestions of the clinicians and the architect's proposal for the design of a new facility or for the remodelling of an available space [21, 45, 47].

The Human Environment

The human environment includes several variables: (a) The type of clients (patients): Age, sex, cultural background, pathology, level of retardation, are all elements which have an impact on the interaction [24]. (b) The staff: the number of staff available, and their functions, as well as their smooth collaboration [68] will be the primary determinants of the human environmental atmosphere. (c) The contact with the neighborhood of residential facilities and the attitude of the community may foster, or destroy, the therapeutic atmosphere of a facility. Small group homes are especially vulnerable to neighborhood rejection and stigmatization [4, 19, 64, 78].

Today, large state institutions are expecting a substantial number of their residents to be discharged and returned to the community for further rehabilitation and reintegration. This trend has led to the need for the establishment of new types of settings for optimal community living. The result is that the community care for a large population of mentally retarded children and adults brings essentially all segments of the population into contact with them. There is a well-known negative reaction in most communities against absorbing mentally or emotionally handicapped persons [38, 71]. Comprehensive surveys show, nonetheless, that group homes are mushrooming in an attempt to absorb adult retardates (and even children), who require different levels of sheltered environment on their way out of the institutes. *Bruininks* et al. [13] reviewed 4,427 community residential facilities in an excellent survey.

The management of group homes includes the counseling, support and rehabilitation of individual clients, and it requires learned skills, not just common sense and good intentions. Hiring skilled staff will increase the success of the client's adaptation and of the acceptance by the community. Through informative meetings and the mass media, the prejudicial fears and the hopeless attitude of most communities can be changed [71] into an actively helpful and resourceful attitude instead of the rejection and discrimination against retardates in the areas of housing [77], jobs and recreational opportunities. The preparation of the community is an administrative skill needed in managing a successful discharge program.

Finances

Financial planning and management is part of any clinical program. The clinician would be inclined to disregard all financial aspects and just treat all patients who need services for as long as they need it. However, such a program would be doomed in a very short time and be unable to meet its payroll. As *Baumeister* [7] has pointed out, more scientific information is available than is translated into policies because the social, political and economic costs are too great. The costs have to be offset by the income in order to keep functioning. Thus, patient selection will depend on the income available to provide the necessary staff and space for the needed services. Income may be generated in different ways: (a) Self-pay; (b) third-party payment for individual patients; (c) general grants from the Federal Government, or the States or from private foundations to cover global operating costs of a facility, and (d) a mixture of different proportions of the above-described revenue sources. Following a careful selection of clients (patients) to be served within a program or facility, depending on the availability of funds, staff and space, it is to be expected that the services will lead to optimal results for that selected client-patient population.

The major item in the budget of any health care operation is the staff salary and fringe benefit category. The number of staff and their salary level depend on the type of services to be rendered and the number of clients to be served. It is not the purpose of this chapter to provide detailed administrative guidelines for budget design and for billing systems to recover expenses. A few remarks will be made about the financial record keeping as it relates to the actual treatment program planning. Some staffing cost factors releated to specialty treatments will also be mentioned since they may point to alternatives in billing methods.

Financial Record Keeping

This function carried out by the administrators can be supported and assisted through the collaboration of the social workers. The patient and/or family will have an opportunity to have a financial interview before admission and discuss with the social worker the relationship of the financial coverage and the extent of services to be provided. In order to keep a realistic level of solvency, accurate financial information must be gathered from patients before admission and updated regularly. Should a change occur in the family's financial status or insurance coverage, a reassessment of the planned length of treatment is in order.

If the coverage for care is insufficient for a specific program the patient may have to be referred elsewhere. In some cases, short-term treatment with limited goals would have to be agreed upon by the staff, the patients and the referring agencies. Instead of aiming at maximum improvement a realistic partial goal can be worked out within the limits of the available financial coverage. For example, priority may be given to drug management for the control of frequent epileptic seizures which are causing emotional maladaptation. In another case the goal may be to extinguish a very disabling symptom, like repeated self-injury or aggression toward others, by a specific behavior modification program. In yet other cases, crisis intervention with careful observation of the effects of psychotropic medication may be sufficient to start the patient on the road to clinical improvement, while detailed guidelines are passed on to other agencies who will provide continued care after the crisis intervention.

A sample of the individual financial data sheet (fig. 14) shows for each patient the types of coverage, maximum coverage, time period of coverage. This information gathered before admission helps in decision-making in the best interest of the family and the patient by planning for the most beneficial services within the contemplated time span in the program. The use of a monthly financial update form (fig. 15) is also advisable. These instruments, if used regularly, can provide an essential link of communication between the clinical program, the financial office and the patient/family.

In order to determine the most appropriate billing method the major cost factor (namely staff salary expenses) has to be taken into consideration. Programs which deliver a large number of specialty treatments (required by multihandicapped retarded patients) would most likely achieve a realistic coverage of expenses by the billing system of fee per service.

The cost factor for each patient's treatment can be analyzed and kept within the parameters of the budget. The staff expenses related to the clin-

Admission financial data sheet

Date: _____   ☐ Inpatient

                                   ☐ Outpatient

Name: _____   Number: _____

Date of admission: _____

Patient information needed: Received: _____

_____   _____

_____   _____

_____   _____

_____   _____

Insurance carrier: _____

Coverage: _____

Group No.: _____   Agreement No.: _____

MMI Deductible: _____

MMI Co insurance: _____

MMI maximum: _____

Second insurance coverage or comments: _____

_____

_____

_____

_____

Fig. 14

ical treatment are prorated per patient based on the following factors: (a) The ratio of staff to patients in each treatment modality (one to one, or group); (b) the frequency of treatment per week; (c) the qualifications of staff who carries out the treatment: MD, board-certified child psychiatrist, resident, registered nurse, physical therapist, speech therapist, social workers, psychiatric aide, psychologist (PhD or MA), etc.; (d) frequency and duration of supervision. This includes the prorated time costs of both supervisee and supervisor. The meaningful collaboration of the administrator and the clinicians regarding a feasible (affordable) treatment and rehabilitation plan will assure the quality of care within the most cost-efficient parameters.

Monthly financial report

Name: _____   ☐ Inpatient

Admission/discharge date: _____   ☐ Outpatient

Service days rendered as of: _____   Days: _____

Charges: _____

Write-offs to interim payment: _____

Net charges: _____

Payment (or write-offs): _____   Received from: _____

_____   _____

_____   _____

 Total: _____

Outstanding balance: _____   Billed to: _____

_____   _____

_____   _____

 Total: _____

Insurance coverage remaining as of: _____   ☐ Confirmed

_____   ☐ Not confirmed

Carrier: _____

Coverage: _____

Group No.: _____   Agreement No.: _____

MMI deductible: _____

MMI Co insurance: _____

MMI maximum: _____

Second coverage or comments: _____

Fig. 15

Professional Education

The question is where do professionals acquire the skills and knowledge necessary to care for retarded persons in the many different settings. Lecture seminars are a time-honored method of continuing education. They provide up-to-date information, however, they fall short on practicum opportunities. Well-organized and functioning programs for the rehabilitation and treatment of multihandicapped retarded patients are the most likely sources of good professional education on mental retardation and associated conditions for many specialists.

There is a need for physicians to become more skillful in the treatment, the management and the counseling of retardates and their families in order to adequately serve this large segment of the population. The physician should be familiar with methods of taking a reliable history from a retarded patient, and assessing the patient's understanding of, and compliance with, the treatment prescription. These are but a few special skills to be mastered by physicians in many fields of medical practice whose case load includes retarded patients. Physicians should also receive information and training in the administration of special or comprehensive programs for retardates, both in institutes and in community-based facilities, since they frequently find themselves facing such responsibilities without the necessary know-how. In the physician's administrative training, emphasis should be placed on the client-screening procedures of agencies, and on fostering outward-bound programs, leading to the discharge of retarded hospital residents to a well-prepared and receptive community.

In facilities engaged in professional education the number of students, interns, residents, and fellows, in training should be determined by the availability of staff. Teaching programs should accept applicants for professional training as long as they can guarantee to provide the trainees with meaningful experience and intensive supervision, without drawing too much staff time away from the clinical services. The trainees should have an opportunity to do practical work in addition to lecture seminars.

The teaching function is a very pleasant and rewarding activity for staff and for students and interns, but it does cost staff time and must be counted as an expense in the budget.

Research

Research topics related to mental retardation can be conducted in almost any setting, however, programs affiliated with, or operated within, an academic department are most likely to get involved in research projects. The director or administrator of research-oriented facilities should recruit clinical staff with research interest. The clinician may conduct research in collaboration with other clinicians on the staff and/or with specialized research personnel. The actual grant management has two distinct aspects: (1) financial accountability and (2) staff management.

The administrator may be instrumental in locating funding sources for research grant applications. The allocation of research budget items includes: the cost of space (in some cases, specially designed and equipped areas) for conducting the research and for staff offices; equipment; support services, and the full-time or prorated salaries of the participating staff. The research project directors should be provided with regularly updated financial reports of their grants whether financed by outside sources or by the institute itself.

The cost accountability of the project director is only one aspect of the interface between the administration and the clinical and research staff. Staff management is the delicate art of administration in research-oriented institutes. An atmosphere has to be created in which the patient's rights are respected while clinical services and research go hand in hand. The whole staff has to feel proud of the ongoing research whether they take active part or not in a given project. The tendency of staff division into clinical service providers and researchers may lead to a detrimental split and competition for power and clout (the old 'town and gown' dichotomy) within the staff which ultimately hurts both the clinical and research functions. This unfortunate splitting of staff may originate from the administrator's methods of handling one or the other staff groups as 'second-class citizens'. The skillful manager will create an atmosphere of mutual respect and reliance on each other between clinician and research staff. It is an art to help the researcher realize that no clinical research is possible without patients and that the patients are there to get services (unless they are paid research volunteers), therefore the research and clinical priorities have to be coordinated through collaboration with the clinical staff. On the other hand the clinician should learn to identify with the aims of a given research project which will ultimately lead to better understanding, prevention or more efficient clinical intervention in the future. It is in such an atmosphere of mutual respect and collaboration that both clinical and research work become most efficient. The administrator will be rewarded for his efforts by the excellent reputation of a well-managed institute or program, which in turn helps to attract the best-qualified staff, students and fellows. Thus, actually a spiraling effect may set in by improving staff quality and consequently improving both the quality of care and of research.

The management of a project with its diverse clinical services and the educational and research components is a challenging and very rewarding task achieved only with the collaboration and enthusiastic support of the whole staff. The high energy level, the intelligence and warm personality of the staff members are the ingredients which account for the excellence of a well-administered project. Such programs will benefit many families, and pave the way for similar projects in the future.

References

1   Alaszewski, A.: Problems in measuring and evaluating the quality of care in mental health handicap hospitals. Health soc. Serv. J. *88:* 9–15 (1978).

2   Anderson, S.E.; Good, L.R.; Hurtig, W.E.: Designing a mental health center to replace a county hospital. Hosp. Community Psychiat. *27:* 807–813 (1976).

3   Atkinson, D.; Broughton, J.; Charlesworth, S.; Furlong, M.; May, A.: A study of mentally handicapped clients in the community. Br. J. ment. Subnorm. *26:* 67–80 (1980).

4   Bachrach, L.: A conceptual approach to deinstitutionalization. Monogr. Am. Ass. ment. Defic. *4:* 51–67 (1981).

5   Bailey, S.: Discussion group 3: psychiatry and architecture. Wld Hosp. *12:* 80–82 (1976).

6   Bakos, M.; Bozic, R.; Chapin, D.; Neuman, S.: Effects of environmental changes on elderly residents' behavior. Hosp. Community Psychiat. *31:* 677–682 (1980).

7   Baumeister, A.A.: Mental retardation policy and research: the unfulfilled promise. Am. J. ment. Defic. *85:* 449–456 (1981).

8   Bell, N.J.; Schoenrock, C.; Bensberg, G.: Change over time in the community: findings of a longitudinal study. Monogr. Am. Ass. ment. Defic. *4:* 195–206 (1981).

9   Bercovici, S.M.: The deinstitutionalization of the retarded: community management of a marginal population; PhD diss. Diss. Abstr. int. *41:* 1667-A (1980); Ann Arbor Univ. Microfilms No. 8023275, 364P (1980).

10 Biklen, D.: The case for deinstitutionalization. Social Policy *10:* 48–54 (1979).

11 Birenbaum, A.: Resettling mentally retarded adults in the community. Almost 4 years later. Am. J. ment. Defic. *84:* 323–329 (1979).

12 Bjannes, A.T.: Placement type and client functional level as factors in provision of services aimed at increasing adjustment. Monogr. Am. Ass. ment. Defic. *4:* 337–350 (1981).

13 Bruininks, R.H.; Hauber, F.A.; Kudla, M.J.: National survey of community residential facilities: a profile of facilities and residents in 1977. Am. J. ment. Defic. *84:* 470–478 (1980).

14 Bruininks, R.H.: Recent growth and status of community residential alternatives. Monogr. Am. Ass. ment. Defic. *4:* 14–27 (1981).

15 Burish, T.G.: A small community model for developing normalizing alternatives to institutionalization. Ment. Retard. *17:* 90–91 (1979).

16 Cheek, F.E.; Maxwell, R.; Weisman, R.: Carpeting the ward; an exploring study in environmental psychiatry. Ment. Hyg. *55:* 109–118 (1971).

17 Chipkin, H.: Deinstitutionalization of the mentally. On the inside, looking out. Fam. Hlth *12:* 40–42 (1980).

18 Conroy, J.W. Trends of deinstitutionalization of mental retardation. Ment. Retard. *15:* 44–46 (1977).

19 Crawford, J.L.: Deinstitutionalization and community placement. Clinical environmental factors. Ment. Retard. *17:* 59–63 (1979).

20 Datel, W.E.; Murphy, J.G.; Pollack, P.L.: Outcome in a deinstitutionalization program employing service integration methodology. J. oper. Psychiat. *9:* 6–24 (1978).

21 Davis, C.; Glick, I.D.; Rosow, I.: The architectural design of a psychotherapeutic milieu. Hosp. Community Psychat. *30:* 453–460 (1979).

22 Dybwad, G.: Planning facilities for severely and profoundly retarded adults. Hosp. Community Psychiat. *19:* 392–395 (1968).

23 Dybwad, G.: Architecture and mental subnormality. Architecture's role in revitalizing the field of M.R. J. ment. Subnorm. *16:* 45–48 (1970).

24 Ellsworth, R.B.; et al.: Some characteristics of effective psychiatric treatment programs. J. consult. clin. Psychol. *47:* 799–817 (1979).

25 Eyman, R.K.; Demain, G.C.; Lei, T.: Relationship between community environments and resident changes in adaptive behavior: a path model. Am. J. ment. Defic. *83:* 330–338 (1979).

26 Foley, A.R.; Lacy, B.N.: On the need for interpersonal collaboration: psychiatry and architecture. Am. J. Psychiat. *123:* 1013–1018 (1967).

27 Frohboese, R.: Parental opposition to deinstitutionalization: a challenge in need of attention and resolution; PhD diss. Diss. Abstr. int. *40:* 5866-B (1980); Ann Arbor Univ. Microfilms No. 8012744 (1979).

28 Gollay, E.; Freedman, R.; Wyngaarden, M.; Kurtz, N.: Coming back: the community experiences of deinstitutionalized mentally retarded people (ABT Books, Cambridge Mass. 1978).

29 Goodman, H.: Architecture and psychiatry. What has been achieved. Wld Hosp. *12:* 52–54 (1976).

30 Gunzburg, A.L.: Architecture and mental subnormality: 2. Sensory experiences in the architecture for the mentally subnormal child. J. ment. Subnorm. *14:* 57–58 (1968).

31 Hackley, J.A.: Long-term care: guidelines for planning a facility. Hospitals *48:* 53–56 (1974).

32 Holahan, C.J.; Saegert, S.: Behavioral and additudinal effects of large-scale variation in the physical environment of psychiatric wards. J. abnorm. Pers. *82:* 454–462 (1973).

33 Intagliata, J.; Kraus, S.; Willer, B.: The impact of deinstitutionalization on a community based service system. Ment. Retard. *18:* 305–307 (1980).

34 Intagliata, J.: Factors related to the quality of community adjustment in family care homes. Monogr. Am. Ass. ment. Defic. *4:* 217–230 (1981).

35 Ittelson, W.H.; Proshansky, H.M.; Rivlin, L.G.: A study of bedroom use of two psychiatric wards. Hosp. Community Psychiat. *21:* 177–181 (1970).

36 Izumi, K.: Perceptual factors in the design of environments for the mentally ill. Hosp. Community Psychiat. *27:* 802–806 (1976).

37 Jones, R.M.: Teamwork, planning keys to success. Hospitals *15:* 249–250 (1979).

38 Kastner, L.S.; Reppucci, N.D.; Pezzoli, J.J.: Assessing community attitudes toward mentally retarded persons. Am. J. ment. Defic. *84:* 137–144 (1979).

39   Klepac, R.L.: Through the looking glass: socio-drama and mentally retarded individual. Ment. Retard. *16:* 343–345 (1978).
40   Lakin, K.C.: Early perspectives on the community adjustment of mentally retarded people. Monogr. Am. Ass. ment. Defic. *4:* 28–50 (1981).
41   Landesman, D.; Berkson, G.; Romer, D.: Affiliation and friendship of mentally retarded residents in group homes. Am. J. ment. Defic. *83:* 571–580 (1979).
42   Landesman, D.: Residential placement and adaptation of severely and profoundly retarded individuals. Monogr. Am. Ass. ment. Defic. *4:* 182–194 (1981).
43   Massachusetts plan for its retarded. A ten-year plan: the report of the Massachusetts mental retardation planning project (Massachusetts Department of Mental Health, 1966).
44   McDevitt, S.C.; Smith, P.M.; Schmidt, D.W.; Rosen, M.: The deinstitutionalized citizen: adjustment and quality of life. Ment. Retard. *16:* 22–24 (1978).
45   McLaughlin, H.P.; Boerger, J.: Recreation areas and skylights bring outdoors into psychiatric unit. Hospitals *55:* 145–146, 148, 171 (1981).
46   Meyer, R.J.: Attitudes of parents of institutionalized mentally retarded individuals toward deinstitutionalization. Am. J. ment. Defic. *85:* 184–187 (1980).
47   Miller, J.A.: Health professionals surveyed for psychiatric-hospital design. Hosp. J. Am. Hosp. Ass. *55:* 129–130 (1981).
48   Moen, M.G.: Eclipse of the family group home concept. Ment. Retard. *17:* 17–19 (1979).
49   Moos, R.H.; Harris, R.S.; Schonborn, K.: Psychiatric patients and staff reaction to their physical environment. J. clin. Psychol. *25:* 322–324 (1969).
50   Morell, B.B.: Deinstitutionalization: those left behind. Social Work *24:* 538–532 (1979).
51   Morisot, M.M.: The psychiatric hospital's liability in cases of neglect of its patient follow-up supervisory and obligations. Responsabilité de l'hôpital psychiatrique pour manquement à ses obligations de surveillance et de renseignement.
52   Nellist, I.: Planning buildings for handicapped children (Thomas, Springfield 1970).
53   Norris, D.: Architecture and mental subnormality. V. The environmental needs of the severely retarded. J. ment. Subnorm. *15:* 45–50 (1969).
54   Pedersen, J.M.: The physical environment of the mentally handicapped: progress in building for the mentally handicapped. J. ment. Subnorm. *16:* 121–125 (1970).
55   Rago, W.V.; Parker, R.M.; Cleland, C.C.: Effect of increased space on the social behavior of institutionalized profoundly retarded adults. Am. J. ment. Defic. *82:* 494–498 (1978).
56   Schalock, R.L.: A systems approach to community living skills training. Monogr. Am. Ass. ment. Defic. *4:* 316–336 (1981).
57   Schalock, R.L.; Harper, R.S.; Genung, T.: Community integration of mentally retarded adults: community placement and program success. Am. J. ment. Defic. *85:* 478–488 (1981).
58   Scheerenberger, R.C.: Deinstitutionalization: trends and difficulties. Monogr. Am. Ass. ment. Defic. *4:* 3–13 (1981).
59   Schroeder, S.R.; Henes, C.: Assessment of progress of institutionalized and deinstitutionalized retarded adults: a matched-control comparison. Ment. Retard. *16:* 147–148 (1978).

60 Schwerdt, J.: Architecture and mental subnormality. 4. Therapeutic variety; a day-to-day basis of design for the subnormal. J. ment. Subnorm. *4:* 101–103 (1968).

61 Seltzer, M.M.: Community adaptation and the impact of deinstitutionalization. Monogr. Am. Ass. ment. Defic. *4:* 82–88 (1981).

62 Shafter, A.: A philosophy of administration: a trilogy. Forum ment. Retard. *10:* 183–185 (1981).

63 Sherwood, S.: Long-term care: issues, perspectives, and directions; in Sherwood, Long-term care (Spectrum, New York 1975).

64 Silperstein, G.N.: Parents' and teachers' attitudes toward mildly and severely retarded children. Ment. Retard. *16:* 321–322 (1978).

65 Spencer, D.A.: Redevelopment of a hospital for the mentally handicapped. Nurse Times *70:* 1172–1173 (1974).

66 Spivack, M.: Psychological implications of mental health center architecture. Hospitals *43:* 39–44 (1969).

67 Sproger, S.R.: Misunderstanding deinstitutionalization: a response to a recent article. Ment. Retard. *18:* 199–201 (1980).

68 Stanton, M.; Schwartz, M.: The mental health hospital: a study of institutional participation in psychiatric illness and treatment (Basic Books, New York 1954).

69 Switzky, H.N.; Rotatori, A.F.; Cohen, H.: Community living skills assessment inventory: an instrument to facilitate deinstitutionalization of the severely developmentally disabled. Psychol. Rep. *43:* 1335–1342 (1978).

70 Sylvester, P.E.: Editorial: Hospital environment for the mentally handicapped. Devl Med. Child Neurol. *18:* 530–533 (1976).

71 Voeltz, L.M.: Children's attitudes toward handicapped peers. Am. J. ment. Defic. *84:* 455–464 (1980).

72 Walker, P.: Recognizing the mental health needs of developmentally disabled people. Social Work *25:* 293–297 (1980).

73 Whitehead, C.E.; Marshal, G.; Kerpen, D.: The aging. Psychiatric hospital. An approach to humanistic redesign. Hosp. Community Psychiat. *27:* 781–788 (1976).

74 Willer, B.: Return of retarded adults to natural families: issues and results. Monogr. Am. Ass. ment. Defic. *4:* 207–216 (1981).

75 Willer, B.: Deinstitutionalization as a crises event for families of MR persons. Ment. Retard. *19:* 28–29 (1981).

76 Wolf, M.: Room size, group size, and density: behavior patterns in a children's psychiatric facility. Environ. Behav. *7:* 199–224 (1975).

77 Wolfensberger, W.: The origin and nature of our institutional models in changing patterns in residential services for the mentally retarded; in Kugel, Shearer, pp. 35–82 (President's Committee on Mental Retardation, Washington, D.C. 1976).

78 Wolpert, J.; Seley, J.E.: Community response to the deinstitutionalization population. J. natn. Ass. private psychiat. Hosps *11:* 31–35 (1980).

79 Wyngaarden, M.: Interviewing mentally retarded persons: issues and strategies. Monogr. Am. Ass. ment. Defic. *4:* 107–113 (1981).

80 Young, L.G.: A model for reinforcing mental health facilities: a student's view. Community ment. Hlth J. *12:* 422–431 (1976).

23 Sociological Implications of Mental Retardation
Lynda Katz-Garris

The Definition

'We shall consider the negative forces that bring about shameful waste of human resources; the economic, apathetic, irrational forces that delay and forestall the application of our accumulative knowledge about the conservation of human resources; the potent negative forces of ignorance, intolerance, prejudice and preconceptions. These are the social and cultural forces that bring about the conditions under which the genetic birthright of children is decried, as they somehow manage to grow – slowly, fortuitously – to an intellectual and physical and motivational realization far below that which might have been possible for them' [*Haywood,* 1970, p. 1].

These words, taken from an opening address delivered by *Haywood* to the Peabody NIMH conference in 1968, are fitting to begin a discussion on the sociological implications of mental retardation. *Adams* [1971] points out that whereas the disciplines of clinical medicine, psychology and education have in previous times successively provided the dominating skills for the study and treatment of the retarded, not until recently has a fourth discipline, sociology and its methodology, been introduced into the field. Its role has been twofold. First, it has thrown into relief the background and current life experiences of the retarded which contribute to the genesis of their handicap. Second, it has demonstrated that ascribing the term 're-tarded' to sections of the population does not depend solely on their characteristics, but also on the characteristics, goals and value system of the society of which they are a part [*Adams,* 1971]. In order to understand the way in which the social scientist views the phenomenon of mental retardation, it is necessary to distinguish the social system view from that of the traditional clinical one.

Role Theory: Clinical versus Sociological

Clinically, mental retardation is viewed as a handicapping condition, which exists in an individual and can be diagnosed by professionals using standardized assessment techniques [*Filler* et al. 1975]. The clinical perspective is a familiar frame of reference which forms the knowledge base for the academic disciplines that train persons in the field of mental retardation. Clinically, there are two models of normalcy, one pathological and one statistical. With the pathological model, one is normal if there is an absence of pathological (abnormal) symptoms. With the statistical model, abnormality is defined as the extent to which an individual varies from the average of the population on a particular trait. Behavioral patterns become translated into pathological signs; that is, a low IQ is bad, and bad is pathological.

Mercer [1973a] writes that with the clinical model, the diagnosis of mental retardation can exist independently from the person, and that it can be viewed as suprasocietal, or transcending cultural differences. For example, pneumonia can be diagnosed with no reference to the culture in which a person lives. The use of a pathological model in mental retardation is most efficient, then, when applied to conditions that show clear evidence of biological dysfunction. It becomes progressively less useful as biological factors become more obscure. At this point a statistical model is likely to be used but it is not suprasocietal and therefore cannot be treated as supracultural. The use of normative and statistical data to make probabilistic generalizations about individual cases has been disputed since the beginning of the mental testing movement and is still unsettled [*Blauton,* 1975]. 'At its core is the ethical issue of making crucial decisions about persons on the basis of probabilities without clear knowledge of the costs of decision errors for the person and for the society' [*Blauton,* 1975, p. 188].

To standardize behavioral norms in terms of the role expectations of the dominant society, to judge them as socially acceptable behavior, and to then structure tests based on them is a quite impossible task in a complex, pluralistic society. Items and procedures used in intelligence tests have inevitably come to reflect the abilities and skills valued by the American 'core culture'. This 'core culture' consists namely of the cultural patterns of that segment of society consisting of white, Anglo-Saxon Protestants whose social status today is predominantly middle and upper class [*Mercer,* 1973b].

'What kinds of abilities and skills does the «core culture» value? Of the 128 intelligence tests listed in Buros' *Mental Measurements Handbook,* 58 were measures of general intelligence with no subtests. Measures of general intelligence are all highly loaded with verbal skills and knowledge. Of the 70 tests that have subtests, 77 % have subtests entitled vocabulary, language or verbal; 51 % have subtests entitled arithmetic, quantitative or numerical, and 53 % have subtests entitled reasoning, logic or conceptual thinking [*Buros,*

1965]. The number of subtests in intelligence tests that measure skills such as manual dexterity or mechanical ability is negligible. The ability to live amicably with other human beings counts not at all in the psychometric test situations' [*Mercer*, 1973b, p. 13].

Having outlined briefly the traditional clinical approach utilized in defining the nature of mental retardation, we will now examine the issue from the perspective of the sociologist. The basic sociological concepts relevant to this discussion are those of status, role expectations or norms, sanctions and socialization.

Sociologists conceptualize society as composed of a network of interlocking social systems. Each social system consists of a group of statuses which are the positions that a person may occupy in that system. The usual statuses in the nuclear family are mother, father, son and daughter. In schools they are teacher, student, principal, custodian, so forth. Some statuses are ascribed at birth, others are acquired. Each status contains a set of prescribed behaviors or rules which the person in that status is expected to observe. If he does, he is rewarded. Such a reward would be a promotion to a more valued status. If he does not meet role expectations, he is punished. One of the more drastic punishments is to be assigned to a less valued status. For example, a child may be held back in a class while his peer group is promoted to the next grade or he may be removed from the regular classroom and placed in the status of an exceptional student.

In summary, for the sociologist, mental retardation is defined as an acquired social status to which individuals are assigned by social systems such as the public schools, diagnostic clinics and welfare agencies. Because their standards and procedures vary, the meaning of mental retardation in one system will differ somewhat from that in another. While the sociological perspective agrees that a disadvantaged social position may result in medical, nutritional and hygienic conditions which could lead to biological damage and the clinical symptoms of mental retardation, such factors alone are not believed sufficient to explain the current differential labeling rate of the economically and socially deprived as mentally retarded. To understand the nature of mental retardation in the community, one must also comprehend the social processes which select out certain persons for labeling while passing over others who may be equally eligible. In the preface to his book, *Sarason and Doris* [1979] writes:

'The day is past when one can write a conventional textbook on mental retardation replete with definitions, descriptions of clinical syndromes, tests and diagnostic criteria, and suggestions for educational and institutional placement and programming. This is not to say that these features are unimportant, but rather that recent changes in our society and public policy have exposed what has always been a function of the nature of our society and its history. Mental retardation is not a "thing" but an invented concept suffused with social values, tradition, intended and unintended prejudice and derogation - all reflecting the dominant characteristics of our society and its history.

Precisely because mental retardation is a socially invented concept, the people who have "it" have to be seen in relation to those who do not have "it". And to understand that relation demands that we come to terms with how we understand our society to be structured; the diverse values that power it; the ways those values are institutionalized; not the cultural "shoulds and oughts" that seem so natural, right, and proper (but may not be); and the threads of continuity that tie the present to the past. Basic to this book is the belief that if we want to understand the concept of mental retardation and those who are called mentally retarded, we have to understand ourselves and our society in historical terms' (p. ix, x).

We therefore conclude that the label 'mental retardation' no longer has meaning unless we have carefully defined the parameters of the context in which the observed behavior is so labeled.

Labeling and Status

Sponsored by a National Institute of Mental Health grant, a study was conducted in Southern California to identify a population of the mentally retarded in a total community population of 130,000 [*Mercer,* 1971]. As part of the case identification, agencies and schools in the community were asked to participate. An analysis of the characteristics of the population nominated by these agencies revealed that: (1) persons 5 through 24 years of age were overrepresented and those under 5 and over 24 were underrepresented; (2) persons from the poorest sections of the community were overrepresented and those from wealthier neighborhoods were underrepresented; (3) when socioeconomic status was held constant, persons of Mexican-American heritage were overrepresented, Blacks appeared in proportionate numbers, and Caucasians from English-speaking homes were underrepresented.

Data from the school system sample indicated that, with respect to the white children who were identified, the clinical and acquired roles' definitions were generally consistent and corresponded closely. However, the discrepancy between definitions for those who were 'eligible' to be labeled as mentally retarded and those who were actually labeled mentally retarded was quite large for the Mexican-American and Black children. Among children from ethnically different backgrounds, a low IQ was necessary, but not sufficient, to place the child in the status of 'mental retardate'. There were almost three times more children with IQs below 80 playing 'normal' roles than there were children playing 'retarded' roles. That is, only 25% of the 'eligibles' were 'actuals' in the sociological sense. Two formulas emerged from the study: (1) Low academic competence + poor adjustment + low competence in English + few friends + perceived low mental ability = mental retardation. (2) Low academic competence + poor adjustment + relative competence in English + being easy to manage + being liked by peers + perceived low mental ability does *not* equal mental retardation [*Mercer, 1971*, p. 29].

A second survey conducted by the Allegheny County Chapter, Pennsylvania Association for Retarded Children on 'Exceptional Dependents Unidentified and Unserved in Allegheny County Public Schools', based on the 1970-71 school year census, supports the California findings. Excluding the city of Pittsburgh, 16,967 births were recorded in Allegheny County in 1966 and of these births, the County reported 84 children known to them as 'exceptional' who were then 5 years of age. In 1959, there were 23,110 births reported in the County, and the schools identified 410 who were 12 years of age. In 1950, 14,053 individual births were recorded who would have been 21 years of age at the time of the survey. The school reported no exceptional individuals in this age group.

National estimates reveal that about 6 million persons in the United States, or roughly 3% of the population, are mentally retarded and 2.3% of the mentally retarded are of school age and in need of special education classes. Total estimates of the prevalence rates of all areas of exceptionality falling in the school age population, that is, between 5 and 17 years of age, amount to 12% of the total age population. Keeping these figures in mind, the highest percentage reported by Allegheny County for any year between 1950 and 1966 for all areas of exceptionality, including the physically handicapped, aurally handicapped, brain-injured, blind, emotionally and socially disturbed, was 1.995%.

The surveyors proceeded to use this figure as a standard minimum percentage which could theoretically be identified for each year of age between 5 and 21. Whether this can be justified as a statistically correct procedure does not negate the fact that this 1.995% estimate for all exceptionalities is below the 2.3% estimate of school age children who are mentally retarded and in need of special education services, not to mention its total lack of relationship to the estimate of 12% which has been applied nationally to all areas of exceptionality.

Taking the rate of incidence then as 1.995% and assuming it to be constant each year, for 1966, the minimum number of 5 year olds to be identified should have been 338 (county reported 84). For the year 1959 the minimum number of identified 12 year olds should have been 461 (county reported 410); while for the year 1950 the minimum number of 21 year olds to be identified should have been 280 (county reported 0) [Allegheny County, PARC, 1972].

In summary, findings extrapolated from the Alegheny County, PARC report indicate that: (1) the heaviest concentration of numbers of exceptional children are between the ages of 12 and 16; (2) those areas which have special county schools for the exceptional child identify the greatest number of exceptional children; (3) those districts representing the lower socioeconomic pockets of the county report the largest number of children identified as educable mentally retarded even if they report no other area of exceptionality; (4) numbers break off drastically at age 18 when the school programs dismiss these children. And finally, as was mentioned earlier, the number of identified exceptional individuals 21 years of age is nonexistent in this survey. Thus, these data appear to corroborate the California study to a great extent.

From a social system perspective, 'mental retardate' is an achieved social status and mental retardation is the role associated with that status. Labeled retardation can then be described as a process, the process of playing the role of 'mental retardate' and meeting the role expectations which others in the system have for those who occupy the status of 'mental retardate'. If a person does not occupy the status of one who is mentally retarded, that is, he does not play the role of 'mental retardate' in any social system, and is not regarded as mentally retarded by any of the significant others in his social world, then he is not mentally retarded, regardless of the level of hiw IQ, the adequancy of his adaptive behaviour, or the extent of his organic impairment. From a social system perspective, a low score on any intelligence test is not a symptom of pathology but rather a behavioral characteristic which is likely to increase the probability that a person will be assigned to the status of 'mental retardate' in some American social systems. Thus, achieving the status of one who is mentally retarded, is a social process and there are many alternative statuses to which persons with comparable biological equipment might be assigned.

Differential diagnosis is the process of social decision making which determines whether a particular person is assigned the status of educationally handicapped, cerebral palsied, autistic, mentally retarded, etc. [MacMillan, 1980; Taylor, 1980]. Mental retardation is not a characteristic of the individual, nor meaning inherent in his behaviour, but a socially determined status, which he may occupy in some social systems and not in others, depending on their norms. It follows that a person may be mentally retarded in one system and not mentally retarded in another. He may change his role by changing his social group. If he plays the role of one who is mentally retarded in every social system in which he participates, he is 'totally' retarded. If he never plays the role of 'mental retardate' in any system, then he is not retarded; he is 'normal'. He is 'situationally retarded' when he plays the role intermittently depending on the social system in which he participates. Thus, individuals can range along a continuum from the 'normals' through the 'situationally' retarded to the 'totally' retarded [*Mercer*, 1971].

To summarize, the meaning of mental retardation from the social system perspective delineates what a person in the field of eligibles must do to acquire the status of 'mental retardate'. Clinical symptoms alone cannot define mental retardation, and when they have done so in the past, the results have had dire consequences for those so diagnosed.

> The relationship between sociocultural factors and mental retardation is at least two-edged. Insofar as the definition of mental retardation carries overtones of adjustment to societal demands and competence in everyday living, the demands made by a given society will to some extent determine the prevalence of mental retardation [*Uzgiris*, 1970, p. 24].

The Institution

Just about a decade ago, *Butterfield* [1969] made the following comments:

> 'While fewer than five percent of the mentally retarded of the nation live in institutions, more money is spent to maintain them than for all of the other public programs serving the remaining 95 percent. Over one-half of all public institutions in this country house more than 1,000 residents and the majority are large, multipurpose facilities.'

Since this publication, a systematic and extensive discharge process has drastically reduced the number of institutional residents by returning them to the community [*Bruininks* et al., 1980; *Crawford* et al., 1979; *Birenbaum and Re*, 1979].

Society's perception of the role of the mentally retarded has historically been reflected in the institutional system which it has established. In sociological terms, a person's social perceptions are profoundly influenced by his basic values and orientation to life. Certain of these values have clear implications for one's perception of the mentally retarded. This same 'social' perception then has definite implications for one's conceptualization of a residential care model for those in the role of the retarded. It has been well established that a person's behavior tends to be greatly affected by the role expectations that are placed upon him. This is the old self-fulfilling prophecy with the unfortunate result that role appropriate behavior will be interpreted to be a person's 'natural' rather than elicited mode of acting. In institutions, role performance is influenced not only by interpersonal stimuli to which a resident is exposed but also by the opportunities and demands of the physical environment [*Repp, 1978*].

Deviancy and Treatment

At this point, it is necessary to examine one last sociological concept, that of deviance. A person can be defined as deviant if he is perceived as being significantly different from others in some overt aspect and if the difference is negatively valued. An overt and negatively valued characteristic is called a 'stigma'. The handicapped person is usually seen as and is expected to play the role of a deviant. The mentally retarded individual, since he is handicapped and often multiply stigmatized, is by definition a deviant [*Rains* et al., 1975].

Historically, societal responses toward the mentally retarded have not been specific but rather were part of a more generalized pattern of response toward deviance. At times, the pervasive societal attitude toward deviance has been one of prevention. Not attaching a negative value to certain types of difference can be thought of as a psychosocial means of prevention. At other times, the deviant have been viewed as capable of change, usually by means such as education, training and treatment. More often than not, the deviant, being perceived as unpleasant, offensive and frightening, have been segregated from the mainstream of society and placed at its periphery; i.e., Blacks, Indians, the deaf, blind, aged, etc. And finally, there have been attempts at destroying those perceived as deviant.

In reviewing the literature, well-defined role preconceptions of the mentally retarded can be found and most of these roles are deviant ones. When he/she is perceived as sick, as a diseased organism, residential facilities have been structured on the medical (hospital) model. This model tends to have the following characteristics: the facility is administered by a medical hierarchy; the residence is labeled or identified as a hospital; living units are referred to as wards or nursing units; residents are referred to as patients and their retardation is identified as being a 'disease' that requires a 'diagnosis' and 'prognosis'; resident care is referred to as nursing care, case records are referred to as charts; hospital routines prevail; and separation between professionals and residents pervades the premises.

A disease conceptualization of retardation tends to result in a management dilemma. On the one hand, such a conceptualization often results in pursuit of treatment hoped to result in cure; on the other hand, unless a 'cure' is seen as likely, the management atmosphere is often permeated with hopeless and treatment nihilism. In other words, the disease conceptualization tends to be correlated with inappropriate extremes of management attitudes [*Wolfensberger,* 1969].

The mentally retarded have also been seen as subhuman organisms. Here the architecture of the facility reflects the perception of the retarded as deviant. The walls, the concrete floors, the barred windows, drains in the middle of the room, locked wards, fences, segregation of the sexes, heat and light controls in the nursing stations and a total lack of privacy are concrete manifestations of such a pervasive belief system. At other times, the retarded have been viewed as a menace, as an object of pity, as a burden of charity, a holy innocent, and finally as a developing person. This perception that the retarded individual is a developing person, is an optimistic one directed at the modifiability of behaviour which does not connote strong negative values. The retarded are seen as capable of growth, development and learning. This would be reflected in the architecture of the facility in terms of a homelike atmosphere; small, self-contained living units; bedrooms for 1–4 residents; family dining facilities; homelike appliances; live-in personnel; doors on rooms and curtained showers.

In the 1850's, institutions for a number of deviant groups in the United States were founded for the purpose of making the deviant less deviant through the process of education. Initially, the institution was seen as a temporary boarding school and efforts were then made to distinguish between the more and less modifiable mentally retarded. The prevalent rationale was that the retarded should be removed from society in order to be trained for return to society.

With the perceived failure of the institution to 'cure large numbers of the retarded' and the inability of many adult residents to adjust to the community, ideologies changed between 1870 and 1880 and the term 'school' began to disappear from the names of institutions and was replaced by the term 'asylum'. This new protective residential care model emphasized benevolent shelter but it bore the seeds of three dangerous trends: isolation, enlargement and economization. Paralleling this isolationist policy was the ever present negative attitude toward the retarded which grew slowly to see them as social menaces.

The peak of the indictment against the retarded came between 1908 and 1915 with the eugenics movement and the focus on 'prevention'. Reactions came in the form of preventive marriage laws, compulsory sterilization laws and preventive segregation. The extreme in segregation was advocated by *Barr* [1897] who proposed the establishment of one or more national institutions or reservations similar to the management of another large group of deviants in America, the Indians [*Wolfensberger and Kugel*, 1969].

As large institutions with massive numbers of segregated retarded individuals began to cost money, the next logical step was the use of the higher functioning among them to reduce costs. Huge farm colonies then developed. One such colony in Massachusetts boasted of covering several thousand square miles of land. As costs were cut, the environment was stripped of amenities and comforts. Education came to be viewed as worthless; those who were taught to read and write were said to cause the most trouble. Even special education classes in the community were seen as a means of identifying the retarded for subsequent institutionalization.

With the late 1920s the alarmist period peaked; the sterilization and segregation movement began to be viewed as a failure. In addition, studies began to show that the retarded adult in the community was not such a menace as once believed. In time it became rather evident that the realities of an institutional approach to the delivery of care for the retarded could not be divorced from the prevailing societal view toward deviancy. Schools became asylums; the institutions became not a paradise but a purgatory; institutional segregation did not contribute to prevention; and institutionalization was not accomplished inexpensively [*Wolfensberger and Kugel*, 1969].

Stigma and Resocialization

Of all the attributes of man, mind is the quintessence; to be found wanting in mental capacity – general intellectual competence – is the most devastating of all possible stigmata [*Edgerton*, 1967, p. 207].

The etymology of the word 'stigma' is revealing for the present discussion. In its archaic sense, a stigma was a mark made on the skin by burning with a hot iron as a token of infamy or subjugation. It is therefore not only a mark of inferiority, but is also a permanent brand from which one never escapes. The word is used pervasively in the literature regarding the mentally retarded [*Han*, 1972; *Blatt*, 1972; *Tuckman*, 1972; *Goldberg*, 1971]. The stigma seems to brand a person entirely inferior, connoting total incapacity and even blame-worthiness.

The error lies in the assumption that a person who lacks the ability to adapt to the particular demands of the schooling system lacks the ability to adapt to most other demands made upon him. We do not say of a person who is incompetent in school: 'He is stupid at *reading.*' Rather we say, 'He is stupid,' meaning, 'He is (or is destined to be) a failure' [*Dexter*, 1964, p. 2]-

If we do not actually believe that intelligence is virtuous, we act as though we do; conversely we treat lack of intelligence with contempt. Although the human tragedy surrounding mental retardation is understood only too well by those persons whose lives have been touched by it, few persons who have not been directly involved are fully aware of the magnitude or the character of the problem that is mental retardation. Even though the estimated prevalence of mental retardation (3% of the population) is not yet confirmed by epidemiological research, some studies have suggested a lower rate, others have suggested a higher one; it is certain that mental retardation is an enormous problem. Thus, it is explicitly recognized that mental retardation is a relative concept, the limits of which have meaning only in terms of social conditions. The essential point is that despite the recognized imperfections of intelligence tests, virtually all diagnoses of mental retardation rely upon these tests. Indeed, legal statutes often require such testing. IQ is the operational tool; and both legal and medical terminologies and classifications of mental retardation are based upon discriminations in intelligence.

No one seriously questions the proposition that experience, especially early experience, affects one's IQ. It is, for example, generally accepted that the longer individuals, especially children, live in conditions of intellectual deprivation or isolation, the lower, on the whole, their IQs will tend to be. Undeniably, then the influence of social and cultural factors upon IQ is great. This point is crucial for an understanding of mental retardation. Most persons who are defined as mentally retarded are not profoundly, severely, or even moderately retarded. Quite the contrary, fully 85% of all the mentally retarded are only mildly retarded. Indeed, *Tarjan and Dingman* [1960], basing their estimates upon a population in the United States of 175 million, concluded that there were 5,276,755 persons in the United States with IQs between 50 and 70 [*Mercer*, 1973b]

Even if we conclude that most, or even all, persons who have IQs in the mildly retarded range suffer some degree of organic impairment of the brain or central nervous system (and this has never been demonstrated), it is nevertheless the case that their disorder is first and foremost an inadequacy in social conduct. Such persons do not become diagnosed as mentally retarded because some specific organic cause has been located. Causal diagnoses of this kind are rare exceptions. Rather, diagnoses are typically made by recourse to IQ testing after some degree of social incompetence has been demonstrated. In short, most mental retardation is mild mental retardation, and mild mental retardation can be perceived as a social phenomenon.

An outstanding void was seen to exist in the sociological knowledge of the mentally retarded outside of custodial or treatment institutions. Neither the details of their everyday life nor their own thoughts and emotions concerning their life circumstances had ever been documented prior to the publication of *Edgerton's* The Cloak of Competence [1967]. His study was an effort to provide information about the life circumstances of a number of mildly retarded persons living in a large city. *Edgerton* and his researchers interviewed a large sample of previously institutionalized mentally retarded persons then living in the community to discuss their behaviour, their thoughts and their feelings as they themselves comprehended and experienced them. Additionally, their goal was to provide a reasonably detailed account of the life circumstances of these persons and the ways in which they perceived and managed their relative incompetence. Finally, the study concentrated upon the critical outcome of concepts such as stigma and passing for an understanding of the lives of these persons.

Edgerton [1967], in summarizing his findings, pointed out that it would be misleading to attempt to bring the lives of these retarded persons into the perspective of 'social deviance'. These former patients were not social deviants who had rejected the normative expectations of the 'outside' normal world. They espoused no countermorality. Quite the contrary, their every effort was directed toward effecting a legitimate entry into the 'outside' world. To do so, they lied and cheated, but they practiced their deceptions in order to claim a place in the 'normal' world, not to deviate from it. Their behavior, in fact, represented the very antithesis of social deviance.

In their review, 'The Mentally Retarded Label: A Theoretical Analysis and Review of Research', *MacMillan* et al. [1974, p. 257] concluded:

> While many accept as fact that labeling children mentally retarded has detrimental effects, conclusive empirical evidence of these effects was not found. The studies that bear on that issue were found to have confounded treatments and shed little light on the debate. An attempt was made to expose the complexity of the problem and to suggest variables that need to be controlled in subsequent research if it is to clarify our understanding of the biasing effect of the label.

Since that time, however, some well-designed research has been undertaken and the results do not support *MacMillan's* conclusion. Among the research is that which focuses on aspects of attribution theory, locus of control and cognitive dissonance. Since we cannot review in detail these studies, the reader is referred to work by *Gibbons* et al. [1979], *Severance and Gasstrom* [1977], *Siperstein* et al. [1980] and *Siperstein and Gottlieb* [1977].

The Community

Epidemiology of Environmental Insult

There have been a number of studies to document the environmental, sociocultural impact on retardation and its prevalence in the community at large. One of the most thorough of these studies is that of *Birch and Richardson* [1970]. The authors conducted a retrospective epidemiological study on 104 children born between the years 1952–1954 in Aberdeen, Scotland, who had previously received a diagnosis of mental subnormality. Their results showed that the greatest proportion of these subnormal children came from the lower social classes with a prevalence rate nine times higher than in the nonmanual segments of the population. There was an excessive representation of cases in which the retardation fell in the mild range, IQ 60 and above, and these were overrepresented in large families existing in overcrowded, substandard housing. No social class gradient was found in children with central nervous system damage and with an IQ below 50. But with those children whose IQs were 50 and above, evidence of central nervous system damage was overrepresented in the lower social classes. In these cases, damage to the central nervous system was more likely to have been accompanied by adverse social-environmental conditions.

The conclusion warranted by our data seems to be that children born to parents who have been themselves inadequately housed, nourished and educated are at risk to a variety of hazards – prenatal, perinatal and postnatal and that the combined weight of such hazards in interaction produces mental subnormality in a substantial proportion of those who survived (p. 163).

A most impressive study of young mentally defective children was reported by *Skeels and Dye* [1939]. These investigators transferred 13 young children under 3 years of age from an orphanage to an institution for retarded children. The average IQ of these children on the Kuhlmann Test of Mental Development at the time of admission to the institution was 64, and the range in IQ was 35–89. These babies were placed in different wards of the institution where older retarded girls were housed. The children received a great deal of attention and stimulation from the attendants and girls on the ward. After a year and a half, the IQs of these children had increased 27.5 points. *Skeels and Dye* [1939] compared these increases in IQs with the changes in IQs of 12 children with somewhat higher original IQs (ranging from 50 to 103) who remained in the orphanage. This group of orphanage children dropped 26.2 points during the same period. These results could not be explained on the basis of the unreliability of infant scales, since a contrast group was used.

In a follow-up study, *Skeels* [1942] retested the experimental and control groups 2½ years following the experimental period. The mean IQ of the 13 experimental children was 95.9, 4 IQ points higher than at he close of the experimental period. 11 of the 13 experimental children had been taken out of the institution and placed in adoptive homes; 1

stayed in the institution and 1 was returned to the orphanage. The mean IQ of the adoptive children was 101.4 with no child having an IQ below 90. The contrast group, which showed an initial IQ of 86.7 and an IQ of 60.3 at the end of the experimental period, now showed a mean IQ of 66.1. There had been a rise of 5.6 IQ points, but, in general, those who remained in the unstimulating environment of the orphanage continued to show retardation.

Perpetuation

Perry [1966], in his 'Notes for a Sociology of Prevention in Mental Retardation', compares society to a production line and the culturally deprived child to one of its products. This is the child who has never seen his mother writing a letter, his father paying a bill by check, whose clothes' colors are always drab and faded. One of the characteristics of this production line to which *Perry* refers is the pattern of inadequate clinical services which then promote the incidence of mental retardation by social means; specifically, (1) the lack of fit between life-styles of clients and professionals, and (2) the actual organization and interrelation of the different kinds of clinical services. The life-style of a mother with a lower socioeconomic status sets up barriers against her even thinking about prenatal and postnatal support. The fact of her successive illegitimate pregnancies may only bring about unintended revulsion on the part of a caretaker. In addition, the fragmentation of services, the number of persons and agencies to be contacted, bullied or seduced by both the professional helper and the patient to obtain a variety of services is in itself a social barrier to adequate clinical care.

The production and maintenance of certain kinds of ideas my also lead to retardation among vulnerable segments of the population, i.e., the premature labeling of the culturally-different child as retarded, the application of sterilization laws on the basis of mental incompetence, prohibition against marriage, permitting the annulment of an adoption if the child is subsequently found to be 'feebleminded'. Finally, *Perry* [1966, p. 161] refers to the middle class bias of both professionals and laymen who have lent support to the problems of the retarded:

I am afraid, however, that today's verbal recognition of the importance of social and other deprivations has not been accompanied by any clear thinking what to do about it. The ignorance of the experts in mental retardation is plastered over with satisfaction that now indeed we recognize an important source of mental retardation in the deprived sociocultural experience of the child. But aside from muttering something about giving the mentally retarded child enough stimulation to overcome the deprivation, the expert worker in the field usually devotes his attention to something else that remains more fashionable today and leaves to newcomers the task of dealing with sociocultural problems.

Alleviation

In the final analysis, any significant gains in the prevention of retardation depend on the effectiveness of measures to reduce mild retardation. The etiology, uncomplicated by central nervous system pathology, remains a controversial issue. The nature-nurture controversy rages on today, but the role of environmental factors is of sufficient magnitude that dramatic changes in a child's daily living experiences can alter his intellectual status. Even where significant IQ changes are not achieved, providing the child with more acceptable adult models to emulate, improving his skills in interpersonal relationships, and promoting his sense of social values can forestall impaired adaptive behavior.

Studies done in such countries as Israel support this view. *Feuerstein* [1970], in his 'A Dynamic Approach to the Causation, Prevention and Alleviation of Retarded Performance', reports that in an 8-year project with relocated youth in Israel, the basic assumption underlying his work was that social institutions dealing with deviant behavior are instrumental in shaping its course, whether this be to perpetuate or remediate such behavior. Accordingly, approaches to retarded performance can be viewed on a continuum of extremes from a passive-acceptant approach to an active-modificational one.

The assumption underlying the active-modificational approach is that given the proper social, cultural and educational policy based on a theoretical framework of the human organism as an open system and further, given an investment in the creation of innovative strategies, retarded performance levels can be raised considerably. The observed low level performance of the retarded is not accepted as a status quo nor perceived as a fixed ceiling of his capacity, nor as a rigid predictor of his future social and occupational adjustment. The retarded child, his family and his educators are helped to realize that society has every expectation that he/she will be able to perform more adequately and further, that society will make every effort to see that these expectations are realized. For this approach, biogenetic or other organic etiologies are held as a basis for only the most extreme cases of retardation.

Feuerstein's project involved itself specifically with 15,000 children of North African origin in a process of acculturation. The children were exposed to a mediated learning experience. An adult interposed himself between the child and the world to frame, select, focus and feedback data to the child in appropriate learnings sets. There was no question that every child involved in the study would have been labeled culturally deprived, and yet there were no children whose level of functioning fell in the retarded range of intelligence or behavioral performance at the end of the project's study.

Another total-environment early intervention project has been underway over a 5-year period in Milwaukee [*Heber* et al., 1972]. A survey was conducted on the residential section of the city with the lowest median family income, greatest population density per living unit and highest rate of dilapidated housing in the city. All families with a newborn infant and at least one other child of the age of 6 were selected for the study. The major finding was that maternal intelligence proved to be the best single predictor of intellectual development in children. Mothers with IQs under 80, while less than one-half of the total group number, had four-fifths of the children with IQs under 80. The measured intellectual level of the offspring of the relatively 'brighter' mothers remained constant over time whereas all of the others declined progressively with age. Implications of maternal-child relationship are self-evident whether one sees it as a prepotency of hereditary factors or the inability of the subnormal mother to create a satisfactory learning environment.

The study then chose 50 newborns whose mothers tested below IQ 70 and randomly assigned them to an experimental and a control group. From 4 weeks of age, infants were given a structured program including sensory and language stimulation, achievement motivation, problem-solving skills and interpersonal skills. Children participated on a full day basis and are now school age enrolled in regular public schools. Mothers received training in homemaking, child care, and rehabilitation services in the form of occupational training and placement. The most striking differences between the two groups were in language skills and measured IQ. At the age of 66 months, the experimental group had a mean IQ of 125 while the mean IQ for the controls was 92. Scores for the controls were higher than for their siblings suggesting that both groups' scores may have reflected practice effects but even so the differences were significant. The project differed from other invervention efforts which have failed to sustain gains in children in the age of enrollment, intensity and duration of stimulus conditions, higher vulnerability of subject population to mental retardation than the poor in general, and the range of rehabilitative services provided the families.

On April 6, 1963, Dr. *Samuel Kirk* spoke to a conference sponsored by the Fund for Perceptually Handicapped Children, Inc. In his speech, Dr. *Kirk* condemned the practice of assigning labels to handicapping conditions. He further introduced the term 'learning disabilities' to describe learning difficulties encountered by children who seemed otherwise nonhandicapped. Apparently those in attendance missed his point, because they used *Kirk's* new term to organize themselves *that very evening* into the Association for Children with Learning Disabilities – ACLD [*Wiederholt, 1973*].

Now, little more than a decade later, it seems ironic that a category designed for certain pseudo-handicapping conditions has become the most commonly assigned designation in special education [*Tucker, 1980*].

Despite disagreement as to who are the learning disabled at least four major aspects consistently emerge in all discussions. A learning disabled child generally has (1) academic retardation, (2) an uneven pattern of development, (3) often times central nervous system dysfunctioning, although emphasis has shifted away from brain damage to behavioral characteristics, and (4) learning problems which cannot be attributed to either environmental disadvantage, mental retardation or emotional disturbance. Although all suggested definitions make it clear that the term 'learning disabled' encompasses more than one narrow type of problem, all learning disabled children share one predominant trait: a significant educational discrepancy between expected academic performance and actual academic achievement [*Levinson*, 1978, p. 257].

In conclusion, we will cite one study done on 50 school districts in the Southwest United States with some 40,000 children enrolled in their school population. Between 1970 and 1977 the percentage of children in special education designated as Learning Disabled rose almost 44%. In addition, the number of black children so labeled rose from less than 0.1 to 6.3% over this same time period. It is important to note that this occurrence parallels the civil litigation of the 70s involving the disproportionate numbers of black children in classes for the educationally mentally retarded. The study's author, Tucker, makes some interesting observations with respect to this trend:

> Is it an accident that at about the same time the civil rights movement began to emphasize the moral ills associated with inappropriate placement of minority students in MR classes that the LD category was waiting in the wings ready to receive these very students – under a new guise, but for the same reasons? If so, then the resulting discrimination (that was so obvious with the socially stigmatizing MR classification) is not so obvious under the new guise because of the popularity of the LD category. Indeed, it is almost a status symbol in some circles. As a result, little concern is expressed that LD can provide an excuse for a lower quality of schooling ... Now that there is an LD category, often with extremely ambiguous and diffuse eligibility requirements, the chances are great that the aberrant learner will be screened quickly into an LD class rather than viewed in terms of what remedial experiences might be provided in the regular setting [*Smith*, 1968].
> ...Placement in a convenient LD class effectively removes much of the responsibility of general education for a child's problem, and with the lowered expectations that come with special class placement there is often significantly less progress [*Ross*, 1976].

Conclusion

The focus of the preceding discussion was to define the problem of mental retardation in terms of its sociological implications. An attempt was made to illustrate and explicate the intermingling of (1) societal attitudes towards its deviant members, (2) the corresponding treatment methodologies employed by society's professional care givers, and (3) the identification procedures employed by the various educational, health and welfare agencies with respect to the mentally retarded. Factors leading to a perpetuation or alleviation of the negative consequences for the individual who bears the label of mental retardation were also discussed. In order to change the delivery of care to the retarded, we are indeed forced to change the prevailing social ideology. In the words of *Tizard* [1966, p. 283]:

> I believe, ..., that it is through the improvement of services, and the study of factors which affect their quality, rather than through biological or psychological research, that the most effective contributions will be made to the social problem of mental retardation during the present century'.

References

Adams, M.: Mental retardation and its social dimensions (Columbia University Press, New York 1971).

Allegheny County Chapter, Pennsylvania Association for Retarded Children Survey. Exceptional dependents unidentified and unserved in Allegheny County public schools by age. Based on Allegheny County School Census 1970–71 School Year and Annual School Reports on Exceptional Children, 1972.

Barr, M.W.: President's Annual Address. J. Psycho-Asthenics 2 (1897); in Wolfensberger, Kugel, Changing patterns in residential services, p. 61 (President's Committee on Mental Retardation, Washington 1969).

Birch, H.G.; Richardson, S.: Mental subnormality in the community (Williams & Wilkins, Baltimore 1970).

Birenbaum, A.; Re, M.: Resettling mentally retarded adults in the community – Almost 4 years later. Am. J. ment. Defic. *83:* 323–329 (1979).

Blatt, B.: Public policy and the education of children with special needs. Exceptional Children *38:* 537–541 (1972).

Blauton, R.L.: Historical perspective on classification of mental retardation; in Hobbs, Issues in the classification of children, vol. 1, pp. 164–193 (Jossey-Bass, San Francisco 1975).

Bruininks, R.; Hauber, T.; Keedla, M.: National survey of community residential facilities: a profile of facilities and residents in 1977. Am. J. ment. Defic. *84:* 470–478 (1980).

Buros, O.K.: The sixth mental measurements yearbook (Gryphon Press, Highland Park 1965).

Butterfield, E.C.: Basic facts about public residential facilities for the mentally retarded; in Kugel, Wolfensberger, Changing patterns in residential services (President's Committee on Mental Retardation, Washington 1969).

Crawford, J.; Aiello, J.; Thompson, D.: Deinstitutionalization and community placement: clinical and environmental factors. Ment. Retard. *17:* 59–63 (1979).

Dexter, A.: The tyranny of schooling: an inquiry into the problem of stupidity, 6–7 (1964).

Dingman, H.F.; Tarjan, G.: Mental retardation and the normal distribution curve. Am. J. ment. Defic. *64:* 991–994 (1960).

Edgerton, R.B.: The cloak of competence: stigma in the lives of the mentally retarded (University of California Press, Berkeley 1967).

Feuerstein, R.; in Haywood, Social-cultural aspects of mental retardation. Proc. Peabody-NIMH Conf. (Appleton Century Crofts, New York 1970).

Filler, J.; Robinson, O.; Smith, R.; Vincent-Smith, L.; Bricker, D.; Bricker, W.: Mental retardation; in Hobbs, Issues in the classification of children, vol. 1, pp. 194–238 (Jossey-Bass, San Francisco 1975).

Gibbons, F.; Sawin, L.; Gibbons, B.: Evaluations of mentally retarded persons: 'Sympathy' or patronization? Am. J. ment. Defic. 84: 124–131 (1979).

Goldberg, I.: Human rights for the mentally retarded in the school system. Ment. Retard. 9: 3–5 (1971).

Han, G.: Special miseducation – the politics of special education. Inequal. Educ. 17 (1972).

Haywood, H.C.: Social-cultural aspects of mental retardation. Proc. Peabody-NIMH Conf. (Appleton Century Crofts, New York 1970).

Heber, R.; Garber, H.; Harrington, S.; Hoffman, C.: Rehabilitation of families of risk for mental retardation. Progress Report (Social Rehabilitation Service, Department of Health, Education and Welfare, 1972).

Levinson, R.: The right to a minimally adequate education for learning disabled children. Valparaiso Univ. Law Rev. 12: 253–287 (1978).

MacMillan, D.: System identification of mildly mentally retarded children: implications for interpreting and conducting research. Am. J. ment. Defic. 85: 108–115 (1980).

MacMillan, D.L.; Jones, R.L.; Aloia, G.P.: The mentally retarded label: a theoretical analysis and review of research. Am. J. ment. Defic. 79: 241–261 (1974).

Mercer, J.R.: The meaning of mental retardation; in Koch, Dobson, The mentally retarded child and his family: a multidisciplinary handbook (Brunner/Mazel, New York 1971).

Mercer, J.R.: Labeling the mentally retarded (University of California Press, Berkeley 1973a).

Mercer, J.R.: The myth of 3 % prevalence; in Eyman, Meyers, Tarjan, Sociobehavioral studies in mental retardation (American Association on Mental Deficiency, 1973b).

Perry, S.E.: in Philips, Prevention and treatment of mental retardation (Basic Books, New York 1966).

Rains, P.; Kituse, J.; Duster, T.; Freidson, E.: The labeling approach to deviance: in Hobbs, Issues in the classification of children, vol. 1, pp. 88–100 (Jossey-Bass, San Francisco 1975).

Repp. A.: On the ethical responsibilities of institutions providing services for mentally retarded people. Ment. Retard. 16: 153–156 (1978).

Ross, A.O.: Psychological aspects of learning disabilities and reading disorders (McGraw-Hill, New York 1976).

Sarason, S.; Doris, J.: Educational handicap, public policy, and social history (MacMillan, New York 1979).

Severance, L.J.; Gasstrom, L.L.: Effects of the label 'mentally retarded' on causal explanations for success and failure outcomes. Am. J. ment. Defic. 81: 547–555 (1977).

Siperstein, G.N.; Budoff, M.; Bak, J.J.: Effects of the labels 'mentally retarded' and 'retard' on the social acceptability of mentally retarded children. Am. J. ment. Defic. 84: 596–601 (1980).

Siperstein, G.N.; Gottlieb, J.: Physical stigma and academic performance as factors affecting children's first impressions of handicapped peers. Am. J. ment. Defic. *81:* 455–462 (1977).

Skeels, H.M.: A study of the effects of differential stimulation on mentally retarded children: a follow-up report. Am. J. ment. Defic. *46* (1942).

Skeels, H.M.; Dye, H.B.: A study of the effects of differential stimulation. Proc. Am. Ass. ment. Defic. *44* (1939).

Smith, R.M.: Clinical teaching (McGraw-Hill, New York 1968).

Taylor, R.: Use of the AAMD classification system: a review of recent research. Am. J. ment. Defic. *85:* 116–119 (1980).

Tizard, M.: in Philips, Prevention and treatment of mental retardation (Basic Books, New York 1966).

Tucker, J.A.: Ethnic proportions in classes for the learning disabled: issues in non-biased assessment. J. Spec. Educ. *14:* 93–105 (1980).

Tuckman, J.: The placement of pseudo-retarded children in classes for mentally retarded. Acad. Ther. *7:* 165–168 (1972).

Uzgiris, I.C.: Sociocultural factors in cognitive development; in Haywood, Socio-cultural aspects of mental retardation. Proc. Peabody-NIMH Conf. (Appleton Century Crofts, New York 1970).

Wiederholt, J.L.: Historical perspectives on the education of the learning disabled; in Mann, Sabatino, The second review of special education (Grune & Stratton, New York 1973).

Wolfensberger, W.: The origin and nature of our institutional models; in Kugel, Wolfensberger, Changing patterns in residential services (President's Committee on Mental Retardation, Washington 1969).

Wolfensberger, W.; Kugel, R.: Changing patterns in residential services (President's Committee on Mental Retardation, Washington 1969).

Subject Index